Adolescents and Young Adults with Hematological Disorders

Challenges and Perspectives

Guest Editors

Martin S. Tallman, New York, N.Y.
Pia Raanani, Petah Tikva

7 figures, 4 in color, and 22 tables, 2014

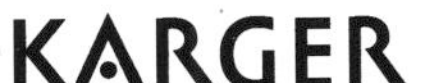

KARGER

Basel · Freiburg · Paris · London · New York · Chennai · New Delhi ·
Bangkok · Beijing · Shanghai · Tokyo · Kuala Lumpur · Singapore · Sydney

Reprint of **Acta Haematologica** (ISSN 0001-5792)
Vol. 132, No. 3–4, 2014

S. Karger
Medical and Scientific Publishers
Basel · Freiburg · Paris · London ·
New York · Chennai · New Delhi ·
Bangkok · Beijing · Shanghai · Tokyo ·
Kuala Lumpur · Singapore · Sydney

Disclaimer
The statements, opinions and data contained in this publication are solely those of the individual authors and contributors and not of the publisher and the editor(s). The appearance of advertisements in the journal is not a warranty, endorsement, or approval of the products or services advertised or of their effectiveness, quality or safety. The publisher and the editor(s) disclaim responsibility for any injury to persons or property resulting from any ideas, methods, instructions or products referred to in the content or advertisements.

Drug Dosage
The authors and the publisher have exerted every effort to ensure that drug selection and dosage set forth in this text are in accord with current recommendations and practice at the time of publication. However, in view of ongoing research, changes in government regulations, and the constant flow of information relating to drug therapy and drug reactions, the reader is urged to check the package insert for each drug for any change in indications and dosage and for added warnings and precautions. This is particularly important when the recommended agent is a new and/or infrequently employed drug.

KARGER

E-Mail karger@karger.com
www.karger.com/aha

Contents

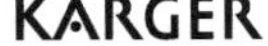

E-Mail karger@karger.com
www.karger.com/aha

Contents

Acta Haematol 2014;132:263
DOI: 10.1159/000363167

Published online: September 10, 2014

The Challenges and Perspectives in Treating Adolescent and Young Adult Patients with Hematological Disorders

Pia Raanani[a, b]   Martin S. Tallman[c]

[a]Institute of Hematology, Davidoff Center, Beilinson Hospital, Rabin Medical Center, Petah Tikva, and
[b]Sackler School of Medicine, Tel Aviv University, Tel Aviv, Israel; [c]Leukemia Service, Memorial Sloan Kettering Cancer Center, Weill Cornell Medical College, New York, N.Y., USA

Adolescent and young adult (AYA) patients constitute a unique group that deserves special attention. There is a marked variability between the definitions of AYAs, ranging from 15–20 to 15–39 years.

The distinct biology of the disease as well as other age-related issues in AYA patients deserve unique psychological and medical attention and emphasize the necessity for a treatment approach taking into consideration their special needs. These include fertility considerations, survivorship issues, psychological support, adherence to treatment difficulties and other dilemmas and problems exclusive to this group of patients.

AYA patients usually tolerate intensive treatments better than older adults do. If possible, they should be referred to special centers and should be encouraged to participate in clinical trials. In recent years, the focus on AYA patients in oncology and hemato-oncology has increased. Nevertheless, a distinct approach to these patients remains an unmet need.

In this special issue, we hope to increase awareness for this group of patients as well as to emphasize the uniqueness of caring for their issues including special therapeutic challenges. The issue covers the wide spectrum of hematological disorders that are pertinent to AYA patients as well as supportive measures relevant to this group.

Thus, Burke and Douer review the clinical and molecular characteristics of acute lymphoblastic leukemia in AYAs as well as the therapeutic approach, while Jachimowicz and Engert address these aspects in AYAs with Hodgkin's lymphoma, and Wolach and Ram concentrate on non-Hodgkin's lymphoma. Other hematological malignancies such as acute myeloid leukemia (reviewed by Ofran and Rowe), chronic myeloid leukemia (by Pemmaraju and Cortes), acute promyelocytic leukemia (by Stein and Tallman), and stem cell transplantation for AYAs with hemato-oncological disorders (by Tewari et al.) were also included. With regard to nononcological disorders, Nowak-Göttl and Kenet reviewed the thrombophilias as well as the bleeding disorders in AYAs, and DeZern and Guinan concentrated on aplastic anemia while Yacobovich and Tamary focused on hemoglobinopathies.

Regarding the supportive and comprehensive aspects of AYAs, Leader and Raanani studied adherence-related issues in AYAs with oncological as well as nononcological disorders. Dreyer and Schwartz-Attias covered the various nursing aspects, including quality of life perspectives, psychosocial aspects and spiritual existential views, while Foster and Stern as well as Kishtagari et al. focused on peer and romantic relationship experiences of AYA survivors of childhood cancer and on survivorship issues in AYAs, respectively.

Finally, the multidisciplinary approach necessary for AYA patients is conveyed in the reviews on cardiotoxicity and fertility in this population covered by Lipshultz et al. and Shapira et al., respectively. And last but not least, Meeneghan and Wood discuss the current and future challenges in delivering quality care to AYA patients as well as the role of clinical trials with this respect.

We believe that at the end of the day instead of being in the quandary of whom, how and where to treat these patients, they will be recognized as an entity in their own right. This issue, we hope, will contribute to the establishment of a new and more structured approach to the treatment of AYAs with hematological disorders.

KARGER

E-Mail karger@karger.com
www.karger.com/aha

Prof. Pia Raanani
Institute of Hematology, Davidoff Center
Beilinson Hospital, Rabin Medical Center
Petah Tikva 49100 (Israel)
E-Mail praanani@012.net.il

Acta Haematol 2014;132:264–273
DOI: 10.1159/000360204

Published online: September 10, 2014

Acute Lymphoblastic Leukemia in Adolescents and Young Adults

Patrick W. Burke   Dan Douer

Leukemia Service, Department of Medicine, Memorial Sloan Kettering Cancer Center, Weill Cornell Medical College, New York, N.Y., USA

Key Words
Acute lymphoblastic leukemia · Acute lymphoblastic leukemia age stratification · Acute lymphoblastic leukemia molecular diversity · Asparaginase · Pediatrics-inspired treatment

Abstract
The cure rate of acute lymphoblastic leukemia (ALL) in children is 80%, compared to less than half in adults. A major proportion of this cure rate drop occurs in adolescents and young adults (AYAs). The age range defining this population varies between studies, biological characteristics are different from both younger children and older adults, and AYAs are treated either by pediatric or adult oncologists, who often apply different treatment approaches to the same ALL patient population. The outcome of AYAs aged 15–21 years treated by more contemporary pediatric protocols is similar to that of younger children but is inferior when using adult regimens. This motivated studying AYA patients, including those above the age of 21 years, with pediatric or 'pediatrics-inspired' regimens that intensified nonmyelosuppressive drugs such as vincristine, steroids and asparaginase, with very promising preliminary results. Discovering new mutations in AYA ALL will help stratify patients into risk subgroups and identify targets for novel agents. This, together with fine-tuning pediatric chemotherapy principles will hopefully finally decrease the cure rate gap between children and AYAs – and even older adults.

© 2014 S. Karger AG, Basel

Introduction

Approximately 6,070 new cases of acute lymphoblastic leukemia (ALL) have been diagnosed in the USA in 2013 [1]. ALL is the most common cancer in children; its incidence increases rapidly after 2 years of age, peaks in young children, declines during adolescence and young adulthood, and gradually increases after the age of 40 years. Approximately 40% of ALL patients are older than 20 years. Clinical outcomes for children with ALL have improved over the past decades, and approximately 80% are now cured [2]. In contrast, the cure rate in adults remains only 35–44% and has not improved over the past 20 years [3–9].

Reviewing ALL in adolescent and young adult (AYA) patients is challenging for several reasons. The age range defining this population varies between studies. Secondly, biological characteristics and chemotherapy pharmacokinetics may differ from those of younger children and older adults [10]. Thirdly, and similar to all AYA cancers,

Dan Douer, MD
Leukemia Service, Department of Medicine
Memorial Sloan Kettering Cancer Center, Weill Cornell Medical College
1275 York Avenue, New York, NY 10065 (USA)
E-Mail douerd@mskcc.org

patients are treated either by pediatric or adult oncologists, who often apply different treatment approaches to the same ALL patient population. And finally, until recently, interaction to unify management approaches at all ages has been limited. However, these factors have recently drawn the attention of investigators to address the special issues of ALL in AYAs, leading to new information with promising clinical implications, which is the focus of this review. The review will be limited to Philadelphia chromosome (Ph)-negative ALL.

Defining the Age Range of AYAs with ALL

Historically, patients with ALL were stratified into 3 age groups: children, who were managed by pediatric oncologists, with an upper age limit that varied by country or institution but generally had an upper limit between puberty and 21 years, 'adults' and 'older adults', who were generally stratified by adult oncologists, mainly due to treatment toxicity concerns and eligibility for clinical trials, with an age cutoff of 60–65 years.

Initially, AYAs were defined as aged 15–21 years and first considered a distinct group in retrospective outcome analyses. Contemporary reviews of AYA ALL still discuss this age range [11]. However, in subsequent studies the upper age limit defining AYAs became 29 years, and the Cancer and Leukemia Group B (CALGB) opened a clinical trial for AYAs aged 16–29 years using a true pediatric regimen. The US National Cancer Institute defined the upper age of AYAs as 39 years, and the CALGB amended its trial to patients aged 16–39 years [12]. Consequently, the National Comprehensive Cancer Network developed different age-specific therapeutic guidelines for Ph-negative ALL for 3 separate adult age groups: AYAs (15–39 years old), adults (from 40 to 60–65 years old) and 'older' adults (older than 60–65 years) [13].

The rationale of combining ALL patients aged 15–39 years into one group is that, by the age of 15, puberty is almost complete and childhood physiology becomes similar to that of adults. Furthermore, 15- to 39-year-olds are becoming independent and share life goals such as education, vocation, establishing careers or starting a family, and are generally in overall good health. Disruption of these developmental aspects can restrict patient time and effort commitment to a complex ALL therapy, making these patients prone to lower adherence. Otherwise, after the age of 40–45, patients are more likely to acquire chronic diseases and comorbidities that require consideration when designing treatment strategies.

Characteristics of ALL in AYAs

Characteristics of ALL AYAs aged 15–39 years differ from those of younger children and older adults in disease-related factors, such as biology and clinical presentation, and patient-related factors, such as treatment tolerance and psychosocial aspects.

For example, T-cell ALL is more common in AYAs, often presenting with a large mediastinal mass. As a result, the clinical presentation is often complicated by superior vena cava syndrome, pleural and pericardial effusions and lung infiltrates, all requiring more intense hemodynamic and respiratory management. T-cell ALL may present with a mediastinal mass but without morphological bone disease (T-cell lymphoblastic lymphoma) that could delay obtaining a diagnostic tissue sample. T-cell ALL should be recognized promptly, leukemia treatment started immediately and – when necessary – cardiopulmonary support initiated. Once recovered, these patients tend to have a better outcome than precursor B-cell (pre-B) ALL [3, 14].

Chromosomal abnormalities are a prominent prognostic factor, and their respective frequencies vary with age. In pre-B ALL, abnormalities associated with very favorable outcomes, such as t(12;21) (ETV6-RUNX1 fusion gene) and high hyperdiploidy (51–65 chromosomes), are common in children but uncommon in adolescents and rarely observed in adults [10]. In contrast, the rate of the unfavorable Ph chromosome, with t(9;22) translocation (BCR-ABL1 fusion gene), is only 5% of children. It increases with age and is the most common chromosomal abnormality in adults; at the ages of 15–39, the incidence of Ph chromosome is 10–25%. The prognosis of Ph-positive ALL is unfavorable for all age groups, although it has improved dramatically by adding imatinib mesylate to chemotherapy with or without allogeneic hematopoietic stem cell transplantation (HSCT). Translocation t(4;11) (MLL-AF4 fusion gene) is the commonest chromosomal abnormality in infant leukemia, occurs in 4–7% of adults and AYAs and is considered the most unfavorable form of ALL [15].

More recently, genome-wide analysis and gene expression profiling have discovered a variety of genomic mutations, not deducible from pre-existing knowledge of the genetic breakpoints of specific chromosomal translocations. Ideally, identifying such DNA alterations would further allow stratifying patients into more homogeneous subgroups that will receive individualized therapeutic approaches. In B-lineage ALL, several early B-cell development genes acquire loss-of-function mutations leading to

Acta Haematol 2014;132:264–273
DOI: 10.1159/000360204

differentiation arrest, such as CDKN2A, PAX5, EBF1, LEF1, IKZF1 and IKZF3 [16]. So far, most published genomic information comes from samples prospectively obtained from pediatric ALL clinical trials that have outcome data. However, preliminary results from a small cohort of AYA and older ALL patients (ages 13–60 years) confirmed similar genetic alterations in this older population [17]. The incidence of genomic alterations and their association with clinical outcomes is being studied in AYA ALL in large national prospective clinical trials, and more complete results are forthcoming.

Genomic information provides several potential practical clinical applications. Recently, a unique subgroup of Ph-negative ALL patients have been defined that lack the BCR-ABL1 fusion gene but share genetic profiles and pathways with Ph-positive ALL [16]. Such 'Ph-like' ALL occurs in approximately 15% of pediatric ALL. Similar to BCR-ABL1-positive ALL, they commonly exhibit IKZF1 deletions, CRLF2 rearrangements, activating JAK mutations and other mutations [16]. Furthermore, similar to Ph-positive cases, 'Ph-like' ALL patients have inferior outcomes when treated with pediatric ALL regimens [18]. It is very likely that AYA and older ALL patients will harbor BCR-ABL1-like genetic profiles, which will likely become part of the routine workup for newly diagnosed patients. Given the poor outcome of 'Ph-like' ALL even with pediatric regimens, clinical trials are currently stratifying these patients to different therapeutic approaches.

Another clinical application of genomic analysis is identifying 'driver' submicroscopic translocations and other gene mutations 'targetable' by drugs already available for other cancers. ALL examples include patients with JAK activation mutations which might benefit from ruxolitinib; ABL1 translocation partnering with non-BCR genes could be treated by an available tyrosine kinase inhibitor or FLT3 inhibitors (mostly studied in acute myeloid leukemia, AML) possibly used in ALL patients with FLT3 overexpression often found with mixed lineage leukemia (MLL) gene rearrangement.

Host Characteristics of AYAs and Older Adults with ALL

Drug clearance of ALL agents may change with increasing age, resulting in an altered toxicity profile in AYAs [19]. Examples are lower clearances of dexamethasone, vincristine, etoposide and methotrexate compared to younger children. New information suggests that pegaspargase pharmacokinetics differ between children and adults, necessitating dose/schedule adjustment for age. The role of asparaginase is further discussed below.

Treatment of Pediatric ALL

The treatment of pediatric ALL evolved over the past 40 years in a series of rationally designed clinical trials, each refined based on the previous results, leading to the cure of most children. The Berlin-Frankfurt-Munster (BFM) Group was among the first that developed a complex multiagent model in children. It has a 2-phase induction; the first includes 4 drugs (daunorubicin, prednisone, vincristine and asparaginase), and the second phase contains cyclophosphamide, cytarabine and 6-mercaptopurine. After remission, several cycles include various drugs plus a cycle of delayed reinduction, which is a truncated form of induction phases I and II. This is followed by maintenance. Other pediatric regimens, structured differently, have been reported [11]; all contain antimetabolites, methotrexate and anthracyclines, and all utilize high cumulative doses of corticosteroids, vincristine and asparaginase, together with early central nervous system (CNS) prophylaxis and prolonged maintenance.

Treatment of Adult ALL

In adult ALL, very few randomized trials compared treatment regimens or individual drugs. The complete remission (CR) rate with any of the more contemporary regimens is approximately 90%, but despite different designs, patient populations, risk factors and upper age limits, overall survival (OS) rates have not changed. In addition, the role of HSCT in first CR is unclear. Thus, no standard regimen has been established for adult ALL, and treatment is generally chosen based on prior training and practice preferences. The current National Comprehensive Cancer Network guidelines recommend a clinical trial as first-line treatment in newly diagnosed adult ALL but do not favor any particular regimen [13].

As in children, adult ALL treatment includes different chemotherapy agents in multiple cycles, together with a long maintenance and CNS prophylaxis. With some exceptions, most regimens fall under one of two models [9, 20]. Some regimens follow principles of the BFM model modified for adults. Several adult variant regimens exist [3–5]. The University of Texas M.D. Anderson Cancer Center developed hyper-CVAD (cyclophosphamide,

Acta Haematol 2014;132:264–273
DOI: 10.1159/000360204

Table 1. Outcome of AYA ALL patients treated by contemporary pediatric regimens

Study	Patients, n	Age, years	5-year Event-free survival	
			AYAs	younger children
COG (CCG 1961) [22]	262	16–21	72% Augmented BFM 82% Standard BFM 67%	
DFCI (91-01 and 95-01) [21]	51	15–18	78%	85% (age 1–10) 77% (age 10–15)
St. Jude (Study XV) [23]	45	15–18	86%	87%

vincristine, Adriamycin, dexamethasone), and it was studied only in adults [7]. It consists of 2 cycles, alternating 4 times, for a total of 8 cycles. Cycle A contains fractionated cyclophosphamide, vincristine, doxorubicin and dexamethasone. Cycle B contains high-dose methotrexate and high-dose cytarabine. Unlike BFM-based regimens, hyper-CVAD contains no asparaginase. The structure of 2 alternating cycles is simpler to follow and widely used in the USA. More recent small, retrospective multi-institutional studies reported longer cytopenias with hyper-CVAD than in those originally reported [20].

Subset Analysis of AYA Patients Treated by Contemporary Pediatric Protocols

Historically, AYAs, aged 15–21, treated by earlier pediatric regimens had a worse outcome than younger children, with event-free survival rates ranging from 46 to 68% [21]. However, subset analyses of AYAs treated by more contemporary pediatric protocols, with more intensive chemotherapy and risk-adjusted approaches, showed improved outcomes (table 1) [21–23]. Specific details of the adjustments in each regimen are reviewed [11]. In all three reported studies the event-free survival rates were excellent and superior to their respective earlier regimens. The largest study (CCG 1961), conducted by the Children's Oncology Group (COG), reported significantly higher event-free survival in the augmented BFM arm [22]. The Dana Farber Cancer Institute (DFCI) consortium and the St. Jude Group reported that outcomes of AYAs treated with more recent regimens were similar to those of younger children and abolished the adverse prognostic impact of older age in pediatric ALL, plus were generally well tolerated [21, 23]. The DFCI reported higher rates of the asparaginase-related toxicities pancreatitis and deep vein thrombosis but not allergies;

St. Jude investigators reported that asparaginase-related toxicities were similar in all age groups, but AYAs had higher rates of infections, osteonecrosis, hyperglycemia and thrombosis, which they partially related to dexamethasone.

However, the unfavorable biological factors in higher age may still impact therapeutic responses in AYAs. For example, poor salvage rates after relapse in AYAs treated with an augmented BFM regimen were reported [24]. After first relapse, children aged 1–9 and 10–15 years still had survival rates of 44 and 39%, respectively, but AYAs initially diagnosed at the ages of 16–20 were without postrelapse survivors.

Retrospective Comparison of AYA ALL Patients Aged 15–21 Treated by Adult versus Pediatric Oncologists

A key observation that encouraged studying AYA ALL patients as a separate age group came from retrospective comparisons of patients aged 15–21 years enrolled in adult clinical trials and treated by adult oncology specialists to those enrolled in pediatric studies and treated by pediatricians. Stock et al. [25] reported that patients aged 16–20 years treated by CCG protocols had significantly better outcomes than patients treated by adult CALGB protocols; at 7 years the OS was 67 versus 46%, respectively. Similar observations were reported from several European groups and have already been extensively reviewed. These reports revealed that biological variations between ages cannot solely account for the difference in outcome. The treatment approaches were different, but other possible explanations are better adherence by both caregivers and patients in pediatric studies and socioeconomic differences between patients referred to pediatricians versus adult specialists [11, 26]. Yet, the complexity of the relationship between age and outcome is illustrated

Acta Haematol 2014;132:264–273
DOI: 10.1159/000360204

by two other retrospective comparisons that reported in AYAs OS rates in the range of 60–70% in protocols designed for adults, while highlighting the role of delivering treatment since patients were treated in large academic referral centers [27, 28].

Prospective Studies with Pediatric Regimens in Adults

Principles

The improved outcome of adolescents (aged 15–21) treated by contemporary pediatric protocols and their inferior outcome on adult regimens motivated studying pediatric regimens in all AYAs, including those older than 21 years. Separating pediatric from adult regimens at the age of 15–21 is arbitrary, and pediatric regimens are likely tolerated beyond this age. Another general treatment concept, not well recognized but well supported by distinct epidemiological, molecular and other ALL properties, is that AML treatment principles may not apply to ALL. For example, the mandatory ALL CNS prophylaxis in all age groups yielded the greatest incremental survival improvement in children but is rarely used in AML; the concept of short periods of very intense myelosuppressive, AML-like chemotherapy may not be essential in ALL [20] but rather longer, less myelosuppressive regimens, as exemplified by mandatory, long-term, low-intensity maintenance that is unique for ALL, may hold greater importance. New pediatric approaches intensified nonmyelosuppressive drugs, such as vincristine, steroids and, in particular, asparaginase, with early CNS prophylaxis.

The Role of Asparaginase

L-Asparaginase is an enzyme, used almost exclusively in ALL, which depletes serum asparagine. Several large, randomized pediatric ALL studies convincingly demonstrated that prolonged and higher cumulative dosing of asparaginase during consolidation significantly improved outcomes. In contrast, oncologists who treat adults have been reluctant to use asparaginase because of toxicity concerns. As a result, until recently, adult ALL regimens contained no asparaginase, or sparingly utilized it in only 1–2 postremission cycles, and the benefit of prolonged asparaginase activity, well documented in children, might have been lost [9].

Improvement of pediatric regimens has generally been attributed to optimizing the dose and schedule of existing chemotherapy drugs, which when adapted to adults might require adjustments for age. This would apply to asparaginase since the rates of asparaginase-related toxicities, such as high-grade hepatotoxicity, hypertriglyceridemia and pancreatitis, were higher in AYAs and adults [29]. The pegylated form, pegaspargase, is now replacing the native *Escherichia coli* form and needs special attention in adults because of its very long activity. The pegaspargase dose in children is 2,500 IU/m^2 at 2-week intervals; this is the dose and schedule approved by the US Food and Drug Administration for all ages, including adults. Recent pharmacokinetic studies in AYAs and older adults demonstrated that a lower, single 2,000 IU/m^2 i.v. pegaspargase dose provided very long and adequate asparaginase activity and serum asparagine depletion, lasting at least 3 weeks in most patients [30]. Therefore, a 2-week interval between pegaspargase doses is probably too short in these patients since overlapping enzymatic activities of 2 successive doses are likely more toxic. A recent report based on these adult pharmacokinetic properties, with multiple doses of 2,000 IU/m^2 i.v. at intervals of 4 weeks or longer, was safe, though not devoid of high-grade side effects [31]. Despite the lower dose, the rate of pegaspargase-related grade 3–4 hyperbilirubinemia and transaminitis was strikingly higher than reported in children. Although no liver failure occurred, high-grade hepatotoxicity was long in duration, often took a month to recover to baseline and delayed subsequent chemotherapy in some patients. Preliminary observations suggest that high-grade hyperbilirubinemia is more common after the first pegaspargase induction dose, and subsequent cycles that included pegaspargase often did not exhibit recurrent hepatotoxicity [32]. Taken together, using multiple doses of pegaspargase, but adjusted for age in AYAs and older adults, would allow more conformity and better implementation of pediatric regimens. However, it is also critical to recognize that pegaspargase-related toxicities are common in adults and should be mitigated by close monitoring, early detection and management using published guidelines [29].

Results of Clinical Trials

Table 2 lists reported clinical trials of pediatric regimens in AYAs and adults with newly diagnosed ALL. The upper age limit for safety is not clear and varied between studies. PETHEMA ALL 96 included only standard-risk patients, demonstrated tolerability in AYAs up to the age of 30 years and significantly improved OS to 63%, without any significant difference between the ages of 15–18 and 19–29 years [33]. In fact, this OS rate compares favorably to that reported by the Eastern Cooperative Oncol-

Acta Haematol 2014;132:264–273
DOI: 10.1159/000360204

Table 2. Pediatric and 'pediatrics-inspired' regimens

	n	Age, years	OS at 3–7 years, %
PETHEMA (standard risk) [33]	46	19–30	63
CALGB 10403 (PEG-ASP)	318	16–39	closed
GRAALL-2003 [34]	172	15–45	64
DFCI [19, 35]	94	18–50	65
USC (PEG-ASP) [31]	51	18–57	58
GMALL (PEG-ASP) [36]	400	15–55	67

ogy Group/Medical Research Council study after HSCT in the same patient population [5].

The CALGB is leading a study in AYAs with a slightly higher age range of 16–39 years, applying one arm of the Children's Oncology Group (AALL0232) pediatric protocol [12]. This study will also address toxicities and protocol adherence by patients and their caregivers, comparing adult specialists versus pediatricians using the same regimen. This study is closed for enrollment, and preliminary reports are forthcoming.

GRAALL-2003 is a large study with a 'pediatrics-inspired' regimen in 225 Ph-negative ALL patients, with a greater age range of 15–60 years. It also investigated the upper age limit for tolerating such an approach [34]. GRAALL-2003 included 8.6-, 3.7- and 16-fold higher cumulative doses of prednisone, vincristine and *E. coli* asparaginase, respectively, than their former LALA-94 adult protocol. The CR rate was 94%, and at 42 months the OS was 61%, significantly higher than the 41% reported in the historic LALA-94 study. Patients eligible for HSCT in first CR showed no difference in outcome. This survival improvement was not seen in patients older than 45 years due to a higher cumulative incidence of treatment-related mortality in first CR (23 vs. 5% in younger patients).

The DFCI consortium used their pediatric ALL regimen that had previously shown equivalent outcomes in AYAs aged 15–18 and younger children and applied it to older patients up to the age of 50 years [19, 35]. This true pediatric regimen included 30 weekly doses of *E. coli* asparaginase. Among 94 patients, the CR rate was 84%; with a median follow-up of 45 months, OS was 65%. Toxicities were not higher than in other protocols.

We recently reported the results of a regimen adopted from the augmented arm of the pediatric protocol CCG 1882, substituting 1 pegaspargase dose in each cycle that contained the native *E. coli* asparaginase. Six doses of pegaspargase were scheduled, and doses were based on pharmacokinetic properties as described above (2,000 IU/m^2/dose i.v.; intervals of ≥4 weeks). Because of pegaspargase's long activity, it was also rationally synchronized with the timing of other chemotherapy drugs, such as anthracyclines and high-dose methotrexate. Among 51 adults aged 18–57 years, CR was achieved in 96%, almost all within 4 weeks, with a 7-year OS of 58% [31].

Although not a true pediatric regimen, GMALL 07/03, with a BFM-like backbone, also attempted to optimize pegaspargase dosing in adult ALL [36]. During the study, the dose of pegaspargase was increased from 1,000 to 2,000 IU/m^2 in induction and from 500 to 2,000 IU/m^2 in consolidation in patients aged 15–55 years. The 91% CR rate was equal among the 826 patients treated with 1,000 IU/m^2 and the 400 patients treated with 2,000 IU/m^2. The OS after 3 years was longer in those receiving more pegaspargase (60 vs. 67%; p > 0.05). OS in AYAs aged 15–45 years was 71 versus 82% (p = 0.02) in those receiving lower versus higher pegaspargase doses, respectively; in older patients, aged 45–55 years, OS was 56 versus 74% (p > 0.05) in patients with lower versus higher pegaspargase dosing, respectively. Overall, intensified pegaspargase was feasible, but the rate of grade III–IV hyperbilirubinemia increased after dose escalation and led to treatment delays in individual patients.

The Princess Margaret Hospital in Toronto, Canada, retrospectively analyzed 85 Ph-negative ALL patients aged 18–60 years treated at a single institution with a modified pediatric DFCI 91-01 regimen [37], which included high doses of *E. coli* asparaginase delivered weekly for 30 weeks during intensification. The CR rate was 89%; 5-year OS was 63%. Most impressively, 3-year OS in adults 35 years or younger was 83%, comparable to the adolescent population using this regimen.

Several conclusions can be drawn from these studies. A CR rate of approximately 90% can be expected with all adult treatment models and remains the same with pediatric regimens or asparaginase intensification, with low rates of both early death and primary resistance. Therefore, a key obstacle in curing adult ALL is not the lack of achieving a morphological CR but rather failing to maintain it, mostly due to relapse. Studies using true pediatric regimens, regimens inspired by pediatric protocols and post-remission asparaginase intensification consistently demonstrated improvement in maintaining remission, with survival rates of 60% or higher. It appears that in AYAs and adults up to their middle 40s, such intensive approaches are safe, but the upper age

Acta Haematol 2014;132:264–273
DOI: 10.1159/000360204

limit still needs determination. The toxicity profile is predictable and acceptable, although pegaspargase-related high-grade hyperbilirubinemia is common in adults.

HSCT in First CR

The Center for International Bone Marrow Transplant Research does not recommend HSCT in first CR in standard-risk ALL patients because it yields outcomes similar to chemotherapy, while for high-risk patients, the data suggests an advantage to HSCT. The Medical Research Council UKALL XII/Eastern Cooperative Oncology Group E2993 trial reported [5] in Ph-negative ALL that 5-year OS was 53% in patients with a donor compared to 45% in patients without a donor. However, in contrast to the Center for International Bone Marrow Transplant Research, the greatest benefit from allogeneic HSCT was observed in standard-risk ALL, with an OS of 62% compared to 52% in patients who received chemotherapy alone. For high-risk ALL, allogeneic HSCT exhibited a more potent antileukemia effect and lower relapse rates than chemotherapy alone, but higher transplant-related mortality resulted in no net survival benefit. The difference between these data sets could emanate from different risk stratification criteria. With promising results of intensive regimens, it is possible that allogeneic HSCT may be needed only for very high-risk disease, such as hyperleukocytosis and very unfavorable chromosomal/molecular abnormalities.

New Agents

The lack of a standard of care for adult ALL and the apparent benefit of prolonged, less myelosuppressive postremission and maintenance therapy present an excellent opportunity to study novel, targeted biological agents; this would certainly apply to AYAs. Several agents have been explored in overt or minimal residual disease-positive relapsed/refractory disease. The more active agents could be incorporated into frontline chemotherapy regimens, though choosing the optimal chemotherapy backbones in such combinations would be challenging [38].

Antibodies

Monoclonal antibodies against precursor B cells targeting CD20, CD19 or CD22 are being studied. Rituximab use is limited by the expression of CD20 in only half of ALL patients. Two studies in CD20-positive ALL using rituximab in combination with different adult chemotherapy backbones showed better survival rates in adults younger than 60 years compared to chemotherapy alone [38, 39]. However, the question of routinely including rituximab in CD20-positive adult ALL therapy is not definitively answered, nor is it answered whether rituximab would benefit pediatric approaches in AYAs. CD22 is more frequently expressed in B-cell ALL, and unlike CD20, CD22 is rapidly internalized upon ligand binding and can be conjugated with a drug toxin [38]. Inotuzumab ozogamicin is an anti-CD22 antibody conjugated to calicheamicin with promising single-agent activity and tolerable side effects in relapsed ALL. A phase III study is currently ongoing. Moxetumomab pasudotox is an anti-CD22 antibody conjugated with truncated *Pseudomonas* exotoxin A that has shown single-agent activity in relapsed ALL. Blinatumomab is a single-chain antibody construct with dual specificity for CD3 and CD19, thereby directing CD3-positive cytotoxic T cells to CD19-positive B cells and ALL lymphoblasts for cell killing. This construct, known as bispecific T-cell engaging or 'BiTE' antibodies, promotes B-cell aplasia. Two small phase II clinical trials showed that single-agent blinatumomab is highly active in minimal residual disease or overt relapse after standard chemotherapy. A larger phase II study is currently ongoing [38]. The Eastern Cooperative Oncology Group will be opening a phase III randomized clinical trial combining blinatumomab with frontline chemotherapy compared to the same chemotherapy given alone, in patients aged 35–70 years; thus, the number of AYAs treated will be rather small.

Cell Therapy

Chimeric antigen receptor (CAR)-modified autologous T cells are an alternative immunotherapy in which a viral vector transduces a CAR gene construct that encodes tumor-specific single-fragment length CD19 antibody, fused to the signal transduction component of the T-cell receptor and T-cell costimulatory domains. This method demonstrated early promising results in pre-B ALL [40]. Like blinatumomab, CAR technology redirects a patient's own T cells to attack CD19-positive cells. Both have shown clinical efficacy in significantly reducing tumor burden in B-cell malignancies. CARs offer the advantage of a potentially sustained antitumor response without repeated cycles of therapy. However, the procedure requires extensive laboratory support and expertise,

Acta Haematol 2014;132:264–273
DOI: 10.1159/000360204

and patients must undergo leukapheresis and conditioning therapy with cyclophosphamide to deplete the endogenous T-cell niche. Blinatumomab, on the other hand, does not require ex vivo engineering of T cells, and the drug's short half-life lessens toxicity concerns to some degree. Both T-cell-recruiting strategies have similar side effect profiles, including tumor lysis and cytokine release syndromes – more often in patients with a high disease burden – as well as neurotoxicity. Limitations to blinatumomab include a cumbersome drug administration schedule, a 28-day continuous infusion, and frequent drug cassette changes.

Targeting Pathways

Tyrosine kinase inhibitors revolutionized the management and outcome in Ph-positive ALL. Several other novel targeted agents are being explored. NOTCH1 pathway and DOT1L inhibitors are novel small molecules already in adult ALL phase I clinical trials [16, 38]. The NOTCH1 signaling pathway regulates the development of normal T lymphocytes and has activating mutations in 50% of T-cell ALL. γ-Secretase inhibitors block the final step of NOTCH1 activation. Targeting DOT1L is intended for chromosomal translocations causing rearrangements of the MLL gene located on chromosome 11q23 that are present in 5–10% of AYA and adult ALL cases. This manifests mostly as t(4;11), which portends a very poor prognosis. Therapy-related acute leukemias, after exposure to cytotoxic agents, also commonly have 11q23/MLL translocations. The MLL gene normally encodes a histone methyltransferase, but when MLL aberrantly fuses with different genes, it recruits another histone methyltransferase named DOT1L, resulting in epigenetic changes and expression of leukemogenic genes. The DOT1L inhibitor decreases expression of target genes and induces apoptosis in MLL-mutated leukemia cell lines [16]. Other novel agents that target other pathways involved in ALL leukemogenesis include: tyrosine kinase inhibitors (e.g. dasatinib) targeting other rearrangements of the ABL1 gene, such as the NUP214/ABL1 oncogene (5% patients with T-cell ALL) [38]; mammalian target of rapamycin inhibitors that synergize with chemotherapy in pre-B ALL; fingolimod used in multiple sclerosis targets PP2A mutations in Ph-positive ALL; JAK mutations may be targeted by JAK inhibitors [41].

Conclusion

In the last decade, AYAs with ALL, defined as patients aged 15–39 years, have been recognized as a subgroup in which empirical observations identified promising opportunities to improve outcomes. Regardless of AYA age range, progress was made at all ages. More intensive pediatric regimens benefited younger AYAs, aged 15–21, by abolishing their inferior outcome compared to younger children, while in the upper AYA age range, such an approach produced overall superior survival rates when replacing adult regimens. In the upper AYA age range, true pediatric regimens' drug dosing may need adjustment but then could possibly be applied to even older adults. Such a dose modification seems particularly germane to pegaspargase, which has historically been underused in adults even though longer administration is key in pediatrics-inspired regimens. AYA host features also include complex psychosocial factors that need to be further addressed. Future challenges include identifying additional genetic alterations that characterize AYA ALL, anticipating that this will provide new targeted therapeutic opportunities. This new biological and treatment outcome information in AYAs could be extended to older adults and advance the ALL field at all ages.

References

1 Siegel R, Naishadham D, Jema A: Cancer statistics. CA Cancer J Clin 2013;63:11–30.
2 Pui CH, Evans WE: Treatment of acute lymphoblastic leukemia. N Engl J Med 2006;354: 166–178.
3 Larson RA, Dodge RK, Burns CP, Lee EL, Stone RM, Schulman P, Duggan D, Davey FR, Sobol RE, Frankel SR, Hooberman AL, Westbrook CA, Arthur DC, George SL, Bloomfield CD, Schiffer CA: A five-drug remission induction regimen with intensive consolidation for adults with acute lymphoblastic leukemia: cancer and leukemia group B study 8811. Blood 1995;85:2025–2037.
4 Stock W, Johnson JL, Stone RM, Kolitz JE, Powell BL, Wetzler M, Westervelt P, Marcucci G, DeAngelo DJ, Vardiman JW, McDonnell D, Mrózek K, Bloomfield CD, Larson RA: Dose intensification of daunorubicin and cytarabine during treatment of adult acute lymphoblastic leukemia: results of Cancer and Leukemia Group B Study 19802. Cancer 2013;119:90–98.
5 Goldstone AH, Richards SM, Lazarus HM, Tallman MS, Buck G, Fielding AK, Burnett AK, Chopra R, Wiernik PH, Foroni L, Paietta E, Litzow MR, Marks DI, Durrant J, McMillan A, Franklin IM, Luger S, Ciobanu N, Rowe JM: In adults with standard-risk acute lymphoblastic leukemia, the greatest benefit is achieved from a matched sibling allogeneic transplantation in first complete remission, and an autologous transplantation is less effective than conventional consolidation/maintenance chemotherapy in all patients: final results of the International ALL Trial (MRC UKALL XII/ECOG E2993). Blood 2008;111:1827–1833.

6 Linker C, Damon L, Ries C, Navarro W: Intensified and shortened cyclical chemotherapy for adult acute lymphoblastic leukemia. J Clin Oncol 2002;20:2464–2471.

7 Kantarjian HM, O'Brien S, Smith TL, Cortes J, Giles FJ, Beran M, Pierce S, Huh Y, Andreeff M, Koller C, Ha CS, Keating MJ, Murphy S, Freireich EJ: Results of treatment with hyper-CVAD, a dose intensive regimen, in adult acute lymphocytic leukemia. J Clin Oncol 2000;18:547–561.

8 Pulte D, Gondos A, Brenner H: Improvement in survival in younger patients with acute lymphoblastic leukemia from the 1980s to the early 21st century. Blood 2009;113:1408–1411.

9 Douer D: Is asparaginase a critical component in the treatment of acute lymphoblastic leukemia? Best Practice Res Clin Haematol 2008;21:647–658.

10 Harrison CJ: Cytogenetics of pediatric and adolescent acute lymphoblastic leukemia. Br J Haematol 2009;144:147–156.

11 Hunger SP, Schafer ES: Optimal therapy for acute lymphoblastic leukemia in adolescents and young adults. Nat Rev Clin Oncol 2011;8:417–424.

12 Wood WA, Lee SJ: Malignant hematologic diseases in adolescents and young adults. Blood 2011;117:5803–5815.

13 Alvarnas JC, Brown PA, Aoun P, Ballen KK, Bellam N, Blum W, Boyer MW, Carraway HE, Coccia PF, Coutre SE, Cultrera J, Damon LE, Deangelo DJ, Douer D, Frangoul H, Frankfurt O, Goorha S, Millenson MM, O'Brien S, Petersdorf SH, Rao AV, Terezakis S, Uy G, Wetzler M, Zelenetz AD, Naganuma M, Gregory KM: Acute lymphoblastic leukemia. J Natl Compr Canc Netw 2012;10:858–914.

14 Hoelzer D, Thiel E, Loffler H, Büchner T, Ganser A, Heil G, Koch P, Freund M, Diedrich H, Ruhl H, Maschmeyer H, Lipp T, Nowrousian MR, Burkert M, Gerecke D, Pralle H, Müller U, Lunsken CH, Fülle H, Ho AD, Küchler R, Busch FW, Schneider W, Görg CH, Emmerich B, Braumann D, Vaupel HA, von Paleske A, Bartels A, Neiss A, Messerer D: Prognostic factors in a multicenter study for treatment of acute lymphoblastic leukemia in adults. Blood 1988;71:123–131.

15 Moorman AV, Harrison CJ, Buck GA, Richards SM, Secker-Walker LM, Martineau M, Vance GH, Cherry AM, Higgins RR, Fielding AK, Foroni L, Paietta E, Tallman MS, Litzow MR, Wiernik PH, Rowe JM, Goldstone AH, Dewald GW: Karyotype is an independent prognostic factor in adult acute lymphoblastic leukemia (ALL): analysis of cytogenetic data from patients treated on the Medical Research Council (MRC) UKALLXII/Eastern Cooperative Oncology Group (ECOG) 2993 trial. Blood 2007;109:3189–3197.

16 Mulligan CG: Molecular genetics of B-precursor acute lymphoblastic leukemia. J Clin Invest 2012;122:3407–3415.

17 Paulsson K, Cazier JB, Macdougall F, Stevens J, Stasevich I, Vrcelj N, Chaplin T, Lillington DM, Lister TA, Young BD: Microdeletions are a general feature of adult and adolescent acute lymphoblastic leukemia: unexpected similarities with pediatric disease. Proc Natl Acad Sci USA 2008;105:6708–6713.

18 Loh ML, Harvey RC, Mullighan CG, Linda SB, Devidas M, Borowitz MJ, Carroll AJ, Chen I-M, Gastier-Foster NM, Heerema NA, Kang H, Raetz EA, Roberts KG, Zhang J, Winick N, Wood BL, Larsen EC, Carroll WL, Willman CL, Hunger SP: A BCR-ABL1-like gene expression profile confers a poor prognosis in patients with high-risk acute lymphoblastic leukemia (HR-ALL): a report from Children's Oncology Group (COG) AALL0232. Blood 2011;118:743.

19 Stock W: Adolescents and young adults with acute lymphoblastic leukemia. Am Soc Hematol Educ Program 2010;2010:21–29.

20 Douer D: Adult lymphoblastic leukemia: a cancer with no standard of care. Acta Haematol 2013;130:196–198.

21 Barry E, DeAngelo DJ, Neuberg D, Stevenson K, Loh ML, Asselin BL, Barr RD, Clavell LA, Hurwitz CA, Moghrabi A, Samson Y, Schorin M, Cohen HJ, Sallan SE, Silverman LB: Favorable outcome for adolescents with acute lymphoblastic leukemia treated on Dana-Farber Cancer Institute Acute Lymphoblastic Leukemia Consortium Protocols. J Clin Oncol 2007:25:813–819.

22 Nachman JB, La MK, Hunger SP, Heerema NA, Gaynon PS, Hastings C, Mattano LA Jr, Sather H, Devidas M, Freyer DR, Steinherz PG, Seibel NL: Young adults with acute lymphoblastic leukemia have an excellent outcome with chemotherapy alone and benefit from intensive postinduction treatment: a report from the Children's Oncology Group. J Clin Oncol 2009;27:5189–5194.

23 Pui CH, Pei D, Campana D, Bowman WP, Sandlund JT, Kaste SC, Ribeiro RC, Rubnitz JE, Coustan-Smith E, Jeha S, Cheng C, Metzger ML, Bhojwani D, Inaba H, Raimondi SC, Onciu M, Howard SC, Leung W, Downing JR, Evans WE, Relling MV: Improved prognosis for older adolescents with acute lymphoblastic leukemia. J Clin Oncol 2010;29:386–391.

24 Freyer DR, Devidas M, La M, Carroll WL, Gaynon PS, Hunger SP, Seibel NL: Postrelapse survival in childhood acute lymphoblastic leukemia is independent of initial treatment intensity: a report from the Children's Oncology Group. Blood 2011;117:3010–3015.

25 Stock W, La M, Sanford B, Bloomfield CD, Vardiman JW, Gaynon P, Larson RA, Nachman J; Children's Cancer Group; Cancer and Leukemia Group B studies: What determines the outcomes for adolescents and young adults with acute lymphoblastic leukemia treated on cooperative group protocols? A comparison of Children's Cancer Group and Cancer and Leukemia Group B studies. Blood 2008;112:1646–1654.

26 Schiffer CA: Differences in outcome in adolescents with acute lymphoblastic leukemia: a consequence of better regimens? Better doctors? Both? J Clin Oncol 2003;21:760–761.

27 Usvasalo A, Räty R, Knuutila S, Vettenranta K, Harila-Saari A, Jantunen E, Kauppila M, Koistinen P, Parto K, Riikonen P, Salmi TT, Silvennoinen R, Elonen E, Saarinen-Pihkala UM: Acute lymphoblastic leukemia in adolescents and young adults in Finland. Haematologica 2008;93:1161–1168.

28 Thomas DA, O'Brien S, Rytting M, Faderl S, Cortes J, Wierda WG, Ravandi F, Kantarjian HM: Acute lymphoblastic leukemia (ALL) or lymphoblastic lymphoma (LL) after frontline therapy with hyper-CVAD regimens. Blood 2008;112:1930.

29 Stock W, Douer D, DeAngelo DJ, Arellano M, Advani A, Damon L, Kovacsovics T, Litzow M, Rytting M, Borthakur G, Bleyer A: Prevention and management of asparaginase/pegasparaginase-associated toxicities in adults and older adolescents: recommendations of an expert panel. Leuk Lymphoma 2011;52:2237–2253.

30 Douer D, Yampolsky H, Cohen LJ, Watkins K, Levine AMJ, Periclou AP, Avramis VI: Pharmacodynamics and safety of intravenous pegaspargase during remission induction in adults aged 55 years or younger with newly diagnosed acute lymphoblastic leukemia. Blood 2007;109:2744–2750.

31 Douer D, Aldoss I, Lunning MA, Ramezani L, Burke P, Mark L, Vrona J, Park JH, Tallman MS, Pullarkat V, Mohrbacher AM, Avramis VI: Pharmacokinetics-based modification of intravenous pegylated asparaginase dosing in the context of a 'pediatric-inspired' protocol in adults with newly diagnosed acute lymphoblastic leukemia (ALL). Synapse 2012;120:1495.

32 Burke PW, Aldoss I, Lunning MA, Avramis VI, Mohrbacher AM, Pullarkat V, Tallman MS, Douer D: High-grade pegylated asparaginase-related hepatotoxicity occurrence in a pediatric-inspired adult acute lymphoblastic leukemia regimen does not necessarily predict recurrent hepatotoxicity in subsequent cycles. Blood 2013;122:2671.

33 Ribera JM, Oriol A, Sanz MA, Tormo M, Fernández-Abellán P, del Potro E, Abella E, Bueno J, Parody R, Bastida P, Grande C, Heras I, Bethencourt C, Feliu E, Ortega JJ: Comparison of the results of the treatment of adolescents and young adults with standard-risk acute lymphoblastic leukemia with the Programa Espanol de Tratamiento en Hematologia pediatric-based protocol ALL-96. J Clin Oncol 2008;26:1843–1849.

34 Huguet F, Leguay T, Raffoux E, Thomas X, Beldjord K, Delabesse E, Chevallier P, Buzyn A, Delannoy A, Chalandon Y, Vernant JP, Lafage-Pochitaloff M, Chassevent A, Lhéritier V, Macintyre E, Béné MC, Ifrah N, Dombret H: Pediatric-inspired therapy in adults with Philadelphia chromosome-negative acute lymphoblastic leukemia: the GRAALL-2003 study. J Clin Oncol 2009;27:911–918.

35 DeAngelo DJ, Dahlberg S, Silverman LB, Couban S, Amrein PC, Seftel MD, Turner AR, Leber B, Howsan-Jan K, Wadleigh M, Sirulnik LA, Supko J, Galinsky I, Sallan SE, Stone RM: A multicenter phase II study using a dose intensified pediatric regimen in adults with untreated acute lymphoblastic leukemia. Blood 2007;110:587.

36 Goekbuget N, Beck J, Brueggemann M: PEG-asparaginase intensification in adult acute lymphoblastic leukemia (ALL): significant Improvement of outcome with moderate increase of liver toxicity in the German Multicenter Study Group for adult ALL (GMALL) Study 07/2003. Blood 2010:116:494.

37 Storring JM, Minden MD, Kao S, Gupta V, Schuh AC, Schimmer AD, Yee KW, Kamel-Reid S, Chang H, Lipton JH, Messner HA, Xu W, Brandwein JM: Treatment of adults with BCR-ABL negative acute lymphoblastic leukaemia with a modified paediatric regimen. Br J Haematol 2009;146:76–85.

38 Douer D: What is the impact, present and future, of novel targeted agents in acute lymphoblastic leukemia? Best Pract Res Clin Hematol 2012;25:453–464.

39 Thomas DA, O'Brien S, Faderl S, Garcia-Manero G, Ferrajoli A, Wierda W, Ravandi F, Verstovsek S, Jorgensen JL, Bueso-Ramos C, Andreeff M, Pierce S, Garris R, Keating MJ, Cortes J, Kantarjian HM: Chemoimmunotherapy with a modified hyper-CVAD and rituximab regimen improves outcome in de novo Philadelphia chromosome-negative precursor B-lineage acute lymphoblastic leukemia. J Clin Oncol 2010;28:3880–3889.

40 Brentjens RJ: CARs and cancers: questions and answers. Blood 2012;119:3872–3873.

41 Deenik W, Beverloo HB, van der Poel-van de Luytgaarde SC, Wattel MM, van Esser JW, Valk PJ, Cornelissen JJ: Rapid complete cytogenetic remission after upfront dasatinib monotherapy in a patient with a NUP214-ABL1-positive T-cell acute lymphoblastic leukemia. Leukemia 2009;23:627–629.

Acta Haematol 2014;132:274–278
DOI: 10.1159/000360205

Published online: September 10, 2014

The Challenging Aspects of Managing Adolescents and Young Adults with Hodgkin's Lymphoma

Ron D. Jachimowicz   Andreas Engert

First Department of Internal Medicine, German Hodgkin Study Group, University of Cologne, Cologne, Germany

Key Words

Biomarker · Hodgkin's lymphoma · Late effects · Treatment

Abstract

Cancer in the adolescent and young adult (AYA) is the second leading cause of nonaccidental death with hematological malignancies spiking during this period. Treatment of AYAs with hematological malignancies usually follows either pediatric or adult protocols with sufficient information lacking on subgroup analyses regarding course and outcome. In this review we will outline up-to-date treatment possibilities for AYAs diagnosed with Hodgkin's lymphoma. Early and late toxicities will be addressed and future directions of research suggested.   © 2014 S. Karger AG, Basel

Definition of Adolescents and Young Adults

A quarter century ago, cancer was generally associated with a better prognosis in adolescents and young adults (AYAs) than in children or older persons. Survival rates since then have increased steadily, but with a more pronounced impact on children and older adults, leaving AYAs behind [1]. Only recently has attention in oncology turned towards AYAs, since these patients are not treated consistently, and standard treatment is poorly defined. Treatment follows either pediatric or adult protocols with information lacking on subgroup analyses regarding the course and outcome of AYA patients. The commonly used age range for AYAs is 15–39 years which is consistent with the National Cancer Institute's Adolescent and Young Adult Oncology Progress Review Group focussing on long-term follow-up. In contrast, the age range used in epidemiological studies on AYAs in the National Cancer Institute Surveillance, Epidemiology and End Results program [1] and the EUROcare registry-based programs on cancer patients was 15–29 years [2]. In this review we will review the data for AYAs in Hodgkin's lymphoma (HL).

Andreas Engert, MD
First Department of Internal Medicine, University Hospital of Cologne
Kerpener Strasse 62
DE–50924 Cologne (Germany)
E-Mail a.engert@uni-koeln.de

Challenging Epidemiology

After suicide, cancer is the second leading cause of nonaccidental death in 20- to 39-year-olds between 2000 and 2005 in the USA and is 4 times more common in this age group when compared to those younger than 20 years of age [1]. Children's cancer is linked to prenatal and congenital factors. In contrast, cancer in older adults is more strongly influenced by environmental factors. AYAs may just display a spontaneous mutation to a malignant phenotype unrelated to environmental or inherited factors, or develop a secondary neoplasm as a result of treatment with chemotherapy and/or radiotherapy for prior cancer. Between 20 and 39 years of age, HL represents 5% of all malignancies [1]. Annual rates for new diagnoses of HL in the USA per 100,000 vary from 0.1–1.2 in children up to the age of 15, 2.9–4.3 in AYAs and 2.4–4.5 in adults over the age of 40 [1].

Challenging Diagnosis

Early detection of cancer in AYAs is more challenging than at other ages. As children become young adults, they are subject to reduced parental surveillance. Together with a general lack of awareness of cancer risk during early adulthood and a higher likelihood to attribute symptoms of cancer to other causes such as trauma or infection, delay in cancer diagnosis can occur [3, 4]. Importantly, unrestricted access to health care is a requirement that is not always met [5].

Furthermore, technical issues can also play an important role in delaying time to diagnosis. Fine-needle aspiration (FNA) is often the first-line approach for diagnosis of lymphadenopathy when a hematological disease is suspected. The rush to employ FNA should be tempered by the need for a clear histological diagnosis. In a study with more than 300 cases of lymphoproliferative disorders, the exact diagnosis was delayed using FNA due to a significant rate of inconclusive findings of up to 28% [6]. Hehn et al. [7] reported that only 29% of new lymphoma cases were diagnosed accurately with FNA alone and, more importantly, 88% of patients were given a diagnosis based on FNA findings that were inadequate to guide treatment. Hence, excisional biopsy is preferable for timely diagnosis. Improving time to diagnosis for AYAs may impact the overall survival (OS). However, survival is not the only measure of outcome relevant to early diagnosis; other measures should include recurrence and survivorship, which includes quality of life and treatment-related late effects.

Treatment of HL in AYAs

Survival rates in HL have improved substantially over the last few decades. Treatment intensification according to stage of disease has led to significant improvement in tumor-free survival in children and adults [8–10]. Cure in these patients however comes at the expense of toxicity and an increased risk of secondary malignancies, leading to diminished long-term survival rates [11]. As compared to adults, different chemotherapy regimens are being used in pediatric oncology due to severer long-term toxicity in children. Whereas male patients are at a higher risk associated with alkylator-based therapy, female patients more often develop secondary malignancies, especially breast cancer within the radiation field [12–15]. Typically used regimens in children are OEPA (vincristine, etoposide, prednisone, Adriamycin) and ABVE-PC (Adriamycin, bleomycin, vincristine, etoposide, prednisone, cyclophosphamide) [16, 17].

In adults, the implementation of interim positron emission tomography in advanced-stage HL aims at reducing short- and long-term side effects by downscaling the intensity of treatment to prevent overtreatment and secondary malignancies [18]. Early response to chemotherapy has been associated with improved freedom from treatment failure and OS resulting in upfront treatment intensification [9]. In an attempt to combine intensive treatment with tailored therapy, Kelly et al. [19] treated 98 patients aged between 4 and 20 years with an upfront treatment intensification using escalated BEACOPP (cyclophosphamide, doxorubicin, etoposide, procarbazine, prednisone, vincristine and bleomycin) followed by a less intensive consolidation in early responders; however, positron emission tomography analysis has not been used. The study demonstrated excellent results with tolerable acute toxicity in children and adolescents suffering from high-risk HL. Importantly, a significant portion of patients included in this trial (48%) were adolescents aged 15–21 years [19].

In a retrospective study, our group evaluated whether adolescents represent a distinct group of patients with HL when treated within German Hodgkin Study Group (GHSG) trials. Adolescent patients aged 15–20 years were compared to young adult patients aged 21–45. Both cohorts displayed similar clinical characteristics with comparable response rates when being treated with stage-adapted protocols developed for adult patients [20]. Complete remission rates were 92.1 and 91.2% in adolescents and young adults, respectively. Outcome at

6 years was also comparable between groups, with an estimated freedom from treatment failure rate of 80.2 and 79.7%. Interestingly, OS was significantly better in adolescent patients with an estimated OS rate of 93.6% compared to 90.9% in young adults, while secondary malignancies were more frequent in the young adult group [20].

In conclusion, treatment of AYA HL patients led to very similar results when treated within prospective risk-adapted trials developed for adult patients. In future studies, downscaling of chemotherapy will still be pursued in order to further decrease late toxicity while maintaining the excellent survival currently observed. Good examples include the GHSG HD10 study in 1,370 early favorable patients [21] and the HD15 trial with a total of 2,182 advanced-stage patients randomized [18].

Short- and Long-Term Toxicities of Treatment

With the intensification of treatment protocols, treatment-related toxicity has increased substantially. Toxicity is generally linked to age. AYAs are in between children and adults, which sets them at a unique position for short-term and long-term treatment side effects. An age-related difference for toxicity in AYAs has been shown for body mass index, hormones and other factors [22]. In adults, anthracycline-related heart failure occurs during or shortly after treatment with doses exceeding 550 mg/m^2. In children however, much lower doses can lead to a decline in cardiac performance and can cause symptoms many years after treatment [23]. The dose threshold is not clear for AYAs and thus warrants attention.

The effort to improve OS with more intensive treatment strategies leads to some concern on late toxicity, quality of life and long-term survival. The development of secondary malignancy is especially important in this respect. In a previous analysis comparing 557 HL patients aged 15–20 years and 3,228 patients aged 21–45 years, treated in prospective randomized trials, we were able to show that the risk of developing a secondary malignancy was significantly higher in the age group 21–45 years with a median observation time of 85 months for OS [20]. The secondary malignancies encountered so far were mainly hematological including secondary acute myeloid leukemia, myelodysplastic syndrome and non-HL. This is to be expected, as these are usually observed in the first years after completing treatment [24, 25]. Secondary solid tumors typically occur with a longer follow-up. Patients treated for HL have an increased relative risk for developing secondary solid tumors for more than 20 years after the initial treatment. Thus, AYA patients must be monitored many years after the initial treatment [26].

With a total of 1,323 HL survivors treated within the GHSG HD13 to HD15 trials, we have previously performed a study on gonadal function and fertility after chemotherapy [27]. Chemotherapy-induced gonadal toxicity was highest in advanced-stage patients treated with the more toxic therapy in both female and male HL survivors. In men, half of the survivors after early-stage treatment had follicle-stimulating hormone and inhibin-B levels corresponding to proven fertility, whereas 88.8% of survivors in advanced stages had levels corresponding to oligospermia. Recovery of a regular cycle in women was reported by more than 90% after early-stage treatment and was mostly completed within 1 year. In contrast, after treatment for advanced-stage HL, age at therapy onset was a decisive factor, and time to resumption of menstrual activity was considerably longer [27]. However, in advanced-stage HL, used here as a role model for aggressive hematological malignancies, aggressive therapy results in the highest OS rates reported in large prospective trials [18, 28]. Fertility in AYAs is of major importance; thus, balancing efficacy and toxicity is a difficult task for both patients and physicians.

Closing the Gap

The differences in survival of AYA patients with hematological malignancies are a potential concern and should be further explored. To date, AYAs have not sufficiently been addressed in clinical trials, with satisfactory data on optimal treatment missing for most entities. Since the 4th study generation of GHSG trials, children were separated from adults at the age of 18, as legally demanded in Germany. We were able to demonstrate that AYA HL patients can be treated within prospective risk-adapted trials developed for adult patients with similar excellent survival rates [20]. The primary goal for further studies in the treatment of HL remains curing HL patients. The secondary goal is to use the least toxic regimen thereby maintaining previous excellent treatment outcomes. However, this aim is not specific for young patients, instead it plays a role for all patients treated for HL. Based on this experience, AYA patients should be enrolled in prospective clinical trials, in order to ensure optimal

Acta Haematol 2014;132:274–278
DOI: 10.1159/000360205

quality and outcomes, and monitor long-term survivorship and quality of life within these trials.

Importantly, identification of hallmarks of HL pathogenesis is needed to develop new treatment approaches for a more specific and less toxic therapy whilst maintaining excellent survival rates. Furthermore, predictive markers such as thymus and activation-regulated chemokine and galectin [29, 30] or genetic profiling [31] need to be implemented in the primary diagnosis of HL to help identify the subset of HL patients at an increased risk of relapse or refractory disease. An adapted up-front therapy for those patients may reduce the need of second-line aggressive therapies, improve survival and downscale toxicities.

References

1   Bleyer A, Budd T, Montello M: Adolescents and young adults with cancer: the scope of the problem and criticality of clinical trials. Cancer 2006;107:1645–1655.
2   Gatta G, Capocaccia R, Coleman MP, Ries LA, Berrino F: Childhood cancer survival in Europe and the United States. Cancer 2002; 95:1767–1772.
3   Haimi M, Perez-Nahum M, Stein N, Ben Arush MW: The role of the doctor and the medical system in the diagnostic delay in pediatric malignancies. Cancer Epidemiol 2011; 35:83–89.
4   Schnurr C, Pippan M, Stuetzer H, Delank KS, Michael JW, Eysel P: Treatment delay of bone tumours, compilation of a sociodemographic risk profile: a retrospective study. BMC Cancer 2008;8:22.
5   Bleyer A: The adolescent and young adult gap in cancer care and outcome. Curr Probl Pediatr Adolesc Health Care 2005;35:182–217.
6   Dong HY, Harris NL, Preffer FI, Pitman MB: Fine-needle aspiration biopsy in the diagnosis and classification of primary and recurrent lymphoma: a retrospective analysis of the utility of cytomorphology and flow cytometry. Mod Pathol 2001;14:472–481.
7   Hehn ST, Grogan TM, Miller TP: Utility of fine-needle aspiration as a diagnostic technique in lymphoma. J Clin Oncol 2004;22: 3046–3052.
8   Nachman JB, Sposto R, Herzog P, Gilchrist GS, Wolden SL, Thomson J, Kadin ME, Pattengale P, Davis PC, Hutchinson RJ, White K; Children's Cancer Group: Randomized comparison of low-dose involved-field radiotherapy and no radiotherapy for children with Hodgkin's disease who achieve a complete response to chemotherapy. J Clin Oncol 2002; 20:3765–3771.
9   Diehl V, Franklin J, Pfreundschuh M, Lathan B, Paulus U, Hasenclever D, Tesch H, Herrmann R, Dorken B, Muller-Hermelink HK, Duhmke E, Loeffler M; German Hodgkin's Lymphoma Study Group: Standard and increased-dose BEACOPP chemotherapy compared with COPP-ABVD for advanced Hodgkin's disease. N Engl J Med 2003;348:2386–2395.
10 Horning SJ, Hoppe RT, Breslin S, Bartlett NL, Brown BW, Rosenberg SA: Stanford V and radiotherapy for locally extensive and advanced Hodgkin's disease: mature results of a prospective clinical trial. J Clin Oncol 2002;20: 630–637.
11 Hodgson DC, Hudson MM, Constine LS: Pediatric Hodgkin lymphoma: maximizing efficacy and minimizing toxicity. Semin Radiat Oncol 2007;17:230–242.
12 Byrne J, Mulvihill JJ, Myers MH, Connelly RR, Naughton MD, Krauss MR, Steinhorn SC, Hassinger DD, Austin DF, Bragg K, et al: Effects of treatment on fertility in long-term survivors of childhood or adolescent cancer. N Engl J Med 1987;317:1315–1321.
13 Wolden SL, Lamborn KR, Cleary SF, Tate DJ, Donaldson SS: Second cancers following pediatric Hodgkin's disease. J Clin Oncol 1998; 16:536–544.
14 Bhatia S, Robison LL, Oberlin O, Greenberg M, Bunin G, Fossati-Bellani F, Meadows AT: Breast cancer and other second neoplasms after childhood Hodgkin's disease. N Engl J Med 1996;334:745–751.
15 Aisenberg AC, Finkelstein DM, Doppke KP, Koerner FC, Boivin JF, Willett CG: High risk of breast carcinoma after irradiation of young women with Hodgkin's disease. Cancer 1997; 79:1203–1210.
16 Mauz-Korholz C, Hasenclever D, Dorffel W, Ruschke K, Pelz T, Voigt A, Stiefel M, Winkler M, Vilser C, Dieckmann K, Karlen J, Bergstrasser E, Fossa A, Mann G, Hummel M, Klapper W, Stein H, Vordermark D, Kluge R, Korholz D: Procarbazine-free OEPA-COPDAC chemotherapy in boys and standard OPPA-COPP in girls have comparable effectiveness in pediatric Hodgkin's lymphoma: the GPOH-HD-2002 study. J Clin Oncol 2010;28:3680–3686.
17 Schwartz CL, Constine LS, Villaluna D, London WB, Hutchison RE, Sposto R, Lipshultz SE, Turner CS, de Alarcon PA, Chauvenet A: A risk-adapted, response-based approach using ABVE-PC for children and adolescents with intermediate- and high-risk Hodgkin lymphoma: the results of p9425. Blood 2009; 114:2051–2059.
18 Engert A, Haverkamp H, Kobe C, Markova J, Renner C, Ho A, Zijlstra J, Kral Z, Fuchs M, Hallek M, Kanz L, Dohner H, Dorken B, Engel N, Topp M, Klutmann S, Amthauer H, Bockisch A, Kluge R, Kratochwil C, Schober O, Greil R, Andreesen R, Kneba M, Pfreundschuh M, Stein H, Eich HT, Muller RP, Dietlein M, Borchmann P, Diehl V; German Hodgkin Study Group; Swiss Group for Clinical Cancer Research; Arbeitsgemeinschaft Medikamentöse Tumortherapie: Reduced-intensity chemotherapy and PET-guided radiotherapy in patients with advanced stage Hodgkin's lymphoma (HD15 trial): a randomised, open-label, phase 3 non-inferiority trial. Lancet 2012;379:1791–1799.
19 Kelly KM, Sposto R, Hutchinson R, Massey V, McCarten K, Perkins S, Lones M, Villaluna D, Weiner M: BEACOPP chemotherapy is a highly effective regimen in children and adolescents with high-risk Hodgkin lymphoma: a report from the Children's Oncology Group. Blood 2011;117:2596–2603.
20 Eichenauer DA, Bredenfeld H, Haverkamp H, Muller H, Franklin J, Fuchs M, Borchmann P, Muller-Hermelink HK, Eich HT, Muller RP, Diehl V, Engert A: Hodgkin's lymphoma in adolescents treated with adult protocols: a report from the German Hodgkin Study Group. J Clin Oncol 2009;27:6079–6085.
21 Engert A, Plutschow A, Eich HT, Lohri A, Dorken B, Borchmann P, Berger B, Greil R, Willborn KC, Wilhelm M, Debus J, Eble MJ, Sokler M, Ho A, Rank A, Ganser A, Trumper L, Bokemeyer C, Kirchner H, Schubert J, Kral Z, Fuchs M, Muller-Hermelink HK, Muller RP, Diehl V: Reduced treatment intensity in patients with early-stage Hodgkin's lymphoma. N Engl J Med 2010;363:640–652.
22 Veal GJ, Hartford CM, Stewart CF: Clinical pharmacology in the adolescent oncology patient. J Clin Oncol 2010;28:4790–4799.
23 Kremer LC, van Dalen EC, Offringa M, Voute PA: Frequency and risk factors of anthracycline-induced clinical heart failure in children: a systematic review. Ann Oncol 2002; 13:503–512.

24 Josting A, Wiedenmann S, Franklin J, May M, Sieber M, Wolf J, Engert A, Diehl V; German Hodgkin's Lymphoma Study Group: Secondary myeloid leukemia and myelodysplastic syndromes in patients treated for Hodgkin's disease: a report from the German Hodgkin's Lymphoma Study Group. J Clin Oncol 2003; 21:3440–3446.

25 Rueffer U, Josting A, Franklin J, May M, Sieber M, Breuer K, Engert A, Diehl V; German Hodgkin's Lymphoma Study Group: Non-Hodgkin's lymphoma after primary Hodgkin's disease in the german Hodgkin's Lymphoma Study Group: incidence, treatment, and prognosis. J Clin Oncol 2001;19: 2026–2032.

26 Dores GM, Metayer C, Curtis RE, Lynch CF, Clarke EA, Glimelius B, Storm H, Pukkala E, van Leeuwen FE, Holowaty EJ, Andersson M, Wiklund T, Joensuu T, van't Veer MB, Stovall M, Gospodarowicz M, Travis LB: Second malignant neoplasms among long-term survivors of Hodgkin's disease: a population-based evaluation over 25 years. J Clin Oncol 2002; 20:3484–3494.

27 Behringer K, Mueller H, Goergen H, Thielen I, Eibl AD, Stumpf V, Wessels C, Wiehlputz M, Rosenbrock J, Halbsguth T, Reiners KS, Schober T, Renno JH, von Wolff M, van der Ven K, Kuehr M, Fuchs M, Diehl V, Engert A, Borchmann P: Gonadal function and fertility in survivors after Hodgkin lymphoma treatment within the German Hodgkin Study Group HD13 to HD15 trials. J Clin Oncol 2013;31:231–239.

28 Von Tresckow B, Plutschow A, Fuchs M, Klimm B, Markova J, Lohri A, Kral Z, Greil R, Topp MS, Meissner J, Zijlstra JM, Soekler M, Stein H, Eich HT, Mueller RP, Diehl V, Borchmann P, Engert A: Dose-intensification in early unfavorable Hodgkin's lymphoma: final analysis of the German Hodgkin Study Group HD14 trial. J Clin Oncol 2012;30:907–913.

29 Sauer M, Plutschow A, Jachimowicz RD, Kleefisch D, Reiners KS, Ponader S, Engert A, von Strandmann EP: Baseline serum TARC levels predict therapy outcome in patients with Hodgkin lymphoma. Am J Hematol 2013;88:113–115.

30 Ouyang J, Plutschow A, Pogge von Strandmann E, Reiners KS, Ponader S, Rabinovich GA, Neuberg D, Engert A, Shipp MA: Galectin-1 serum levels reflect tumor burden and adverse clinical features in classical Hodgkin lymphoma. Blood 2013;121:3431–3433.

31 Scott DW, Chan FC, Hong F, Rogic S, Tan KL, Meissner B, Ben-Neriah S, Boyle M, Kridel R, Telenius A, Woolcock BW, Farinha P, Fisher RI, Rimsza LM, Bartlett NL, Cheson BD, Shepherd LE, Advani RH, Connors JM, Kahl BS, Gordon LI, Horning SJ, Steidl C, Gascoyne RD: Gene expression-based model using formalin-fixed paraffin-embedded biopsies predicts overall survival in advanced-stage classical Hodgkin lymphoma. J Clin Oncol 2013;31:692–700.

Acta Haematol 2014;132:279–291
DOI: 10.1159/000360212

Published online: September 10, 2014

Adolescents and Young Adults with Non-Hodgkin's Lymphoma: Slipping between the Cracks

Ofir Wolach   Ron Ram

Institute of Hematology, Davidoff Cancer Center, Beilinson Hospital, Rabin Medical Center and the Sackler Faculty of Medicine, Tel Aviv University, Tel Aviv, Israel

Key Words

Adolescents and young adults · Non-Hodgkin's lymphoma

Abstract

Adolescents and young adults (AYAs) with cancer have inferior survival as compared to children. The reasons for this survival gap are multifactorial and related to psychosocial aspects, patient- and disease-related biological characteristics as well as to therapeutic approaches within this age span. Non-Hodgkin's lymphoma (NHL) comprises approximately 7% of cancer among AYAs, and patient allocation and therapy vary between health systems. In this systematic review we focus on the current biological and clinical knowledge relevant to AYAs with NHL applying these data to the clinical approach and practice. Data are insufficient to recommend a pediatric or an adult approach for AYAs with diffuse large B-cell lymphoma and anaplastic large cell lymphoma. Dose-adjusted EPOCH-R seems to be a promising, radiation-free approach for AYAs with primary mediastinal B-cell lymphoma. Limitations in data interpretation include the lack of interventional trials tailored specifically for the AYA population and the lack of uniform criteria for staging and response assessment in pediatric and adult trials.

© 2014 S. Karger AG, Basel

Introduction

Non-Hodgkin's lymphoma (NHL) encompasses a heterogeneous set of malignancies. Within this diverse group, wide variations exist in disease histology, biology and in the clinical approach to each lymphoma subtype [1]. Analysis of the Surveillance, Epidemiology and End Result (SEER) data set demonstrates that the incidence of NHL increases with age [2, 3]. Annual rates of new NHL diagnoses range from 0.5–1.2/100,000 in children up to the age of 15 years to 1.8–7.2 in adolescents and young adults (AYAs) and 10.5–116.4/100,000 in adults over 40 years of age [4]. Survival of patients with NHL is affected by age with a significant decrease in patient outcome with older age. Data emerging from German and American population-based registries demonstrate a striking age-related survival difference. The 5-year relative survival of patients with NHL in the years 2002–2006 in a large German registry was reported to be 82% in the 15- to 49-year-old and decreased to 46% in the >75-year-old group [5].

AYAs, commonly defined as patients aged 16–39 years [4], have become the focus of basic and clinical investigation in recent years. Inferior survival of this patient group as compared to younger patients was demonstrated across various hematological and nonhematological malignancies [6]. The reasons for this survival gap are not com-

Ofir Wolach, MD
Institute of Hematology
Davidoff Cancer Center, Rabin Medical Center
Petah Tikva (Israel)
E-Mail tammyof@smile.net.il

pletely understood and may be related to patient-related factors, disease-related factors and to therapeutic strategies. Patient-related factors that may affect survival include psychosocial aspects unique to this age group, insurance barriers and delays in diagnosis [4]. Furthermore, in contrast to pediatric populations, a low recruitment rate to clinical trials is characteristic of the AYA population [7], and thus data analyzed for this group are less robust and mainly based on clinical experience.

Therapeutic strategies and treatment intensity significantly vary between pediatric and adult approaches and may affect patient outcome. A recent report from the Children's Oncology Group showed clear age-related differences in the pattern of treatment toxicity in older (aged 16–21 years) and younger patients [6], pointing to age-related pharmacokinetic differences in the tolerability of intensive therapy. There are no clear guidelines as to the proper allocation of AYA patients with malignancies, and local referral patterns may significantly differ.

The frequency of different lymphoma subtypes varies within the AYA group of patients. According to SEER data, NHL comprises 7% of cancer in the 15- to 29-year-old group with the most prevalent histological subtype being diffuse large B-cell lymphoma (DLBCL). This is in contrast to younger patients in whom Burkitt's lymphoma and lymphoblastic lymphoma are the commonest variants. Follicular and mantle cell lymphoma appear in the 15- to 20-year-old group but are uncommon in younger patients [2]. The major histological subtypes among adolescents were reported from French (age 15–20 years) and German (age 15–18 years) cooperative trials and demonstrated the following frequencies: DLBCL in 37 and 15%, Burkitt's lymphoma in 22 and 27%, anaplastic large cell lymphoma (ALCL) in 18 and 20% and lymphoblastic lymphoma in 17 and 15%, respectively [8, 9]. Primary mediastinal B-cell lymphoma (PMBCL) comprised 6% of patients in 1 study [8].

In this systematic review we focus on the current biological and clinical knowledge relevant to AYAs with 3 NHL subtypes applying these data to the clinical approach and practice.

Materials and Methods

Data Sources and Search
We followed the published recommendations for systematic reviews to search the literature and report the results [10]. A comprehensive search strategy was employed to identify both published and unpublished studies, with no restriction on language, type of publication or study years. We searched Medline from 1971 through June 2013 and the proceedings of the relevant conferences (American Society of Hematology, American Society of Clinical Oncology and European Hematology Association) from 2004 to 2012. We used the following search terms: (adolescent or young adults) and (lymphoma [MeSH]) and crossed them with a highly sensitive search for trials: prospective or longitudinal or cohort or randomized controlled trial [pt] or controlled clinical trial [pt] or randomized controlled trials [mh] or random allocation [mh] NOT (animals [mh] NOT human [mh]). The references of all identified articles were inspected for more studies.

Study Selection
To be eligible for inclusion in this review, publications had to include original data from randomized controlled trials, cohort studies, case-control or nested case-control studies. Two reviewers (R.R. and O.W.) inspected the title and, when available, the abstract of each reference identified in the search and applied the inclusion criteria. Where relevant articles were identified, the full article was obtained and inspected independently by the above two reviewers, and inclusion criteria were applied. The quality of design and strength of evidence were used to grade authors' recommendations [11].

Diffuse Large B-Cell Lymphoma

DLBCL is the most common histological subtype of NHL. It accounts for over 30% of all NHL with an incidence that increases with age [12, 13]. The median age for diagnosis of DLBCL is between the sixth and seventh decades [14], but it is still the most common lymphoma encountered in AYAs with NHL [2]. Analysis of SEER registries from 1992 through 2001 demonstrated that DLBCL comprised 28% of NHL diagnoses in patients aged 0–19 years as compared to 49% of diagnoses in the 20–29 years age group [3]. Patient age at diagnosis significantly affects survival in DLBCL [5]. Pediatric and adolescent patients were previously shown to have higher survival rates than young adults with DLBCL. Analysis of SEER data during the years 1999–2001 demonstrated an estimated 5-year survival rate of 92.2% for patients aged 0–19 years as compared to 84.7% for patients aged 20–29 years [3].

The systematic evaluation of different treatment approaches in AYAs is a complex challenge. Randomized controlled trials designed specifically for AYAs are lacking, and thus most data regarding the efficacy of different therapeutic approaches stems from analysis of subgroups within pediatric and adult studies. Different approaches to classification, staging and treatment and the lack of consensus definition for response among pediatric and adult approaches make comparison of factors that affect outcome extremely difficult.

Children usually treated within cooperative studies are grouped with other mature B-cell lymphomas and are treated with risk-adapted and intensive approaches [15, 16]. The number of treatment cycles as well as dose intensity are related to the estimated risk for relapse of the patient [17]. The evidence regarding adolescents with DLBCL largely comes from those treated within cooperative pediatric trials, but off-trial allocation may be influenced by local referral patterns.

Recently, Cairo et al. [18] presented their analysis on 1,111 pediatric and adolescent patients with mature B-lineage NHL treated in the FAB LMB96 trial. This was a French, American and British cooperative effort recruiting patients up to the age of 21 years. Therapy was risk adapted and generally followed as such: low-risk patients (limited stage, resected disease) received 2 treatment courses (COPAD: cyclophosphamide, vincristine, prednisone, doxorubicin), and high-risk patients (bone marrow involvement >25% and/or central nervous system involvement) received acute lymphoblastic leukemia-type therapy. The intermediate-risk group (non-low- and non-high-risk patients) included most patients with DLBCL, and therapy included a prephase (COP: low-dose cyclophosphamide, vincristine and prednisone) followed by 2 induction courses (COPDM: cyclophosphamide, vincristine, prednisone, doxorubicin, high-dose methotrexate and intrathecal therapy), 2 consolidation courses (CYM: cytarabine/high-dose methotrexate) and a single maintenance course (cyclophosphamide, vincristine, prednisone, doxorubicin and high-dose methotrexate) [18–20]. Randomization for an intensified second induction and for maintenance therapy was part of the study design. Such an approach yielded a 3-year overall survival (OS) and event-free survival (EFS) of 90 and 88%, respectively. The EFS rates for low-, intermediate- and high-risk patients were 99, 89 and 79%, respectively [21]. As expected, Burkitt's and Burkitt-like lymphomas were more frequent in the pediatric group, and DLBCL was more prevalent in the adolescent group. Interestingly, the estimated 3-year EFS in this study was similar for children under the age of 15 and for adolescents over the age of 15 (89 and 84%, respectively). Multivariate analysis demonstrated that age, prognostic group, stage and pathology did not affect EFS while primary site, elevated lactate dehydrogenase (LDH) and concomitant involvement of the bone marrow and central nervous system did [21]. Recently the addition of rituximab to the FAB LMB96 protocol for patients with advanced NHL demonstrated even better outcomes for this patient population [22].

Other groups did however demonstrate inferior outcomes for adolescents as compared to children treated under identical conditions. Patte et al. [23] studied 561 patients with various types of mature B-cell lymphoma treated with the LMB89 protocol and demonstrated that age between 15 and 18 years is an independent risk factor for shortened EFS as compared to younger patients (relative risks 6.7 and 1.4 as compared to patients aged <8 years and 8–15 years, respectively; p = 0.01). Burkhardt et al. [24] studied the impact of age on patient outcome by analyzing 3 Berlin-Frankfurt-Munster (BFM) multicenter protocols from 1986 to 2007. These studies included 2,915 evaluable patients up to the age of 18 years with aggressive NHL. Of these, 242 patients were diagnosed with DLBCL, centeroblastic subtype. Patients received a pulse-type therapy according to protocol consisting of 5-day courses based on dexamethasone, cyclophosphamide, ifosphamide, methotrexate, cytarabine, doxorubicin, etoposide and intrathecal therapy. Within the DLBCL population, a 5-year EFS of 85% was reported for adolescents over the age of 15 years as compared to 96% in children under 15 years of age (p = 0.0019). Further analysis of the DLBCL subgroup demonstrated a striking gender effect. While no difference in EFS was noted among younger and older male patients, adolescent females fared significantly worse compared with younger females (5-year EFS for male and female adolescents 97 and 71%, respectively). This gender effect remained significant in multivariate analysis [8, 24].

Adult patients with DLBCL are generally treated with rituximab and CHOP (cyclophosphamide, vincristine, doxorubicin and prednisone)-based therapy. Most adult studies use the age of 60–65 years as the watershed line to study 'older' versus 'younger' patients with DLBCL, thus grouping AYAs with patients up to the age of 60 years. Although patients are stratified by clinical scores that predict outcome, notably the International Prognostic Index (IPI) and the age-adjusted IPI [25], and despite recently identified biological and genetic markers associated with outcome [14], risk-adapted therapy in adults with DLBCL is not generally practiced outside of clinical trials.

Randomized controlled trials treating low-risk patients under the age of 60 years (age-adjusted IPI 0–1) demonstrated inferior outcomes to those reported in pediatric studies. The combination of rituximab and CHOP-like therapy was reported to achieve a 3-year EFS and OS of 79 and 93%, respectively, for low-risk young patients [26, 27]. In a phase III study comparing a more intensive R-ACVBP (rituximab, doxorubicin, cyclophosphamide,

Acta Haematol 2014;132:279–291
DOI: 10.1159/000360212

vindesine, bleomycin and prednisone) to R-CHOP, the EFSs for low-risk patients treated with R-ACVBP and R-CHOP were 81 and 67%, respectively. The 3-year OS for the two groups were 92 and 84%, respectively [28]. In both studies cited above, the median patient age was 47 years. Cunningham et al. [29] recently demonstrated in a randomized prospective manner that R-CHOP given every 21 days is comparable in terms of progression-free survival and OS to the dose-dense R-CHOP given every 14 days in AYA and adult patients and that even patients with high-risk IPI and patients under the age of 60 did not benefit from such an intensive therapy.

As opposed to the more favorable groups, adults with an age-adjusted IPI of 2–3 compose a high-risk population with one third of patients having refractory disease [14]. A high-intensity, transplantation-based approach as part of first-line therapy did not provide a survival benefit in the prerituximab era [30]. Recent studies that incorporated rituximab into dose-dense and dose-intense regimens followed by transplantation demonstrated a better progression-free survival with no OS benefit [31, 32]. Current treatment approaches are not satisfactory in the young high-risk patients, and various high-intensity, transplantation-based approaches are under evaluation [14].

Age-specific differences in disease biology may account at least in part for survival differences between younger and older patients with DLBCL. Klapper et al. [33] recently demonstrated that the frequency of adverse molecular signatures in DLBCL increases with age. The pivotal studies by Alizadeh et al. [34] and Rosenwald et al. [35] defined subgroups within the adult DLBCL population based on the pattern of gene expression, mainly the germinal center B-cell type (GCB) and the activated B-cell type (ABC) subgroups, and demonstrated superior outcome for the former [34, 35]. A classification based on immunohistochemistry expression pattern of CD10, BCL6 and MUM1 was later developed by Hans et al. [36] and was shown to correlate with GCB and ABC phenotypes. In the pediatric and adolescent population, the GCB phenotype is more common than in the adult population. Applying the Hans classifier to patients with DLBCL enrolled to the FAB LMB96 and the BFM trials demonstrated a GCB phenotype in 75 and 82% of patients, respectively [37, 38], a significantly higher incidence compared with the adult frequency of 40–50% [37]. Of note, the GCB phenotype did not confer superior EFS in these studies. Analysis of pediatric and adolescent patients enrolled in the FAB LMB96 trial also demonstrated high proliferation rates (83% of cases), increased c-Myc

protein expression (84%) and decreased Bcl2 protein expression (28%) [37].

Deffenbacher et al. [39] studied molecular distinctions between pediatric and adult mature B-cell NHL through genetic expression profiling. The frequencies of GCB and ABC subgroups were in line with results from immunohistochemistry-based classification studies demonstrating a predominance of GCB signature among the 21 pediatric DLBCL cases studied. Comparing molecularly classified pediatric and adult cases of DLBCL identified only 132 differentially expressed genes between adult and pediatric GCB with adult samples demonstrating enrichment in the expression of genes involved in B-cell receptor signaling and altered T- and B-cell signaling pathways as compared to children [39]. Higher rates of *myc* rearrangement as well as characteristic chromosomal abnormalities were demonstrated in pediatric cases as compared to adults [37, 39–41]. Recently, a novel translocation resulting in an IG/IRF4 fusion was described in germinal center-derived B-cell lymphoma. This genetic signature was associated with young age and a favorable outcome [42].

A dose-adjusted (DA)-EPOCH-R (etoposide, prednisone, vincristine, cyclophosphamide, doxorubicin and rituximab) protocol may be of special interest for the AYA population. This protocol was developed at the National Cancer Institute based on the observation that continuous low-dose drug exposure enhances cell killing of rapidly proliferating tumor cells in vitro. Oral prednisone is given with a 96-hour infusional protocol of vincristine, doxorubicin and etoposide in combination with bolus administration of cyclophosphamide and rituximab. A pharmacodynamic dosing based on the neutrophil nadir is applied since the efficacy of infusional schedules is limited by subthreshold steady-state concentrations, below which a drug is ineffective [43–45]. The use of DA-EPOCH-R in patients with untreated DLBCL seems to be effective with an acceptable toxicity profile. In a recent Cancer and Leukemia Group B trial, 69 patients over the age of 18 (median age 58; range 23–83) were treated with DA-EPOCH-R, and at a median follow-up of 62 months OS was 84%. The 5-year EFS and OS for the low/low-intermediate, high-intermediate and high IPI risk groups were 85 and 95%, 85 and 92%, and 43 and 43%, respectively. When patients were stratified by the GCB and non-GCB phenotype based on the Hans classifier [36], a survival benefit for the GCB group was noted. EFSs at 62 months for the GCB and non-GCB groups were 94 and 58%, respectively (p = 0.008) [45]. The superior outcome of patients in the GCB phenotype group treated with DA-

Acta Haematol 2014;132:279–291
DOI: 10.1159/000360212

EPOCH-R may be of interest for the AYA population since the frequency of the GCB phenotype is significantly higher in the pediatric and adolescent population as compared to the adult population [37, 38]. These differences between the immunohistochemistry-defined GCB and non-GCB groups in terms of outcome are noteworthy. While a clear survival difference between GCB and non-GCB patients was demonstrated when gene expression profiling was used [34, 35], no difference in outcome between the GCB and non-GCB groups was shown in the majority of trials using immunohistochemistry-based classifiers to discriminate both pediatric/adolescent [37, 38] and adult patients [46, 47]. Modulation of the key germinal center B-cell transcription factor BCL6 may play a significant role in the superior protocol efficacy in the GCB group. The potent inhibition of topoisomerase II in this protocol by continuous exposure to two topoisomerase II inhibitors, etoposide and doxorubicin, may lead to downregulation of BCL6 expression and ameliorate its effects [43–45].

Bouabdallah et al. [48] recently presented the first matched control analysis of AYA and older patients with large B-cell lymphoma. Fifty-five AYA patients aged 16–30 years were compared to 165 patients aged 31–65 years. Groups were fully matched for IPI, chemotherapy regimen and rituximab delivery. The AYA patients demonstrated higher rates of mediastinal mass, LDH and PMBCL subtype. No differences between the two groups were observed in terms of complete remission, OS or EFS [48]. Patte et al. [9] analyzed patients 15–20 years old treated in pediatric or adult trials in France. Of 341 patients with NHL, 37% (126 patients) were diagnosed with DLBCL. EFS at 3 years for patients with DLBCL treated with pediatric and adult approaches was 77 and 83% (nonsignificant), respectively [9].

In summary, the AYA population with DLBCL is an 'at-risk' population that is underrepresented in clinical trials. Unique biological characteristics may allow a more tailored therapeutic approach towards this population. Current data demonstrate superior outcomes for pediatric and adolescent patients with DLBCL as compared to adults, but no prospective controlled comparison has yet been published. Based on the current data, both pediatric and adult regimens are reasonable and allocation may be largely based on the local policy (level of evidence 2+, grade of recommendation C). Randomized controlled trials focused on the AYA population are needed to assess therapeutic interventions in this population. Studies assessing a pediatric inspired approach in the AYA population similar to the effort undertaken in AYAs with acute lymphoblastic leukemia [49] may be needed in order to improve the outcome of AYA patients with high-risk DLBCL.

Primary Mediastinal B-Cell Lymphoma

PMBCL is a distinct clinical and pathological entity that is thought to stem from asteroid B cells of the thymus. Disease is more often encountered in young women and presents with a large mediastinal mass that frequently invades adjacent structures [14]. The typical histological presentation consists of tumor cells with a pale cytoplasm and a diffuse growth pattern associated with variable degrees of sclerosis. PMBCL has a distinct molecular signature that interestingly shares molecular features with classical Hodgkin's lymphoma [50]. This entity is reported to comprise 10% of DLBCL cases [51] and may be of special interest for AYAs since it is more often recorded in young women [14]. A report from the BFM group showed that PMBCL comprises 1% of NHL among patients under the age of 15 years as compared to 6% in patients in the 15- to 18-year age group [8]. In the Mabthera International Trial Study, which enrolled patients from the age of 18 to 60 years, 12% of the 714 evaluable patients with aggressive lymphoma had PMBCL. Younger age (median 36 years) and female predominance (59% of the cohort) characterized this subgroup [52]. In the RICOVER-60 trial that enrolled patients with aggressive NHL between the ages of 61 and 80 years, only 13 of the 1,222 patients (1%) were diagnosed with PMBCL [53]. In contrast to the excellent responses of the majority of children and adolescents with mature B-cell lymphoma enrolled in large cooperative trials (refer to the DLBCL section), patients with PMBCL fare less well in terms of survival. Early reports from the Children's Cancer Group and BFM study groups demonstrated in relatively small cohorts of patients a 5-year EFS of 75 and 70%, respectively [54, 55]. A later analysis of the BFM experience (n = 51) demonstrated a nonsignificant difference in outcome between the pediatric and adolescent populations: 5-year EFS of 70% for patients up to the age of 15 years as compared to 57% in patients over 15 years of age (p = 0.41) [8]. Forty-two patients with PMBCL were recently presented in an analysis of the FAB LMB96 protocol and demonstrated a 5-year EFS and OS of 66 and 73%, respectively. [56]. Of note, according to the pediatric Murphy staging system [57], PMBCL is considered a stage III disease and is thus treated as an intermediate-risk disease (refer to DLBCL section).

Acta Haematol 2014;132:279–291
DOI: 10.1159/000360212

The approach to young-adult and adult patients with PMBCL has significantly changed in recent years with dramatic improvements in patient outcome, resulting from both the introduction of rituximab and novel escalated dose-dense therapies. There is no standard of care for PMBCL in adults and various therapeutic approaches evolved over the years. The use of intensified protocols such as MACOP-B (methotrexate, doxorubicin, cyclophosphamide, vincristine, prednisone and bleomycin) or VACOP-B (etoposide instead of methotrexate) were investigated and demonstrated conflicting efficacy as compared to CHOP or CHOP-like regimens [58, 59]. Moreover, most protocols add radiotherapy to disease bulk to improve disease control and may expose by this the relatively young patients to potential toxicities associated with this combined modality approach [60]. The advent of rituximab significantly improved outcomes with CHOP-based therapies. An analysis of 87 patients with PMBCL in the Mabthera International Trial (median age 36 years) demonstrated a 3-year EFS of 78% with the addition of rituximab to CHOP as compared with 52% in the CHOP arm (p = 0.012). Rituximab virtually eliminated progressive disease and improved OS from 78 to 89% (p = 0.158). Of note, 78% of patients in the R-CHOP arm received adjuvant radiotherapy [52]. Recently, Dunleavy et al. [51] published a prospective phase II study on the National Cancer Institute experience with the DA-EPOCH-R protocol for patients with PMBCL (refer to DLBCL section for details on this protocol). Fifty-one patients, half of whom were younger than 30 years (range 19–52 years), were included in the analysis. The 5-year EFS and OS for this cohort were 93 and 97%, respectively. Only 2 patients of the 3 nonresponders in this cohort were consolidated with radiotherapy while all responders were not exposed to radiotherapy. These excellent outcomes were similar in a retrospective cohort of 16 patients presented in the same publication [51]. Dose intensity as well as the infusional nature of this protocol may contribute to these outstanding outcomes. Moreover, the topoisomerase II inhibitory properties of this protocol (as discussed in the DLBCL section) may modulate BCL6 activity and lead to downregulation of this protein, thus ameliorating its effects. Indeed, BCL6 is highly expressed in PMBCL malignant cells and was expressed in 89% of patients in the above study [51]. The DA-EPOCH-R offers a highly effective approach for treating patients with PMBCL and importantly abates the need for consolidative radiotherapy in most patients. Following these promising results, DA-EPOCH-R was adopted for pediatric and adolescent patients in the B-cell NHL-BFM04 study in 2010. Variations from the original

protocol included limiting the cumulative exposure to doxorubicin and the administration of intrathecal prophylaxis. Recently 15 patients with a median age of 16 years (range 11.5–17.8 years) were reported. The 2-year EFS and OS in this group were both 92% [61].

In summary, a significant fraction of patients affected with PMBCL are AYAs. As such, most patients with PMBCL in the pediatric cooperative trials are adolescents, and young adults comprise much of the patient cohort in adult trials. Patient outcomes are somewhat disappointing in pediatric protocols thus far but recent publications demonstrate promising results for adults treated with DA-EPOCH-R. PMBCL may be the unusual case of adopting a so-called adult-inspired protocol for adolescents and perhaps pediatric patients. Based on the current data, we recommend DA-EPOCH-R for all AYA patients (level of evidence 2+, grade of recommendation C). Further randomized controlled trials comparing DA-EPOCH-R with standard R-CHOP are warranted.

Anaplastic Large Cell Lymphoma

ALCL is characterized by large anaplastic cells which stain positive for CD30 [62]. The majority of cases are associated with the nonrandom translocation t(2;5)(p23;q35). This unique chromosomal translocation fuses the anaplastic lymphoma kinase *(ALK)* gene on chromosome 2 with the nucleophosmin *(NPM)* gene on chromosome 5 resulting in a fusion gene that encodes for an 80-kDa NPM-ALK chimeric protein with constitutive tyrosine kinase activity [63]. Based on the ALK expression, distinct subgroups have been specified in the 2008 version of the WHO classification: primary cutaneous CD30-positive T-cell lymphoproliferative disorders, ALK-positive ALCL, and ALK-negative ALCL [62].

ALCL occurs more commonly in adolescents with lymphoma than in other ages [8]. The incidence of ALCL increases from 11% in the younger adolescent group and approaches 20% in those older than 15 years [8].

The clinical presentation of ALCL is heterogeneous and can vary greatly between individual patients. Of note, extranodal manifestations mainly involving the skin, soft tissue and bone are reported more frequently than in other adolescent subgroups of NHL [64, 65]. The majority of the patients have a prolonged period of nonspecific symptoms and most are diagnosed at an advanced stage [66]. Bone marrow and central nervous system involvement at diagnosis is rare, while B symptoms are common. As in other forms of malignancies, adolescents, compared to children, are usually diagnosed at a more advanced stage (80 vs. 68%, p = 0.06) [66]. As in other subtypes of malignancies, compliance and sociological challenges are of main importance contributing to the relatively late diagnosis [4]. Outcomes for adolescents compared with children with ALCL show no differences between the two age groups (70 ± 3 vs. 70 ± 6%) and, within the adolescent age group, there is no significant difference in outcome according to sex [8]. Most of the adolescent patients exhibit ALK1 protein expression and only a minority have an ALK1-negative disease. This is true for both adolescents and younger patients with 12% versus 10% ALK1-negative ALCL, respectively [8]. Similarly, another multicenter trial of the European Intergroup Cooperation NHL group recruiting patients up to the age of 22 years, demonstrated a frequency of ALK-positive cases of 96% [67]. Apart from the ALK1 status, CD56 expression was also identified as an independent predictor of outcome, regardless of ALK expression status [68].

Contrary to other NHL subtypes, adolescent age at diagnosis does not affect prognosis [8, 64]. Similarly, age >10 years was of no prognostic relevance for 72 pediatric ALCL patients treated with a UKCCSG (United Kingdom Children's Cancer Study Group) chemotherapy regimen. The pooled BFM-SFOP (Société Française d'Oncologie Pédiatrique)-UKCCSG analyses of prognostic parameters in ALCL reported on 117 of 225 patients >10 years of age at diagnosis [69] and showed that age >10 years was not associated with outcome. Concerning the ALK1 status, ALK1-negative ALCL was reported to occur more frequently with increasing age and was associated with inferior outcome [70, 71]. Within the BFM-SFOP-UKCCSG series, the frequency of ALK1-negative ALCL did not differ between pediatric and adolescent patients. In fact, the comparison of current outcome data in adolescents with published data on adult ALCL patients trends toward inferior survival in adults with ALCL, which might be, at least in part, related to the higher rates of ALK-negative ALCL in adult patients [63, 72, 73].

No clinical trials specifically focused on adolescents with ALCL have been reported to date. Treatment of adolescent ALCL patients therefore follows either pediatric or adult protocols, and the criteria for the allocation of adolescents to pediatric or adult departments vary within study groups. For the purpose of comparing pediatric and adult protocols, studies were separated accordingly.

Several pediatric clinical trials recruited patients up to the age of 18 or 21 years at diagnosis and thus included a substantial number of adolescent patients. Both ALL-based regimen and B-NHL-based therapy have resulted in comparable EFS rates of 70–93%. The largest pediatric series of ALCL patients reported on 352 patients enrolled in the EICNHL trial ALCL 99 [67]. This trial enrolled patients up to the age of 22 years. The chemotherapy regimen was based on the BFM-90 protocol [74]. The largest series of adolescents with ALCL treated according to the pediatric protocols was reported by the NHL-BFM group. This recent analysis included all patients registered in NHL-BFM studies between 1986 and 2007 [8] and reported the outcome of 74 adolescent ALCL patients who were 15–18 years of age at diagnosis. There was no difference in disease risk between children and adolescents. All these trials, as shown in table 1, showed similar outcomes, and the outcome for adolescents compared to children with ALCL enrolled during the same period was also similar. Treatment-related mortality was uncommon occurring in 1% of the adolescents, and secondary malignancies were documented in 3% [8]. Overall, survival of patients with ALK-positive lymphoma was better than that of patients with ALK-negative ALCL (71 vs. 15%, respectively). It is hard to draw strict conclusions regarding the success of the different regimens in adolescents; however, several conclusions can be made: first, outcomes for patients older than 10 years are similar to those <10 years; second, both continuous ALL-like protocols and B-NHL pulse intensive chemotherapy regimen are equal in terms of OS.

In contrast to the pediatric studies, most of the adult studies utilized doxorubicin-based or CHOP-based regimens for the treatment of adult ALCL patients. In the study by Gascoyne et al. [72] all patients were treated with a doxorubicin-based regimen. Although no subgroup analysis of adolescent patients was done, the median age of the 36 patients in the ALK-positive group was 30 years, thus the overall results of this group may apply to adolescent patients. The 5-year OS was 79% in this group. Normal LDH, good performance status, <2 extranodal sites and IPI <3 were all found to be associated with better survival. A recent report of the International Peripheral T-Cell Lymphoma Project reported on 87 patients with ALK-positive and 72 patients with ALK-negative ALCL. For patients with ALK-positive disease, the median age was 34 years [63]. Treatment was an anthracycline-based regimen and 5-year survival for the ALK-positive patients was 70%. Interestingly this report claimed that survival below the age of 40 years was not statistically different between the ALK-positive and the ALK-negative groups, suggesting that age is a prominent factor driving outcome differences. Patte et al. [9] compared between pediatric and adult protocols that were

Acta Haematol 2014;132:279–291
DOI: 10.1159/000360212

Table 1. Main characteristics and outcomes in selected studies that included AYA patients

Study group	Publication	Age, years	Patients, n	Outcome	Comments
DLBCL					
NHL-BFM (p)	Burkhardt et al. [8], 2011	15–18	55	5-year EFS 85%	Female sex associated with worse prognosis in the adolescent group (5-year EFS for males 97% and for females 71%; p = 0.0067)
FAB/LMB96 (p)	Patte et al. [20], 2007	Median 10.2 (range 2.5–20.5)	102 patients aged 15–21 years (total n = 637)	4-year EFS 93%	Treated as intermediate-risk patients per protocol (refer to text)
MInT trial (a)	Pfreundschuh et al. [26, 27], 2011	Median 47 (range 36–55)	413	6-year EFS 74% 6-year OS 90%	Low-risk patients (aaIPI ≤1); phase III trial comparing CHOP-like to R-CHOP-like therapy (results presented for R-CHOP arm)
LNH03-2B (a)	Recher et al. [28], 2011	Median 47 (range 18–59)	379	3-year EFS/OS: R-CHOP 67%/84% R-ACVBP 81%*/92%*	Low-risk patients (aaIPI ≤1); phase III trial comparing R-CHOP-like to more intensive R-ACVBP therapy
UK NCRI Lymphoma Clinical Study Group (a)	Cunningham et al. [29], 2013	Median 61 (range 19–85)	1,080	2-year PFS/OS: R-CHOP14 75%/83% R-CHOP21 75%/81%	R-CHOP21 equivalent to R-CHOP14 across all pre-specified subgroups including age and IPI
SWOG S9704 (a)	Stiff et al. [31], 2013	15–65	253	2-year PFS/OS: ASCT-based 69%*/74% CHOP/R-CHOP alone 56%/71%	High-risk patients attaining at least partial response randomized to ASCT or CHOP/R-CHOP alone
PMBCL					
NHL-BFM (p)	Burkhardt et al. [8], 2011	15–18	24	5-year EFS 57%	
FAB/LMB96 (p)	Gerrard et al. [56], 2013	Median 15.7 (range 12.5–19.7)	42	5-year EFS 66% 5-year OS 73%	Treated as intermediate-risk patients per protocol (refer to text)
CCG (p)	Lones et al. [54], 2000	Median 12.5 (range 4–19)	20	5-year EFS 75% 5-year OS 85%	
NHL-BFM04 (p)	Woessman et al. [61], 2013	Median 16 (range 11.5–17.8)	15	2-year EFS 92%	Treated with DA-EPOCH-R
MInT (a)	Rieger et al. [52], 2011	Median 36 (range 27–43)	87	3-year EFS/OS: R-CHOP (like) 78%*/89% CHOP (like) 52%/78%	Subgroup analysis of the phase III MinT trial
NCI (a)	Dunleavy et al. [51], 2013	Median 30 (range 19–52)	51	5-year EFS 93% 5-year OS 97%	Phase II, DA-EPOCH-R
ALCL					
EICNHL 99 (p)	Brugieres et al. [67], 2009	Median 11 (range 0.3–19.5)	25 patients <16 years	2-year OS 92.5%	Phase III study assessing different doses of methotrexate
SFOP HM89 and HM91 (p)	Brugieres et al. [64], 1998	Median 10 (range 1.5–17)	38 patients >10 years	3-year OS 83% 3-year EFS 66% 3-year EFS 69% for AYAs	Data from 2 prospective phase II studies
NHL-BFM90 (p)	Seidemann et al. [74], 2001	Median 10.5 (range 0.8–17.3)	Not reported	5-year EFS 76%	A single-arm phase II study assessing a BFM regimen
CCG-5491 (p)	Lowe et al. [80], 2009	Not reported	18 patients >14 years	5-year OS 80% 5-year EFS 68%	
NHL-BFM90 (p)	Burkhardt et al. [8], 2011	15–18	74	5-year EFS 70%	
BCCA/UNMC (a)	Gascoyne et al. [72], 1999	15–75	18 with ALK positive <30 years	5-year OS 65% (ALK-positive 79%; ALK-negative 46%)	Cohort of 70 patients treated in 2 centers with different regimens; risk factors associated with OS were analyzed
International PTCL Project (a)	Savage et al. [63], 2008		44 with ALK positive <34 years	5-year OS ALK-positive 70%; ALK-negative 49%	A multicenter study designed to assess lymphoma risk factors

* p ≤ 0.05: statistically significant as compared to comparator arm. (p) = Pediatric oncology study group; (a) = adult oncology study group; PFS = progression-free survival; R-CHOP = rituximab, cyclophosphamide, vincristine, doxorubicin and prednisone; aaIPI = age-adjusted International Prognostic Index; R-ACVBP = rituximab, doxorubicin, cyclophosphamide, vindesine, bleomycin and prednisone; ASCT = autologous stem cell transplantation; DA-EPOCH-R = dose-adjusted etoposide, prednisone, vincristine, cyclophosphamide, doxorubicin and rituximab; PTCL = peripheral T-cell lymphoma.

Acta Haematol 2014;132:279–291
DOI: 10.1159/000360212

Wolach/Ram

given in several different studies to patients at ages of 15–20 years. They found no difference in 3-year EFS between the two groups (77 vs. 74%, respectively).

The common practice in many adult protocols is to further consolidate patients with ALCL (mainly those who have an ALK-negative disease) with autologous transplantation [75]. None of the studies reported specifically on the outcomes of adolescent patients given autografts; however, this approach, at least in patients with ALK-negative disease, is reasonable to date. The outcome of patients who do not respond to first-line therapy is dismal. The subgroup of patients with CD30-positive ALCL can be salvaged with brentuximab (a novel antibody-drug conjugate targeting CD30). This approach, when successful, is associated with only short response and should serve as a bridging to allogeneic hematopoietic cell transplantation [76]. The success of allogeneic hematopoietic cell transplantation for refractory or high-risk pediatric ALCL also suggests the potential immunotherapeutic benefit of a graft-versus-lymphoma effect [77]. A different novel agent, crizotinib, is a targeted inhibitor of ALK that has been shown to possess a substantial activity in a variety of malignancies harboring ALK translocation, specifically in ALK-positive ALCL [78]. Recently, a second-generation ALK inhibitor (AP26113) has shown promising results among patients progressing or not responding to crizotinib [79].

In conclusion, the outcome for ALCL patients treated according to pediatric protocols is similar for adolescents and younger children. Moreover, results are comparable, at least for the ALK-positive group when treated with adult protocols. Thus, ALK-positive adolescents can be treated with either adult or pediatric protocols (level of evidence 2+, grade of recommendation C). For the ALK-negative group (consisting only of 10% of adolescent patients) data are scarce. It is not clear whether the prognosis in this group, similarly to adult patients, is dismal. Future studies are encouraged to focus on this group to identify risk factors, outcomes and preferable therapy.

Conclusions

AYAs with NHL comprise a unique population with distinct psychosocial and biological features and with no standard of care for therapy. In this systematic review we highlighted several biological and clinical aspects characteristic of AYAs with NHL. Based on the review of data there are several points to be raised regarding future research goals in this age span. First, the lack of prospective trials designed specifically for this population coupled with a lack of uniform staging and response criteria between pediatric and adult cooperative groups preclude well-controlled comparisons of therapeutic strategies. Second, subgroup analysis of AYAs within prospective trials, specifically in young adults, is lacking and most of the data are analyzed by means of extrapolation from existing adult and pediatric trials. Furthermore, identifying biological properties that are characteristic of lymphoma in AYAs may enable a more tailored therapeutic approach towards this population Future trials should separately report outcomes on this group, and a multicenter collaborative effort focusing on therapeutic interventions in AYAs with NHL, perhaps in designated AYA centers, is a medical need. Only upon completion of these studies will we be able to answer the question whether AYAs should be treated as older children or as young adults.

Disclosure Statement

The authors have no conflicts of interest to declare.

References

1 Shankland KR, Armitage JO, Hancock BW: Non-Hodgkin lymphoma. Lancet 2012;380: 848–857.

2 O'Leary M, Sheaffer J, Keller F, Shu X, Cheson B: Lymphomas and reticuloendothelial neoplasmas; in Bleyer A, O'Leary M, Barr R, Ries L (eds): Cancer Epidemiology in Older Adolescents and Young Adults 15–29 Years of Age. Including SEER Incidence and Survival: 1975–2000. Bethesda, National Cancer Institute, 2006, pp 25–38.

3 Tai E, Pollack LA, Townsend J, Li J, Steele CB, Richardson LC: Differences in non-Hodgkin lymphoma survival between young adults and children. Arch Pediatr Adolesc Med 2010; 164:218–224.

4 Wood WA, Lee SJ: Malignant hematologic diseases in adolescents and young adults. Blood 2011;117:5803–5815.

5 Pulte D, Jansen L, Gondos A, Emrich K, Holleczek B, Katalinic A, Brenner H; Group GCSW: Survival of patients with non-Hodgkin lymphoma in Germany in the early 21st century. Leuk Lymphoma 2013;54:979–985.

6 Freyer DR, Felgenhauer J, Perentesis J; Adolescent COG, Young Adult Oncology Discipline C: Children's Oncology Group's 2013 blueprint for research: adolescent and young adult oncology. Pediatr Blood Cancer 2013; 60:1055–1058.

7 Bleyer A, Budd T, Montello M: Adolescents and young adults with cancer: the scope of the problem and criticality of clinical trials. Cancer 2006;107:1645–1655.

8 Burkhardt B, Oschlies I, Klapper W, Zimmermann M, Woessmann W, Meinhardt A, Landmann E, Attarbaschi A, Niggli F, Schrappe M, Reiter A: Non-Hodgkin's lymphoma in adolescents: experiences in 378 adolescent NHL patients treated according to pediatric NHL-BFM protocols. Leukemia 2011;25:153–160.

9 Patte C, Auperin A, Sebban C, Bergeron C, Gisselbrecht C, Ribrag V, Reyes F, Brugieres L: The 15–20 year old patients with NHL treated in France: data of childhood and adult database (abstract 85). Ann Oncol 2005;16(suppl 5):61.

10 Stroup DF, Berlin JA, Morton SC, Olkin I, Williamson GD, Rennie D, Moher D, Becker BJ, Sipe TA, Thacker SB: Meta-analysis of observational studies in epidemiology: a proposal for reporting. Meta-analysis of observational studies in epidemiology (MOOSE) group. JAMA 2000;283:2008–2012.

11 Harbour R, Miller J: A new system for grading recommendations in evidence based guidelines. BMJ 2001;323:334–336.

12 Morton LM, Wang SS, Devesa SS, Hartge P, Weisenburger DD, Linet MS: Lymphoma incidence patterns by WHO subtype in the United States, 1992–2001. Blood 2006;107:265–276.

13 Shenoy PJ, Malik N, Nooka A, Sinha R, Ward KC, Brawley OW, Lipscomb J, Flowers CR: Racial differences in the presentation and outcomes of diffuse large B-cell lymphoma in the United States. Cancer 2011;117:2530–2540.

14 Martelli M, Ferreri AJ, Agostinelli C, Di Rocco A, Pfreundschuh M, Pileri SA: Diffuse large B-cell lymphoma. Crit Rev Oncol Hematol 2013;87:146–171.

15 Hochberg J, Waxman IM, Kelly KM, Morris E, Cairo MS: Adolescent non-Hodgkin lymphoma and Hodgkin lymphoma: state of the science. Br J Haematol 2009;144:24–40.

16 Sandlund JT: Should adolescents with NHL be treated as old children or young adults? Hematol Am Soc Hematol Educ Program 2007, pp 297–303.

17 Lange J, Burkhardt B: Treatment of adolescents with aggressive B-cell malignancies: the pediatric experience. Curr Hematol Malig Rep 2013;8:226–235.

18 Cairo MS, Gerrard M, Sposto R, Auperin A, Pinkerton CR, Michon J, Weston C, Perkins SL, Raphael M, McCarthy K, Patte C; FAB LMB96 International Study Committee: Results of a randomized international study of high-risk central nervous system B non-Hodgkin lymphoma and B acute lymphoblastic leukemia in children and adolescents. Blood 2007;109:2736–2743.

19 Gerrard M, Cairo MS, Weston C, Auperin A, Pinkerton R, Lambilliote A, Sposto R, McCarthy K, Lacombe MJ, Perkins SL, Patte C; FAB LMB96 International Study Committee: Excellent survival following two courses of COPAD chemotherapy in children and ado-lescents with resected localized B-cell non-Hodgkin's lymphoma: results of the FAB/LMB 96 international study. Br J Haematol 2008;141:840–847.

20 Patte C, Auperin A, Gerrard M, Michon J, Pinkerton R, Sposto R, Weston C, Raphael M, Perkins SL, McCarthy K, Cairo MS; FAB LMB96 International Study Committee: Results of the randomized international FAB/LMB96 trial for intermediate risk B-cell non-Hodgkin lymphoma in children and adolescents: it is possible to reduce treatment for the early responding patients. Blood 2007;109:2773–2780.

21 Cairo MS, Sposto R, Gerrard M, Auperin A, Goldman SC, Harrison L, Pinkerton R, Raphael M, McCarthy K, Perkins SL, Patte C: Advanced stage, increased lactate dehydrogenase, and primary site, but not adolescent age (≥15 years), are associated with an increased risk of treatment failure in children and adolescents with mature B-cell non-Hodgkin's lymphoma: results of the FAB LMB 96 study. J Clin Oncol 2012;30:387–393.

22 Goldman S, Smith L, Anderson JR, Perkins S, Harrison L, Geyer MB, Gross TG, Weinstein H, Bergeron S, Shiramizu B, Sanger W, Barth M, Zhi J, Cairo MS: Rituximab and FAB/LMB 96 chemotherapy in children with stage III/IV B-cell non-Hodgkin lymphoma: a Children's Oncology Group report. Leukemia 2013;27:1174–1177.

23 Patte C, Auperin A, Michon J, Behrendt H, Leverger G, Frappaz D, Lutz P, Coze C, Perel Y, Raphael M, Terrier-Lacombe MJ; Société Française d'Oncologie Pédiatrique: The Société Française d'Oncologie Pédiatrique LMB89 protocol: highly effective multiagent chemotherapy tailored to the tumor burden and initial response in 561 unselected children with B-cell lymphomas and L3 leukemia. Blood 2001;97:3370–3379.

24 Burkhardt B, Zimmermann M, Oschlies I, Niggli F, Mann G, Parwaresch R, Riehm H, Schrappe M, Reiter A, Group BFM: The impact of age and gender on biology, clinical features and treatment outcome of non-Hodgkin lymphoma in childhood and adolescence. Br J Haematol 2005;131:39–49.

25 A predictive model for aggressive non-Hodgkin's lymphoma. The International Non-Hodgkin's Lymphoma Prognostic Factors Project. N Engl J Med 1993;329:987–994.

26 Pfreundschuh M, Kuhnt E, Trumper L, Osterborg A, Trneny M, Shepherd L, Gill DS, Walewski J, Pettengell R, Jaeger U, Zinzani PL, Shpilberg O, Kvaloy S, de Nully Brown P, Stahel R, Milpied N, Lopez-Guillermo A, Poeschel V, Grass S, Loeffler M, Murawski N; MabThera International Trial Group: CHOP-like chemotherapy with or without rituximab in young patients with good-prognosis diffuse large-B-cell lymphoma: 6-year results of an open-label randomised study of the Mab-Thera International Trial (MInT) group. Lancet Oncol 2011;12:1013–1022.

27 Pfreundschuh M, Trumper L, Osterborg A, Pettengell R, Trneny M, Imrie K, Ma D, Gill D, Walewski J, Zinzani PL, Stahel R, Kvaloy S, Shpilberg O, Jaeger U, Hansen M, Lehtinen T, Lopez-Guillermo A, Corrado C, Scheliga A, Milpied N, Mendila M, Rashford M, Kuhnt E, Loeffler M; MabThera International Trial Group: CHOP-like chemotherapy plus rituximab versus CHOP-like chemotherapy alone in young patients with good-prognosis diffuse large-B-cell lymphoma: a randomised controlled trial by the MabThera International Trial (MInT) group. Lancet Oncol 2006;7:379–391.

28 Recher C, Coiffier B, Haioun C, Molina TJ, Ferme C, Casasnovas O, Thieblemont C, Bosly A, Laurent G, Morschhauser F, Ghesquieres H, Jardin F, Bologna S, Fruchart C, Corront B, Gabarre J, Bonnet C, Janvier M, Canioni D, Jais JP, Salles G, Tilly H; Groupe d'Etude des Lymphomes de l'Adulte: Intensified chemotherapy with ACVBP plus rituximab versus standard CHOP plus rituximab for the treatment of diffuse large B-cell lymphoma (LNH03-2b): an open-label randomised phase 3 trial. Lancet 2011;378:1858–1867.

29 Cunningham D, Hawkes EA, Jack A, Qian W, Smith P, Mouncey P, Pocock C, Ardeshna KM, Radford JA, McMillan A, Davies J, Turner D, Kruger A, Johnson P, Gambell J, Linch D: Rituximab plus cyclophosphamide, doxorubicin, vincristine, and prednisolone in patients with newly diagnosed diffuse large B-cell non-Hodgkin lymphoma: a phase 3 comparison of dose intensification with 14-day versus 21-day cycles. Lancet 2013;381:1817–1826.

30 Greb A, Bohlius J, Schiefer D, Schwarzer G, Schulz H, Engert A: High-dose chemotherapy with autologous stem cell transplantation in the first line treatment of aggressive non-Hodgkin lymphoma (NHL) in adults. Cochrane Database Syst Rev 2008;1:CD004024.

31 Stiff PJ, Unger JM, Cook JR, Constine LS, Couban S, Stewart DA, Shea TC, Porcu P, Winter JN, Kahl BS, Miller TP, Tubs RR, Marcellus D, Freidberg JW, Barton KP, Mills GM, LeBlanc M, Rimza LM, Forman SJ, Fisher RI: Autologous transplantation as consolidation for aggressive non-Hodgkin's lymphoma. N Engl J Med 2013;369:1681–1690.

32 Vitolo U, Chiappella C, Brusamolino E, Angelucci E, Rossi GC, Carella AM, Evangelista A, Stelitano C, Balzarotti M, Merli F, Gaidano G, Pavone V, Rigacci L, Zaja F, Cascavilla N, D'Arco A, Rusconi C, De Renzo A, Pinotti G, Spina M, Pregno P, Russo E, Gotti M, Tucci A, Cabras M, Pileri S, Levis A, Martelli M: Rituximab dose-dense chemotherapy followed by intensified high-dose chemotherapy and autologous stem cell transplantation (HDC + ASCT) significantly reduces the risk of progression compared to standard rituximab dose-dense chemotherapy as first line treatment in young patients with high-risk (aa-IPI 2–3) diffuse large B-cell lymphoma (DLBCL): final results of phase III randomized trial DLCL04 of the Fondazione Italiana Linfomi (FIL). American Society of Hematology Meeting, Chicago, 2012, abstract 2688.

33 Klapper W, Kreuz M, Kohler CW, Burkhardt B, Szczepanowski M, Salaverria I, Hummel M, Loeffler M, Pellissery S, Woessmann W, Schwanen C, Trumper L, Wessendorf S, Spang R, Hasenclever D, Siebert R; Molecular Mechanisms in Malignant Lymphomas Network Project of the Deutsche Krebshilfe: Patient age at diagnosis is associated with the molecular characteristics of diffuse large B-cell lymphoma. Blood 2012;119:1882–1887.

34 Alizadeh AA, Eisen MB, Davis RE, Ma C, Lossos IS, Rosenwald A, Boldrick JC, Sabet H, Tran T, Yu X, Powell JI, Yang L, Marti GE, Moore T, Hudson J Jr, Lu L, Lewis DB, Tibshirani R, Sherlock G, Chan WC, Greiner TC, Weisenburger DD, Armitage JO, Warnke R, Levy R, Wilson W, Grever MR, Byrd JC, Botstein D, Brown PO, Staudt LM: Distinct types of diffuse large B-cell lymphoma identified by gene expression profiling. Nature 2000;403: 503–511.

35 Rosenwald A, Wright G, Chan WC, Connors JM, Campo E, Fisher RI, Gascoyne RD, Muller-Hermelink HK, Smeland EB, Giltnane JM, Hurt EM, Zhao H, Averett L, Yang L, Wilson WH, Jaffe ES, Simon R, Klausner RD, Powell J, Duffey PL, Longo DL, Greiner TC, Weisenburger DD, Sanger WG, Dave BJ, Lynch JC, Vose J, Armitage JO, Montserrat E, Lopez-Guillermo A, Grogan TM, Miller TP, LeBlanc M, Ott G, Kvaloy S, Delabie J, Holte H, Krajci P, Stokke T, Staudt LM; Lymphoma/Leukemia Molecular Profiling Project: The use of molecular profiling to predict survival after chemotherapy for diffuse large-B-cell lymphoma. N Engl J Med 2002;346:1937–1947.

36 Hans CP, Weisenburger DD, Greiner TC, Gascoyne RD, Delabie J, Ott G, Muller-Hermelink HK, Campo E, Braziel RM, Jaffe ES, Pan Z, Farinha P, Smith LM, Falini B, Banham AH, Rosenwald A, Staudt LM, Connors JM, Armitage JO, Chan WC: Confirmation of the molecular classification of diffuse large B-cell lymphoma by immunohistochemistry using a tissue microarray. Blood 2004;103:275–282.

37 Miles RR, Raphael M, McCarthy K, Wotherspoon A, Lones MA, Terrier-Lacombe MJ, Patte C, Gerrard M, Auperin A, Sposto R, Davenport V, Cairo MS, Perkins SL; Group SLCUNS: Pediatric diffuse large B-cell lymphoma demonstrates a high proliferation index, frequent c-Myc protein expression, and a high incidence of germinal center subtype: report of the French-American-British (FAB) International Study Group. Pediatr Blood Cancer 2008;51:369–374.

38 Oschlies I, Klapper W, Zimmermann M, Krams M, Wacker HH, Burkhardt B, Harder L, Siebert R, Reiter A, Parwaresch R: Diffuse large B-cell lymphoma in pediatric patients belongs predominantly to the germinal-center type B-cell lymphomas: a clinicopathologic analysis of cases included in the German BFM (Berlin-Frankfurt-Munster) multicenter trial. Blood 2006;107:4047–4052.

39 Deffenbacher KE, Iqbal J, Sanger W, Shen Y, Lachel C, Liu Z, Liu Y, Lim MS, Perkins SL, Fu K, Smith L, Lynch J, Staudt LM, Rimsza LM, Jaffe E, Rosenwald A, Ott GK, Delabie J, Campo E, Gascoyne RD, Cairo MS, Weisenburger DD, Greiner TC, Gross TG, Chan WC: Molecular distinctions between pediatric and adult mature B-cell non-Hodgkin lymphomas identified through genomic profiling. Blood 2012;119:3757–3766.

40 Dave BJ, Weisenburger DD, Higgins CM, Pickering DL, Hess MM, Chan WC, Sanger WG: Cytogenetics and fluorescence in situ hybridization studies of diffuse large B-cell lymphoma in children and young adults. Cancer Genet Cytogenet 2004;153:115–121.

41 Poirel HA, Cairo MS, Heerema NA, Swansbury J, Auperin A, Launay E, Sanger WG, Talley P, Perkins SL, Raphael M, McCarthy K, Sposto R, Gerrard M, Bernheim A, Patte C; FAB LMB96 International Study Committee: Specific cytogenetic abnormalities are associated with a significantly inferior outcome in children and adolescents with mature B-cell non-Hodgkin's lymphoma: results of the FAB/LMB 96 international study. Leukemia 2009;23:323–331.

42 Salaverria I, Philipp C, Oschlies I, Kohler CW, Kreuz M, Szczepanowski M, Burkhardt B, Trautmann H, Gesk S, Andrusiewicz M, Berger H, Fey M, Harder L, Hasenclever D, Hummel M, Loeffler M, Mahn F, Martin-Guerrero I, Pellissery S, Pott C, Pfreundschuh M, Reiter A, Richter J, Rosolowski M, Schwaenen C, Stein H, Trumper L, Wessendorf S, Spang R, Kuppers R, Klapper W, Siebert R; Molecular Mechanisms in Malignant Lymphomas Network Project of the Deutsche Krebshilfe, German High-Grade Lymphoma Study Group, Berlin-Frankfurt-Munster NHL Trial Group: Translocations activating IRF4 identify a subtype of germinal center-derived B-cell lymphoma affecting predominantly children and young adults. Blood 2011;118: 139–147.

43 Wilson WH, Dunleavy K, Pittaluga S, Hegde U, Grant N, Steinberg SM, Raffeld M, Gutierrez M, Chabner BA, Staudt L, Jaffe ES, Janik JE: Phase II study of dose-adjusted EPOCH and rituximab in untreated diffuse large B-cell lymphoma with analysis of germinal center and post-germinal center biomarkers. J Clin Oncol 2008;26:2717–2724.

44 Wilson WH, Grossbard ML, Pittaluga S, Cole D, Pearson D, Drbohlav N, Steinberg SM, Little RF, Janik J, Gutierrez M, Raffeld M, Staudt L, Cheson BD, Longo DL, Harris N, Jaffe ES, Chabner BA, Wittes R, Balis F: Dose-adjusted EPOCH chemotherapy for untreated large B-cell lymphomas: a pharmacodynamic approach with high efficacy. Blood 2002;99: 2685–2693.

45 Wilson WH, Jung SH, Porcu P, Hurd D, Johnson J, Martin SE, Czuczman M, Lai R, Said J, Chadburn A, Jones D, Dunleavy K, Canellos G, Zelenetz AD, Cheson BD, Hsi ED; Cancer Leukemia Group B: A Cancer and Leukemia Group B multi-center study of DA-EPOCH-rituximab in untreated diffuse large B-cell lymphoma with analysis of outcome by molecular subtype. Haematologica 2012;97:758–765.

46 Gutierrez-Garcia G, Cardesa-Salzmann T, Climent F, Gonzalez-Barca E, Mercadal S, Mate JL, Sancho JM, Arenillas L, Serrano S, Escoda L, Martinez S, Valera A, Martinez A, Jares P, Pinyol M, Garcia-Herrera A, Martinez-Trillos A, Gine E, Villamor N, Campo E, Colomo L, Lopez-Guillermo A; Grup per l'Estudi dels Limfomes de Catalunya i Balears: Gene-expression profiling and not immunophenotypic algorithms predicts prognosis in patients with diffuse large B-cell lymphoma treated with immunochemotherapy. Blood 2011;117:4836–4843.

47 Ott G, Ziepert M, Klapper W, Horn H, Szczepanowski M, Bernd HW, Thorns C, Feller AC, Lenze D, Hummel M, Stein H, Muller-Hermelink HK, Frank M, Hansmann ML, Barth TF, Moller P, Cogliatti S, Pfreundschuh M, Schmitz N, Trumper L, Loeffler M, Rosenwald A: Immunoblastic morphology but not the immunohistochemical GCB/non-GCB classifier predicts outcome in diffuse large B-cell lymphoma in the RICOVER-60 trial of the DSHNHL. Blood 2010;116:4916–4925.

48 Bouabdallah R, Coso D, Esterni B, Vey N, Chetaille B, Blaise D: Adolescents and young adults versus adult patients with large cell lymphoma: a matched control analysis on 55 patients (E18526). Program Abstr 2013 Am Soc Clin Oncol Annu Meet, Chicago, 2012.

49 Ram R, Wolach O, Vidal L, Gafter-Gvili A, Shpilberg O, Raanani P: Adolescents and young adults with acute lymphoblastic leukemia have a better outcome when treated with pediatric-inspired regimens: systematic review and meta-analysis. Am J Hematol 2012; 87:472–478.

50 Savage KJ, Monti S, Kutok JL, Cattoretti G, Neuberg D, De Leval L, Kurtin P, Dal Cin P, Ladd C, Feuerhake F, Aguiar RC, Li S, Salles G, Berger F, Jing W, Pinkus GS, Habermann T, Dalla-Favera R, Harris NL, Aster JC, Golub TR, Shipp MA: The molecular signature of mediastinal large B-cell lymphoma differs from that of other diffuse large B-cell lymphomas and shares features with classical Hodgkin lymphoma. Blood 2003;102:3871–3879.

51 Dunleavy K, Pittaluga S, Maeda LS, Advani R, Chen CC, Hessler J, Steinberg SM, Grant C, Wright G, Varma G, Staudt LM, Jaffe ES, Wilson WH: Dose-adjusted EPOCH-rituximab therapy in primary mediastinal B-cell lymphoma. N Engl J Med 2013;368:1408–1416.

52 Rieger M, Osterborg A, Pettengell R, White D, Gill D, Walewski J, Kuhnt E, Loeffler M, Pfreundschuh M, Ho AD; MabThera International Trial Group: Primary mediastinal B-cell lymphoma treated with CHOP-like chemotherapy with or without rituximab: results of the MabThera International Trial Group Study. Ann Oncol 2011;22:664–670.

53 Pfreundschuh M, Schubert J, Ziepert M, Schmits R, Mohren M, Lengfelder E, Reiser M, Nickenig C, Clemens M, Peter N, Bokemeyer C, Eimermacher H, Ho A, Hoffmann M, Mertelsmann R, Trumper L, Balleisen L, Liersch R, Metzner B, Hartmann F, Glass B, Poeschel V, Schmitz N, Ruebe C, Feller AC, Loeffler M; German High-Grade Non-Hodgkin Lymphoma Study Group: Six versus eight cycles of bi-weekly CHOP-14 with or without rituximab in elderly patients with aggressive CD20+ B-cell lymphomas: a randomised controlled trial (RICOVER-60). Lancet Oncol 2008;9:105–116.

54 Lones MA, Perkins SL, Sposto R, Kadin ME, Kjeldsberg CR, Wilson JF, Cairo MS: Large-cell lymphoma arising in the mediastinum in children and adolescents is associated with an excellent outcome: a children's cancer group report. J Clin Oncol 2000;18:3845–3853.

55 Seidemann K, Tiemann M, Lauterbach I, Mann G, Simonitsch I, Stankewitz K, Schrappe M, Zimmermann M, Niemeyer C, Parwaresch R, Riehm H, Reiter A; NHL Berlin-Frankfurt-Munster Group: Primary mediastinal large B-cell lymphoma with sclerosis in pediatric and adolescent patients: treatment and results from three therapeutic studies of the Berlin-Frankfurt-Munster group. J Clin Oncol 2003;21:1782–1789.

56 Gerrard M, Waxman IM, Sposto R, Auperin A, Perkins SL, Goldman S, Harrison L, Pinkerton R, McCarthy K, Raphael M, Patte C, Cairo MS; French-American-British/Lymphome Malins de Burkitt 96 International Study Committee: Outcome and pathologic classification of children and adolescents with mediastinal large B-cell lymphoma treated with FAB/LMB96 mature B-NHL therapy. Blood 2013;121:278–285.

57 Murphy SB: Classification, staging and end results of treatment of childhood non-Hodgkin's lymphomas: dissimilarities from lymphomas in adults. Semin Oncol 1980;7:332–339.

58 Fisher RI, Gaynor ER, Dahlberg S, Oken MM, Grogan TM, Mize EM, Glick JH, Coltman CA Jr, Miller TP: Comparison of a standard regimen (CHOP) with three intensive chemotherapy regimens for advanced non-Hodgkin's lymphoma. N Engl J Med 1993;328:1002–1006.

59 Zinzani PL, Martelli M, Bertini M, Gianni AM, Devizzi L, Federico M, Pangalis G, Michels J, Zucca E, Cantonetti M, Cortelazzo S, Wotherspoon A, Ferreri AJ, Zaja F, Lauria F, De Renzo A, Liberati MA, Falini B, Balzarotti M, Calderoni A, Zaccaria A, Gentilini P, Fattori PP, Pavone E, Angelopoulou MK, Alinari L, Brugiatelli M, Di Renzo N, Bonifazi F, Pileri SA, Cavalli F; International Extranodal Lymphoma Study Group: Induction chemotherapy strategies for primary mediastinal large B-cell lymphoma with sclerosis: a retrospective multinational study on 426 previously untreated patients. Haematologica 2002;87:1258–1264.

60 Travis LB, Ng AK, Allan JM, Pui CH, Kennedy AR, Xu XG, Purdy JA, Applegate K, Yahalom J, Constine LS, Gilbert ES, Boice JD Jr: Second malignant neoplasms and cardiovascular disease following radiotherapy. J Natl Cancer Inst 2012;104:357–370.

61 Woessmann W, Lisfeld J, Burkhardt B; NHL-BFM Study Group: Therapy in primary mediastinal B-cell lymphoma. N Engl J Med 2013; 369:282.

62 Jaffe ES: The 2008 WHO classification of lymphomas: implications for clinical practice and translational research. Hematol Am Soc Hematol Educ Program 2009, pp 523–531.

63 Savage KJ, Harris NL, Vose JM, Ullrich F, Jaffe ES, Connors JM, Rimsza L, Pileri SA, Chhanabhai M, Gascoyne RD, Armitage JO, Weisenburger DD, International Peripheral T-Cell Lymphoma Project: ALK– anaplastic large-cell lymphoma is clinically and immunophenotypically different from both ALK+ ALCL and peripheral T-cell lymphoma, not otherwise specified: report from the International Peripheral T-Cell Lymphoma Project. Blood 2008;111:5496–5504.

64 Brugieres L, Deley MC, Pacquement H, Meguerian-Bedoyan Z, Terrier-Lacombe MJ, Robert A, Pondarre C, Leverger G, Devalck C, Rodary C, Delsol G, Hartmann O: CD30(+) anaplastic large-cell lymphoma in children: analysis of 82 patients enrolled in two consecutive studies of the French Society of Pediatric Oncology. Blood 1998;92:3591–3598.

65 Reiter A, Schrappe M, Tiemann M, Parwaresch R, Zimmermann M, Yakisan E, Dopfer R, Bucsky P, Mann G, Gadner H: Successful treatment strategy for Ki-1 anaplastic large-cell lymphoma of childhood: a prospective analysis of 62 patients enrolled in three consecutive Berlin-Frankfurt-Munster Group studies. J Clin Oncol 1994;12:899–908.

66 Laver JH, Kraveka JM, Hutchison RE, Chang M, Kepner J, Schwenn M, Tarbell N, Desai S, Weitzman S, Weinstein HJ, Murphy SB: Advanced-stage large-cell lymphoma in children and adolescents: results of a randomized trial incorporating intermediate-dose methotrexate and high-dose cytarabine in the maintenance phase of the APO regimen: a Pediatric Oncology Group phase III trial. J Clin Oncol 2005;23:541–547.

67 Brugieres L, Le Deley MC, Rosolen A, Williams D, Horibe K, Wrobel G, Mann G, Zsiros J, Uyttebroeck A, Marky I, Lamant L, Reiter A: Impact of the methotrexate administration dose on the need for intrathecal treatment in children and adolescents with anaplastic large-cell lymphoma: results of a randomized trial of the EICNHL group. J Clin Oncol 2009;27:897–903.

68 Suzuki R, Kagami Y, Takeuchi K, Kami M, Okamoto M, Ichinohasama R, Mori N, Kojima M, Yoshino T, Yamabe H, Shiota M, Mori S, Ogura M, Hamajima N, Seto M, Suchi T, Morishima Y, Nakamura S: Prognostic significance of CD56 expression for ALK-positive and ALK-negative anaplastic large-cell lymphoma of T/null cell phenotype. Blood 2000;96:2993–3000.

69 Le Deley MC, Reiter A, Williams D, Delsol G, Oschlies I, McCarthy K, Zimmermann M, Brugieres L, European Intergroup for Childhood Non-Hodgkin Lymphoma: Prognostic factors in childhood anaplastic large cell lymphoma: results of a large European intergroup study. Blood 2008;111:1560–1566.

70 Falini B, Pileri S, Zinzani PL, Carbone A, Zagonel V, Wolf-Peeters C, Verhoef G, Menestrina F, Todeschini G, Paulli M, Lazzarino M, Giardini R, Aiello A, Foss HD, Araujo I, Fizzotti M, Pelicci PG, Flenghi L, Martelli MF, Santucci A: ALK+ lymphoma: clinico-pathological findings and outcome. Blood 1999;93:2697–2706.

71 Stein H, Foss HD, Durkop H, Marafioti T, Delsol G, Pulford K, Pileri S, Falini B: CD30(+) anaplastic large cell lymphoma: a review of its histopathologic, genetic, and clinical features. Blood 2000;96:3681–3695.

72 Gascoyne RD, Aoun P, Wu D, Chhanabhai M, Skinnider BF, Greiner TC, Morris SW, Connors JM, Vose JM, Viswanatha DS, Coldman A, Weisenburger DD: Prognostic significance of anaplastic lymphoma kinase (ALK) protein expression in adults with anaplastic large cell lymphoma. Blood 1999;93:3913–3921.

73 Thomas DA, Faderl S, Cortes J, O'Brien S, Giles FJ, Kornblau SM, Garcia-Manero G, Keating MJ, Andreeff M, Jeha S, Beran M, Verstovsek S, Pierce S, Letvak L, Salvado A, Champlin R, Talpaz M, Kantarjian H: Treatment of Philadelphia chromosome-positive acute lymphocytic leukemia with hyper-CVAD and imatinib mesylate. Blood 2004;103:4396–4407.

74 Seidemann K, Tiemann M, Schrappe M, Yakisan E, Simonitsch I, Janka-Schaub G, Dorffel W, Zimmermann M, Mann G, Gadner H, Parwaresch R, Riehm H, Reiter A: Short-pulse B-non-Hodgkin lymphoma-type chemotherapy is efficacious treatment for pediatric anaplastic large cell lymphoma: a report of the Berlin-Frankfurt-Munster Group trial NHL-BFM 90. Blood 2001;97:3699–3706.

75 Nademanee A, Palmer JM, Popplewell L, Tsai NC, Delioukina M, Gaal K, Cai JL, Kogut N, Forman SJ: High-dose therapy and autologous hematopoietic cell transplantation in peripheral T cell lymphoma (PTCL): analysis of prognostic factors. Biol Blood Marrow Transplant 2011;17:1481–1489.

76 Gibb A, Jones C, Bloor A, Kulkarni S, Illidge T, Linton K, Radford J: Brentuximab vedotin in refractory CD30+ lymphomas: a bridge to allogeneic transplantation in approximately one quarter of patients treated on a named patient programme at a single UK center. Haematologica 2013;98:611–614.

77 Woessmann W, Peters C, Lenhard M, Burkhardt B, Sykora KW, Dilloo D, Kremens B, Lang P, Fuhrer M, Kuhne T, Parwaresch R, Ebell W, Reiter A: Allogeneic haematopoietic stem cell transplantation in relapsed or refractory anaplastic large cell lymphoma of children and adolescents – a Berlin-Frankfurt-Munster Group report. Br J Haematol 2006;133:176–182.

78 Mosse YP, Lim MS, Voss SD, Wilner K, Ruffner K, Laliberte J, Rolland D, Balis FM, Maris JM, Weigel BJ, Ingle AM, Ahern C, Adamson PC, Blaney SM: Safety and activity of crizotinib for paediatric patients with refractory solid tumours or anaplastic large-cell lymphoma: a Children's Oncology Group phase 1 consortium study. Lancet Oncol 2013;14:472–480.

79 Camidge R, Bazhenova L, Salgia R, Weiss G, Langer C, Tsang Shaw A, Narasimhan N, Dorer D, Rivera V, Zhang J, Clackson T, Haluska F, Gettinger S: First-in-human dose-finding of the ALK/EGFR inhibitor AP26113 in patients with advanced malignancies: updated results (abstract 8031). Program Abstr 2013 Am Soc Clin Oncol Annu Meet, Chicago 2013.

80 Lowe EJ, Sposto R, Perkins SL, Gross TG, Finlay J, Zwick D, Abromowitch M; Children's Cancer Group Study: Intensive chemotherapy for systemic anaplastic large cell lymphoma in children and adolescents: final results of Children's Cancer Group Study 5941. Pediatr Blood Cancer 2009;52:335–339.

Acta Haematol 2014;132:292–297
DOI: 10.1159/000360200

Published online: September 10, 2014

Acute Myeloid Leukemia in Adolescents and Young Adults: Challenging Aspects

Yishai Ofran[a, b]   Jacob M. Rowe[a–c]

[a]Department of Hematology and Bone Marrow Transplantation, Rambam Health Care Campus, and
[b]Bruce Rappaport Faculty of Medicine, Technion, Israel Institute of Technology, Haifa, and [c]Department of
Hematology, Shaare Zedek Medical Center, Jerusalem, Israel

Key Words

Acute myeloid leukemia · Adolescents · Young adults

Abstract

Treating adolescents and young adults (AYAs) diagnosed with cancer is a challenge. Acute myeloid leukemia (AML) which is usually diagnosed in a previously healthy kid, requiring immediate aggressive chemotherapy, brings difficulties and conflicts associated with severe illness to extremes. The incidence of AML in adolescents aged 15–19 years approaches 8.5 per million. Only in recent years has it become evident that the prognosis of AYAs diagnosed with AML is poorer compared to younger children diagnosed with AML with similar characteristics. No specific genetic aberration or other known poor risk factor was found to explain the inferior prognosis of AYAs. In acute lymphoblastic leukemia the contribution of differences between adult and pediatric protocols to AYA outcome is established. It has been suggested that pediatric protocols should also apply to AYAs with AML; however, data supporting this are vague. Herein, existing evidence regarding special considerations in treating AYAs with AML is discussed. Mental and psychological age-specific aspects important to consider when treating AYAs with AML are overviewed. Awareness for adolescent special needs, adherence to protocols and intensive supportive care are important. Multidisciplinary adolescent-oriented staff should be involved in the therapy of any AYA with AML escorting this special patient population on the road to cure.

© 2014 S. Karger AG, Basel

Introduction

Acute myeloid leukemia (AML) is the most common leukemia in adults. The prevalence of AML strongly correlates with age. AML is a relatively rare disease during childhood, and its incidence rises exponentially over the age of 60 [1]. AML characteristics and prognosis change with age and most significantly between pediatric and adult patients. Adolescents and young adults (AYAs) with AML face a significantly worse prognosis compared to younger pediatric AML patients [2, 3]. Differences in the frequency of leukemia subtypes and common molecular aberrations between adult and pediatric patients are well known (table 1). Age is an established independent poor risk factor in adult patients and is associated with higher rates of poor risk cytogenetics and secondary leukemia [1]. Yet, the disease characteristics of AYA and pe-

Yishai Ofran, MD
Department of Hematology and Bone Marrow Transplantation
Rambam Health Care Campus
Haifa 31096 (Israel)
E-Mail y_ofran@rambam.health.gov.il

diatric AML patients are very similar; thus, the reason for the poorer outcome of AYAs is not obvious. Herein, evidence for a distinct biological behavior and practical questions regarding treatment protocol selection in AYAs will be discussed. Special challenges in the management of AYA patients will also be reviewed.

Special Considerations during Diagnosis and Primary Evaluation in AYAs

In acute lymphoblastic leukemia, it has been shown not only that AYAs have a poorer prognosis than younger children, but also that this can be overcome if pediatric protocols are applied and strictly executed [4, 5]. Whether a similar attitude should be applied to AYAs with AML is not known. In children and AYAs, AML is almost exclusively de novo [6], abruptly diagnosed in a previously healthy individual. Clinical and laboratory evaluation at diagnosis is similar to the regular adult workup with some specifically pediatric considerations [7]. Leukemia diagnosis and characteristics in AYAs should include morphology evaluation of bone marrow smears, immunophenotyping, cytogenetics, fluorescence in situ hybridization and specific molecular genetic markers. A complete blood count, biochemistry, coagulation tests and chest X-ray are indicated to rule out life-threatening emergencies or infection. In addition and unlike adults, all AYAs should undergo a cerebrospinal diagnostic tap even in the absence of neurological symptoms, due to a high reported risk for asymptomatic central nervous system (CNS) infiltration by leukemic cells in children [8, 9]. CNS involvement approaches 30% in some pediatric AML series, but most cases are of infants and children younger than 4 years [10]. In such a young pediatric population, CNS involvement was reported not to be associated with poorer outcome, but it should be emphasized that most protocols that are in use for this age group contain a routine CNS-directed therapy and prophylaxis. Whether or not a newly diagnosed AYA with a clear CNS spinal fluid requires CNS prophylaxis is debatable.

Fertility preservation is challenging in AYA patients newly diagnosed with AML. Time constraints and the high frequency of emergencies are a barrier since therapy should often not be delayed even for few days [11]. Optimal collection for sperm banking requires the collection of multiple samples to maximize the amount of sperm available for cryopreservation prior to chemotherapy initiation [12]. However, male AYAs require quiet and relaxing conditions for sperm collection and often fail when being asked to masturbate few hours after being diagnosed with leukemia. If therapy is indicated before a sufficient amount of semen has been collected, it should be noted that following a single induction cycle, most healthy males will maintain adequate sperm quality, and a second collection is indicated prior to the consolidation cycle.

Female AYAs diagnosed with AML face other challenges for fertility preservation. Since most female AYAs have no spouse or partner with whom they were planning to become parents, and due to the need for immediate antileukemic therapy, in vitro fertilization and embryo preservation are usually not an option. Time also limits the possibility for preservation of stimulated oocytes because a full hormonal stimulation cycle cannot be conducted prior to chemotherapy [13]. Of special consideration is the fact that, at diagnosis, ovaries may be infiltrated with leukemic cells. It was recently reported that using molecular diagnostic markers, leukemic infiltration was identified in 6/8 cryopreserved ovary cortexes, collected at leukemia diagnosis [14]. Thus, freezing ovary wedge biopsies for future reimplantation carries the risk for iatrogenic reintroduction of leukemic cells into a leukemia survivor. A progress in ex vivo stimulation of frozen ovary sections gives hope to young female AML patients. It might be that in the future a simple and rapid laparoscopic ovary biopsy will be sufficient, and with further ex vivo oocyte stimulation, in vitro fertilization and embryo implantation the parenthood dream can become real for leukemia survivors. Usage of gonadotropin-releasing hormone agonist therapy may protect female patients exposed to chemotherapy in lymphoma protocols [15, 16]. However, AML protocols are much more intensive, and gonadotropin-releasing hormone agonists may not be sufficient in preserving fertility in leukemia survivors.

Treating AYAs with chemotherapy is associated with specific psychological, social and body image challenging aspects [17, 18]. In case of AML, these challenges are amplified by the abrupt onset of disease and the immediate need of very intensive therapies. Prolonged hospitalization, especially if isolation is required, may aggravate psychosocial difficulties and even the risk for depression, since for AYAs individuality, independence and social connections are of particular importance at this age. It is essential to create a patient-oriented support network, balancing and collaborating between family and friends synergizing all support sources. Enlistment of immediate family members to help and be involved in the care of AML patients is always encouraged. In addition, the possibility that allogeneic stem cell

Acta Haematol 2014;132:292–297
DOI: 10.1159/000360200

transplantation will be indicated requires commencing tissue typing tests for patients' siblings and parents as soon as possible. AYA siblings may be very young; thus, parents should be provided a specific psychological counseling helping them, informing and dealing with siblings' needs, especially in cases when young kids are required to become hematopoietic cell donors for their sick brother or sister.

Risk Stratification in AYAs – Adults or Children?

Stratification and prognostication of AML differ between adult and pediatric patients (table 1). For example, AML preceded by myelodysplasia is common among patients with advanced age and is very rare among pediatric patients. The frequency of some cytogenetic and molecular abnormalities significantly differs between adults and pediatric patients. For example, core binding leukemia with either t(8:21) or inv16 cytogenetic aberrations is identified in 20–22% of pediatric and only in 13% of adult AML patients [4]. The NPM1 mutation is more frequent among adults identified in 27.5% [19] compared to 8% of pediatric AML patients [20, 21]. Few studies analyzed the clinical value of genetic aberration frequencies specifically in AYAs. One important source of evidence is an analysis of cytogenetic results from the Medical Research Council (MRC) 10 trial [22]. The MRC 10 was a large prospective study for both children and adults up to the age of 55 years that recruited 1,612 patients. Looking at cytogenetic risk group frequencies, it is clear that standard risk cytogenetics is less frequent over the age of 35 years (table 2). Cytogenetic group distributions among AYAs aged 14–35 equal the distribution among younger children. Interestingly, the prognosis for all cytogenetic groups declines over age and for most in the adverse risk group where the 3-year survival rate dropped from 42% in children to 19% in AYAs (table 2).

Some genetic aberrations were reported to have a different prognostic power in adult and pediatric patients. For example, in adults the c-KIT mutation is considered to override the good prognosis associated with t(8:21) [23]. In contrast, among pediatric and adolescent patients, the 5-year event-free survival was equal for c-KIT mutated and wild-type patients presenting with core-binding leukemia [24].

FLT3-ITD and NUP98/NSD1 translocations are genetic aberrations that are associated with poor prognosis in AML patients. FLT3-ITD is present in 30% of adults [25] but only in 15–18% of pediatric AML patients [26], and NUP98/NSD1 translocation is almost exclusively present under the age of 30 years [27]. It has been reported that the combination of FLT3-ITD and NUP98/NSD1 translocation carries a special deleterious effect and is common among AYAs [28].

Whether AYA AML patients have more in common with adult or pediatric patients is not clear. In a large survey evaluating the age effect on AML biology and response to therapy among pediatric patients [29], a clearly defined pattern was reported in the infancy age, but a distinct biology of AYAs could not be clearly identified. Large prospective studies that included both pediatric and adult patients did not report any special consideration or outcome for AYAs [30, 31]. Evidence from adult and pediatric studies established the significance of older age as a poor prognostic factor in each group independently. The age effect is probably a continuum making prognosis in AYAs better than that in adults but worse than in younger children. How aging per se and through which biological mechanisms age affects leukemia prognosis is still a mystery.

Table 1. AML characterization in adult and pediatric patients

	Adult patients		Pediatric patients	
	frequency, %	prognosis	frequency, %	prognosis
Second AML	17	adverse	1	adverse
CBF: t(8:21) or inv16	13	favorable	20–22	favorable
MLLT3-MLL t(9:11)	2	intermediate	7	favorable
NPM1 mutation	27–35	favorable	8	favorable
FLT3-ITD	30	adverse	15	adverse

CBF = Core-binding factor.

Table 2. Age-related AML risk group distribution (%) and overall survival (OS)

Risk		0–14 years	14–35 years	>35 years
Standard	prevalence	25.8	30.5	18.2
	3-year OS	78	66	65
Intermediate	prevalence	64.4	59.2	71.5
	3-year OS	55	51	37
Poor	prevalence	9.7	10.1	10.2
	3-year OS	42	19	5

Acta Haematol 2014;132:292–297
DOI: 10.1159/000360200

Ofran/Rowe

Table 3. Major differences between AML adult and pediatric protocols

	Induction I	Induction II	Consolidation	Intensification	CNS prophylaxis
Typical adult protocol	D1–7: AraC 100 mg/m^2 D1–3: Dauno 60–90 mg/m^2	On D14, only if residual disease	HIDAC	HIDAC	No
Typical pediatric protocol	D1–6: AraC 100 mg/m^2 D1, 3, 5: Dauno 50–60 mg/m^2 D1–5: VP16 100 mg/m^2	As early as D8 to all patients	MiDAC VP16 150 mg/m^2 for 5 days or mitoxantrone 12 mg/m^2 for 3 days	MiDAC L-asparaginase	Yes

D = Day; AraC = cytarabine; Dauno = daunorubicin; HIDAC = high-dose cytarabine; VP16 = etoposide; MiDAC = modified intermediate-dose cytarabine.

Therapy of AML in AYAs

AYAs are cared for by both adult and pediatric hemato-oncologists. Since no AYA-specific protocols have been established, AYAs may be receiving either adult or pediatric regimens according to local preferences. In the nontransplant setting, adult AML protocols contain 1 or 2 cycles for induction of remission followed by risk-adapted postremission therapy. Most commonly, consolidation therapy is based on recurring cycles of high-dose cytarabine. Pediatric protocols are intensified by sequential multiagent chemotherapies (table 3). There are no prospective randomized comparisons of AYAs treated with adult or pediatric protocols. Recently, the outcome of 517 AYA AML patients was compared between those treated with adult and those with pediatric protocols. The 10-year event-free and overall survivals of patients treated in pediatric Children's Oncology Group studies were superior to those treated in adult Cancer and Leukemia Group B and Southwest Oncology Group trials (45 vs. 34%, 38 vs. 23%, respectively; p = 0.006) [32]. However, the better prognosis may be attributed to the fact that patients on Children's Oncology Group protocols were significantly younger (median, 17.2 vs. 20.1 and 19.8 years, p < 0.001).

When consecutive St. Jude- and MD Anderson-joined pediatric protocols were compared, the most recent AML02 protocol which is more intensive than previous protocols yielded a better outcome for AYAs [33]. This is worth mentioning because timed sequential therapy was shown to be superior for pediatric [34] but not for adult AML patients [35].

Confounding Factors Specific to AYAs

Potential explanations for the worse outcome of AYAs compared to younger pediatric AML patients may be other than the biology of leukemia. Leukemic patients treated within clinical trials usually do better than the average real-world patients. This may reflect the effect clinical trials have on the quality of participating centers [36], or the benefit patients gain from the rigidity of timelines within clinical trials. In the USA, the percentage of AYAs included in clinical trials is much lower than the participating rate among younger children [37]. In Europe, across almost all malignancies survival rates of AYAs are poor, but in the UK, AML is an exception which may be related to the high participation rate in the national MRC trials [38]. AYAs often fail to adhere to intensive prolonged therapies such as AML protocols [39]. It may be suggested that confounding factors between AYAs treated in pediatric wards and those treated in regular adult programs are the involvement of their parents and adherence to the protocol schedule, supportive care and infection prevention rules.

Conclusion

Treating AYA patients with AML is challenging. The abrupt onset and the immediately required aggressive therapies aggravate the difficulties and challenges that are generally evident in all AYA patients diagnosed with cancer. The prognosis of AYAs diagnosed with AML is inferior to that of younger pediatric patients. However, no genetic or phenotypic aberrations were found to be specific to myeloid leukemia in AYAs. It is controversial whether this poor prognosis is derived from an as yet unknown difference in disease biology which may be in accordance with the general deleterious effect of age in AML patients. In addition, some psychosocial difficulties which are specific to adolescence may contribute to the lower adherence to protocols, and a reduced compliance with supportive care instructions may also hamper the outcome in AYAs. The question whether the next AYA AML patient should be referred to pediatric or adult leukemia programs has not yet been answered. Regardless of referral destination, the treating staff should be aware of age-specific needs and concerns for supportive care. It is recommended that the referral decision considers the patient's individual fitness to local available pediatric or adult leukemia programs. Participation in clinical trials or in national protocols should be encouraged. Special efforts are required to ensure adherence to a selected protocol. AML is curable for 50% of AYAs, and by enlistment of multidisciplinary adolescent-oriented staff the road to cure can be made with the lowest short- and long-term consequences.

References

1 Juliusson G, Lazarevic V, Horstedt AS, Hagberg O, Hoglund M: Acute myeloid leukemia in the real world: why population-based registries are needed. Blood 2012;119:3890–3899.
2 Horibe K, Saito AM, Takimoto T, Tsuchida M, Manabe A, Shima A, Ohara A, Mizutani S: Incidence and survival rates of hematological malignancies in Japanese children and adolescents (2006–2010): based on registry data from the Japanese Society of Pediatric Hematology. Int J Hematol 2013;98:74–88.
3 Bleyer A, O'Leary M, Barr R, Ries LAG (eds): Cancer Epidemiology in older adolescents and Young Adults 15 to 29 Years of Age, Including SEER Incidence and Survival: 1975–2000. NIH publ No 06-5767. Bethesda, National Cancer Institute, 2006.
4 Boissel N, Auclerc MF, Lheritier V, Perel Y, Thomas X, Leblanc T, Rousselot P, Cayuela JM, Gabert J, Fegueux N, Piguet C, Huguet-Rigal F, Berthou C, Boiron JM, Pautas C, Michel G, Fiere D, Leverger G, Dombret H, Baruchel A: Should adolescents with acute lymphoblastic leukemia be treated as old children or young adults? Comparison of the French FRALLE-93 and LALA-94 trials. J Clin Oncol 2003;21:774–780.
5 De Bont JM, Holt B, Dekker AW, van der Does-van den Berg A, Sonneveld P, Pieters R: Significant difference in outcome for adolescents with acute lymphoblastic leukemia treated on pediatric vs adult protocols in the Netherlands. Leukemia 2004;18:2032–2035.
6 Rubnitz JE, Inaba H: Childhood acute myeloid leukaemia. Br J Haematol 2012;159:259–276.
7 Creutzig U, van den Heuvel-Eibrink MM, Gibson B, Dworzak MN, Adachi S, de Bont E, Harbott J, Hasle H, Johnston D, Kinoshita A, Lehrnbecher T, Leverger G, Mejstrikova E, Meshinchi S, Pession A, Raimondi SC, Sung L, Stary J, Zwaan CM, Kaspers GJ, Reinhardt D: Diagnosis and management of acute myeloid leukemia in children and adolescents: recommendations from an international expert panel. Blood 2012;120:3187–3205.
8 Creutzig U, Zimmermann M, Ritter J, Reinhardt D, Hermann J, Henze G, Jurgens H, Kabisch H, Reiter A, Riehm H, Gadner H, Schellong G: Treatment strategies and long-term results in paediatric patients treated in four consecutive AML-BFM trials. Leukemia 2005;19:2030–2042.
9 Webb DK, Harrison G, Stevens RF, Gibson BG, Hann IM, Wheatley K: Relationships between age at diagnosis, clinical features, and outcome of therapy in children treated in the Medical Research Council AML 10 and 12 trials for acute myeloid leukemia. Blood 2001;98:1714–1720.
10 Johnston DL, Alonzo TA, Gerbing RB, Lange BJ, Woods WG: The presence of central nervous system disease at diagnosis in pediatric acute myeloid leukemia does not affect survival: a Children's Oncology Group study. Pediatr Blood Cancer 2010;55:414–420.
11 Zuckerman T, Ganzel C, Tallman MS, Rowe JM: How I treat hematologic emergencies in adults with acute leukemia. Blood 2012;120:1993–2002.
12 Lass A, Akagbosu F, Abusheikha N, Hassouneh M, Blayney M, Avery S, Brinsden P: A programme of semen cryopreservation for patients with malignant disease in a tertiary infertility centre: lessons from 8 years' experience. Hum Reprod 1998;13:3256–3261.
13 Levine J, Canada A, Stern CJ: Fertility preservation in adolescents and young adults with cancer. J Clin Oncol 2010;28:4831–4841.
14 Rosendahl M, Andersen MT, Ralfkiaer E, Kjeldsen L, Andersen MK, Andersen CY: Evidence of residual disease in cryopreserved ovarian cortex from female patients with leukemia. Fertil Steril 2010;94:2186–2190.
15 Beck-Fruchter R, Weiss A, Shalev E: GnRH agonist therapy as ovarian protectants in female patients undergoing chemotherapy: a review of the clinical data. Hum Reprod Update 2008;14:553–561.
16 Blumenfeld Z, Avivi I, Eckman A, Epelbaum R, Rowe JM, Dann EJ: Gonadotropin-releasing hormone agonist decreases chemotherapy-induced gonadotoxicity and premature ovarian failure in young female patients with Hodgkin lymphoma. Fertil Steril 2008;89:166–173.
17 Epelman CL: The adolescent and young adult with cancer: state of the art – psychosocial aspects. Curr Oncol Rep 2013;15:325–331.
18 Zebrack BJ, Mills J, Weitzman TS: Health and supportive care needs of young adult cancer patients and survivors. J Cancer Surviv 2007;1:137–145.
19 Thiede C, Koch S, Creutzig E, Steudel C, Illmer T, Schaich M, Ehninger G: Prevalence and prognostic impact of NPM1 mutations in 1,485 adult patients with acute myeloid leukemia (AML). Blood 2006;107:4011–4020.
20 Brown P, McIntyre E, Rau R, Meshinchi S, Lacayo N, Dahl G, Alonzo TA, Chang M, Arceci RJ, Small D: The incidence and clinical significance of nucleophosmin mutations in childhood AML. Blood 2007;110:979–985.
21 Hollink IH, Zwaan CM, Zimmermann M, Arentsen-Peters TC, Pieters R, Cloos J, Kaspers GJ, de Graaf SS, Harbott J, Creutzig U, Reinhardt D, van den Heuvel-Eibrink MM, Thiede C: Favorable prognostic impact of NPM1 gene mutations in childhood acute myeloid leukemia, with emphasis on cytogenetically normal AML. Leukemia 2009;23:262–270.
22 Grimwade D, Walker H, Oliver F, Wheatley K, Harrison C, Harrison G, Rees J, Hann I, Stevens R, Burnett A, Goldstone A: The importance of diagnostic cytogenetics on outcome in AML: analysis of 1,612 patients entered into the MRC AML 10 trial. The Medical Research Council adult and children's leukaemia working parties. Blood 1998;92:2322–2333.
23 Park SH, Chi HS, Min SK, Park BG, Jang S, Park CJ: Prognostic impact of c-KIT mutations in core binding factor acute myeloid leukemia. Leuk Res 2011;35:1376–1383.

Acta Haematol 2014;132:292–297
DOI: 10.1159/000360200

24 Pollard JA, Alonzo TA, Gerbing RB, Ho PA, Zeng R, Ravindranath Y, Dahl G, Lacayo NJ, Becton D, Chang M, Weinstein HJ, Hirsch B, Raimondi SC, Heerema NA, Woods WG, Lange BJ, Hurwitz C, Arceci RJ, Radich JP, Bernstein ID, Heinrich MC, Meshinchi S: Prevalence and prognostic significance of KIT mutations in pediatric patients with core binding factor AML enrolled on serial pediatric cooperative trials for de novo AML. Blood 2010;115:2372–2379.

25 Patel JP, Gonen M, Figueroa ME, Fernandez H, Sun Z, Racevskis J, Van Vlierberghe P, Dolgalev I, Thomas S, Aminova O, Huberman K, Cheng J, Viale A, Socci ND, Heguy A, Cherry A, Vance G, Higgins RR, Ketterling RP, Gallagher RE, Litzow M, van den Brink MR, Lazarus HM, Rowe JM, Luger S, Ferrando A, Paietta E, Tallman MS, Melnick A, Abdel-Wahab O, Levine RL: Prognostic relevance of integrated genetic profiling in acute myeloid leukemia. N Engl J Med 2012;366:1079–1089.

26 Balgobind BV, Hollink IH, Arentsen-Peters ST, Zimmermann M, Harbott J, Beverloo HB, von Bergh AR, Cloos J, Kaspers GJ, de Haas V, Zemanova Z, Stary J, Cayuela JM, Baruchel A, Creutzig U, Reinhardt D, Pieters R, Zwaan CM, van den Heuvel-Eibrink MM: Integrative analysis of type-I and type-II aberrations underscores the genetic heterogeneity of pediatric acute myeloid leukemia. Haematologica 2011;96:1478–1487.

27 Hollink IH, van den Heuvel-Eibrink MM, Arentsen-Peters ST, Pratcorona M, Abbas S, Kuipers JE, van Galen JF, Beverloo HB, Sonneveld E, Kaspers GJ, Trka J, Baruchel A, Zimmermann M, Creutzig U, Reinhardt D, Pieters R, Valk PJ, Zwaan CM: NUP98/NSD1 characterizes a novel poor prognostic group in acute myeloid leukemia with a distinct HOX gene expression pattern. Blood 2011;118:3645–3656.

28 Ostronoff F, Alonzo TA, Gerbing RB, Loken MR, Pardo L, Aplenc R, Sung L, Raimondi SC, Hirsch BA, Kahwash S, Heerema-McKenney A, Winter L, Glick K, Byron P, Lavey RS, Davies SM, Smith FO, Gamis AS, Meshinchi S: Cryptic NUP98/NSD1 translocations are highly prevalent in FLT3/ITD-positive acute myeloid leukemia and lead to high rate of induction failure. Report from Children's Oncology Group. Blood 2012;120:529a.

29 Creutzig U, Buchner T, Sauerland MC, Zimmermann M, Reinhardt D, Dohner H, Schlenk RF: Significance of age in acute myeloid leukemia patients younger than 30 years: a common analysis of the pediatric trials AML-BFM 93/98 and the adult trials AMLCG 92/99 and AMLSG HD93/98A. Cancer 2008;112:562–571.

30 Hann IM, Stevens RF, Goldstone AH, Rees JK, Wheatley K, Gray RG, Burnett AK: Randomized comparison of DAT versus ADE as induction chemotherapy in children and younger adults with acute myeloid leukemia. Results of the Medical Research Council's 10th AML trial (MRC AML10). Adult and childhood leukaemia working parties of the Medical Research Council. Blood 1997;89:2311–2318.

31 Burnett AK, Russell NH, Hills RK, Hunter AE, Kjeldsen L, Yin J, Gibson BE, Wheatley K, Milligan D: Optimization of chemotherapy for younger patients with acute myeloid leukemia: results of the Medical Research Council AML15 trial. J Clin Oncol 2013;31:3360–3368.

32 Woods WG, Franklin AR, Alonzo TA, Gerbing RB, Donohue KA, Othus M, Horan J, Appelbaum FR, Estey EH, Bloomfield CD, Larson RA: Outcome of adolescents and young adults with acute myeloid leukemia treated on COG trials compared to CALGB and SWOG trials. Cancer 2013;119:4170–4179.

33 Rubnitz JE, Pounds S, Cao X, Jenkins L, Dahl G, Bowman WP, Taub JW, Pui CH, Ribeiro RC, Campana D, Inaba H: Treatment outcome in older patients with childhood acute myeloid leukemia. Cancer 2012;118:6253–6259.

34 Woods WG, Kobrinsky N, Buckley JD, Lee JW, Sanders J, Neudorf S, Gold S, Barnard DR, DeSwarte J, Dusenbery K, Kalousek D, Arthur DC, Lange BJ: Timed-sequential induction therapy improves postremission outcome in acute myeloid leukemia: a report from the children's Cancer Group. Blood 1996;87:4979–4989.

35 Moore JO, George SL, Dodge RK, Amrein PC, Powell BL, Kolitz JE, Baer MR, Davey FR, Bloomfield CD, Larson RA, Schiffer CA: Sequential multiagent chemotherapy is not superior to high-dose cytarabine alone as postremission intensification therapy for acute myeloid leukemia in adults under 60 years of age: Cancer and Leukemia Group B study 9222. Blood 2005;105:3420–3427.

36 Boros L, Chuang C, Butler FO, Bennett JM: Leukemia in Rochester (NY). A 17-year experience with an analysis of the role of cooperative group (ECOG) participation. Cancer 1985;56:2161–2169.

37 Bleyer WA: Cancer in older adolescents and young adults: epidemiology, diagnosis, treatment, survival, and importance of clinical trials. Med Pediatr Oncol 2002;38:1–10.

38 Gatta G, Capocaccia R, De Angelis R, Stiller C, Coebergh JW: Cancer survival in European adolescents and young adults. Eur J Cancer 2003;39:2600–2610.

39 Butow P, Palmer S, Pai A, Goodenough B, Luckett T, King M: Review of adherence-related issues in adolescents and young adults with cancer. J Clin Oncol 2010;28:4800–4809.

Acta Haematol 2014;132:298–306
DOI: 10.1159/000363434

Published online: September 10, 2014

Chronic Myeloid Leukemia in Adolescents and Young Adults: Patient Characteristics, Outcomes and Review of the Literature

Naveen Pemmaraju   Jorge Cortes

Department of Leukemia, M.D. Anderson Cancer Center, University of Texas, Houston, Tex., USA

Key Words

Adolescent and young adult · Chronic myeloid leukemia

Abstract

Over the past two decades, many improvements have been made in the management of patients with leukemia. Research in this field most often focuses on the youngest and oldest patient age groups. However, the population of patients in between those age groups has received relatively little attention with few studies specifically focusing on them. This important 'age gap' has demonstrated a unique, difficult-to-treat group of patients known as adolescents and young adults, or AYAs. Variably defined in the literature as patients from late teenage years to the age of up to 40 years, the AYA group of patients represents a vulnerable subset of patients now identified to require its own focus, development of therapeutic strategies and parallel emphasis on special support systems involving multidisciplinary psychosocial care. Despite the great advancements that have been realized for patients with chronic myeloid leukemia (CML), the AYA group has seldom been the focus of specific reports and studies, and the outcome appears to lag behind the general population. This review focuses on this subset of AYA patients with CML and summarizes the available data and recent developments, challenges and treatment options for this group of patients.

© 2014 S. Karger AG, Basel

Introduction

Over the past two decades, significant improvement has been demonstrated in treatment outcomes for many patients with hematological malignancies. Notably, outcomes in children with acute leukemia have experienced a remarkable improvement in a relatively short time. Most notably, this has been demonstrated in pediatric acute lymphoblastic leukemia (ALL) where historically poor outcomes have now been successfully improved to a cure rate approximating 90% of patient cases [1]. At the other end of the spectrum, older adults have been the focus of much research in recent years although progress to date has been much more modest [2].

The history and progress of therapy among chronic myeloid leukemia (CML) patients is notable, because

Jorge Cortes, MD
Department of Leukemia, University of Texas
M.D. Anderson Cancer Center
1515 Holcombe Boulevard, Unit 428, Houston, TX 77030 (USA)
E-Mail jcortes@mdanderson.org

overall, patients with CML are experiencing some of the best outcomes in all of leukemia and a dramatic transformation of the natural history of the disease that is unparalleled in cancer and most dramatically showcased in the modern era of tyrosine kinase inhibitors (TKIs) [3]. CML has been historically thought of as a disease of older adults with a reported median age of 67 years in national registries [4]. However, a growing subset of patients with CML are being diagnosed at younger ages [5]. In fact, the median age of the CML patients reported in most trials in the literature is at least a decade younger.

Recently, there is growing attention being placed on a subset of patients with cancer that are diagnosed in between the two extremes of life: the adolescents and young adults (AYAs). This subgroup of patients represents an emerging, dynamic group of patients with unique features related to their disease, psychosocial needs and therapeutic challenges [6]. The field of AYA oncology has recognized an 'age gap' phenomenon in which AYA patients are having a 'lag time' in terms of improvements in outcomes among many different tumor types, including those with hematological malignancies [7]. In the field of leukemia research, this phenomenon has been most (and almost exclusively) studied among ALL patients, the so-called AYA ALL patients [8], as this subtype of leukemia is classically the most common to affect younger patients. Little is known about patient characteristics and outcomes in the other leukemias, including CML. The focus of this review article is to summarize the available information regarding CML AYAs and to discuss future directions for study in this emerging field.

Definition of AYA

The age range for definition of AYA patients with malignancies is highly variable and has been in flux as more awareness develops in this unique field [7, 9, 10]. Various age ranges have been proposed, such as ages between 12 and 24 years [11] or between 15 and 25 [11], or 15 and 29 [5, 12]. Most recently the AYA Oncology Progress Review Group and National Comprehensive Cancer Network guidelines [7] proposed an age range of 15–39 years, similar to the proposed Surveillance Epidemiology and End Results (SEER) age range of 16–39 years [2]. This review will focus on studies including patients with the widest age range, from 15 to 39 years, in order to include a broader range of studies pertaining to the CML AYA field. Importantly, most of these studies represent a subanalysis of larger series where patients of all ages or mostly adults are included.

Outcomes

Little is known about outcomes in the CML AYA population. Since CML is generally regarded as a disease of patients aged in their 60s and 70s, patients in the AYA group constitute a small subset of patients with CML enrolled on clinical trials or described in population studies. Only a few reports have analyzed specifically the characteristics and outcome of this patient population.

Two different epidemiological studies have been reported analyzing the SEER database over different time periods [13, 14]. In the study conducted by Brunner et al. [13], the authors demonstrated that all age ranges examined had overall improvement in outcomes in time (cut-off date of year 2000) when compared to results prior to the TKI era versus after the TKI era, including the lowest age range included (age 15–44 years). This age group, which approximates the AYA age range, included 1,356 patients, or 27% of the total CML population analyzed (5,138 patients in the SEER database from 2000 to 2005) [13]. Another SEER database study, performed by Chen et al. [14], retrospectively reviews data on CML patients of all ages back to 1975. In this study, the authors found an improvement in relative survival in all age groups except for pediatric patients under the age of 15, including improvement in the AYA age group (defined here as ages 15–29 years) [14]. Of importance, in the analysis by Chen et al., patients were included who received therapy prior to the TKI era (going back to 1975) and therefore includes patients who received interferon and allogeneic stem cell transplantation as part of their standard of care, which was prior to the TKI era. These analyses thus demonstrate that the introduction of TKI into the therapeutic algorithms of patients with CML, including AYA patients, considerably improves the outcome with the suggestion that the survival may be approaching that of the general population for age-matched individuals [15]. The question then arises whether the outcome of AYA patients with CML may be similar or not to that of older patients.

Tables 1 and 2 summarize baseline characteristics and results, respectively, of the two large reports focusing on CML AYAs. One such analysis by Pemmaraju et al. [5] retrospectively examined CML patients who were enrolled in prospective clinical trials at one institution. In this report, among 468 adult CML patients treated in 4 prospective clinical trials for newly diagnosed patients treated with TKI as initial therapy, with a median age for the overall cohort of 47 years (range 15–85 years), AYA patients (defined in that report as patients aged 15–29 years) made up 13% (61 patients) of the total population.

Importantly, in this analysis, AYA patients had a lower rate of complete cytogenetic, major molecular and complete molecular response compared to the older patients. There was a trend for an inferior event-free survival for the AYA population compared to their older counterparts. Although the rates for overall survival and transformation-free survival were not statistically significantly different, the follow-up may not have been long enough and the population not large enough to demonstrate the difference expected based on response. Still, these results highlighted an unexpected trend towards worse overall outcomes in the AYA CML population [5].

More recently, Kalmanti et al. [16] performed an analysis on the German CML study IV data set, which includes 1,520 CML patients of all ages enrolled in a randomized trial. The authors subdivided the CML patients by age, describing 120 patients aged 16–29 years that made up the AYA group for this analysis. Similar to Pemmaraju et al. [5], Kalmanti et al. [16] found that CML AYA patients made up 8% of the overall CML population studied and exhibited more splenomegaly and also a higher white blood cell count as compared to older CML patients, thus suggesting that AYAs may have more aggressive features. An additional finding of this study demonstrated that AYA CML patients had a higher rate of BCR-ABL transcript levels greater than 10% on the international scale at the 3-month time point as compared to older patients, a feature recognized as an early indicator of poor long-term outcome. However, in this analysis there was no difference in the rates of cytogenetic or molecular response between the AYA and the older age groups, and no difference in overall survival could be identified. The conclusions from this study include the confirmation that CML AYA patients indeed represent a unique group of CML patients who exhibit unique clinical features and suggest that some of these patients may have a more aggressive disease course requiring closer monitoring and further investigation, but that overall these patients have no worse outcomes in terms of overall survival compared to older CML patients.

These two reports, the most relevant in defining the outcome of AYA CML patients in the TKI era, are thus somewhat contrasting in their results. There is likely a multifactorial set of factors that explain the apparent discrepancies between these studies. First, this is a rare subgroup of patients, making up only 13–27% of the total CML population (with CML already itself a rare disease to begin with, as estimated to be only 5,920 cases in the USA in 2013) [4]. Furthermore, both analyses are retrospective reviews of a subset of patients included in larger trials rather than prospective studies of this particular subset of patients. Definitive conclusions are difficult to make based on small numbers of patients available for analysis under these circumstances. Secondly, the impor-

Table 1. Comparison of baseline characteristics of two studies that included analysis of CML AYA patients

	Pemmaraju et al. [5]	Kalmanti et al. [16]
AYAs, n	61 (13)	120 (8)
CML initial therapy, n		
Imatinib 400 mg	11 (18)	25 (21)
Imatinib 800 mg	24 (39)	35 (29)
Nilotinib	13 (21)	0
Dasatinib	13 (21)	0
Imatinib + interferon α	0	39 (32)
Imatinib + cytarabine	0	13 (11)
Imatinib (previous interferon)	0	8 (7)
Males	38 (62)	80 (67)
Median spleen size (below costal margin), cm	8 [1–23]	5 [0-38]
Median WBC count, ×10^9/l	30.5 [1.0–283]	144 [9–571]
Median hemoglobin, g/dl	12.2 [6.7–15.5]	11.1 [6.9–16.2]
Median platelets, ×10^9/l	332 [73–1,769]	430 [59–2,590]
Sokal risk, n		
Low	51 (84)	64 (54)
Intermediate	8 (13)	23 (19)
High	2 (3)	31 (26)

WBC = White blood cell. Figures in parentheses indicate the percentage of the study population, those in square brackets the range.

Table 2. Comparison of results of two studies that included analysis of CML AYA patients

	Pemmaraju et al. [5]	Kalmanti et al. [16]
Responses, n		
CCyR	48/57 (84)	109/120 (91)
MMR	43/57 (75)	114/120 (95)
CMR	13/57 (23)	104/120 (87)
Overall 5-year survival, %	93	97
Deaths, n	3	4
Progression to AP/BP	1	1
SCT-related	1	2
Car accident	1	0
Cardiopulmonary complication	0	1

Figures in parentheses indicate percentages. CCyR = Complete cytogenetic response; MMR = major molecular response; CMR = complete molecular response; AP/BP = accelerated phase/blast phase; SCT = stem cell transplantation.

tance of and widespread utilization of allogeneic stem cell transplantation, especially as salvage therapy in many of these AYA patients, has changed and evolved over time and might be a factor defining outcome. In particular, the survival rate of patients may be greatly affected by the use, timing and type of stem cell transplant used in CML. The utilization and circumstances under which transplantation was used in these patients are not clearly defined in these analyses. Third, the study of Pemmaraju et al. [5] is a single-institution-based experience of patients referred for clinical trials, and therefore has inherent biases of a tertiary-based referral population, as compared to the German series that comes from a multicenter clinical trial. Fourth, the question of adherence over time periods and across age ranges is a topic of great importance across various demographic and socioeconomic groups [17]. This is especially relevant, since adherence rates have been correlated with achievement of molecular responses among CML patients [18, 19]. In addition, changing health care coverage and cost schemas which influence the nature of AYA patients' interaction with and subsequent utilization of the complex and ever-changing US health care system could be major factors in patient outcomes over time [20, 21]. In Texas for example, where the majority of the patients included in the study from Pemmaraju et al. [5] is derived from, there is a large percentage of uninsured patients that have difficulties accessing care even if the mediation itself may be provided by the study. In other parts of the world, the access to health care is more universal and widely available. It will be of great interest in future studies, for example, to explore this issue of adherence vis-à-vis a patient's health care system further, and to observe differences among AYA CML patients in various health care systems across the world, in nationalized/one-payor systems (such as some European nations) versus the multi-payor private insurance-based system of the USA. Finally, other socioeconomic factors not analyzed in these series may have an impact on the outcome of patients. For example, young patients who are more educated or those that are still being supported or cared for by their parents may have a better outcome than those with lower education and who may have a weaker support system (e.g. no family members, not speaking the language, etc.). Cultural differences (e.g. active participation in their management, aversion to traditional medications, etc.) may also play an important role. Clearly, more focused studies on AYA CML patients measuring outcomes and correlating them to all these factors to directly explore their influence on response and rates of discontinuation are warranted.

Treatment Strategies for the CML AYA Patient

There are no current standards or recommendations proposed specifically for CML AYA patients. Thus, the recommendations for adult patients are usually proposed as they are not felt to require a unique medical approach. Standard therapy with upfront TKI, whether first-generation TKI (imatinib) [22] or second-generation TKI (dasatinib [23], nilotinib [24]) should be offered to AYA patients and older adults alike. Salvage therapy in second-line settings and beyond for AYA patients should again include all therapies available to older patients with CML, with no known age restrictions for younger patients in the AYA group, including the other TKI therapies not yet used from frontline setting, several newer CML drugs recently Food and Drug Administration approved (ponatinib [25], bosutinib [26], omacetaxine [27]), enrollment in a clinical trial or allogeneic stem cell transplantation (SCT). With particular attention for the AYA group, as compared to the older group of CML patients (especially those aged 70 and above), allogeneic SCT has historically been put forward to represent a more readily available option in some younger patients' cases (especially those with molecular mutations such as the T315I mutation) in appropriately selected CML patients [28, 29]. One SCT study for patients with CML conducted by Saussele et al. [28] based on the interim analysis of the German CML Study IV (total n = 1,272) analyzed 84 consecutive CML patients who had undergone SCT. Criteria for SCT in this study included: low European Group for Blood and Marrow Transplantation score, advanced CML or imatinib failure. The median age of the 84 patients was 37 years (range 16–62 years). Transplantation-related mortality was reported as 8%. The 3-year survival posttransplantation rates for patients with chronic phase CML (n = 56) was 91% and for advanced phase CML (n = 28) 59%. A total of 88% of the CML patients who underwent SCT went on to achieve complete molecular remission. There was no overall survival difference noted between the SCT group and the non-SCT group (via matched-pair comparison analysis). In this study, there was no specific breakdown in terms of younger AYA patients only (age 16–29), as the median age of this report was 37 years (range 16–62). Despite the belief that AYA patients might represent a group of patients for which SCT may be considered earlier on in the disease course, it should be noted that there is as yet no available data that SCT yields better long-term outcomes when compared to standard second-line TKI therapy. Importantly, SCT continues to have a risk of morbidity and mortality that, even in this population with lower transplant-related mortality and morbidity, exceeds that of the use of TKI. Conversely, the possible adverse consequences of a prolonged use of TKI for many years constitute an argument in favor of SCT. In our opinion, AYA patients who have experienced resistance or intolerance to frontline therapy with TKI should be offered a second-line TKI and followed closely. Initiating a stem cell consultation and possibly a search for sibling donors might be appropriate, but we do not recommend SCT on these patients unless they have experienced failure to at least 2 and possibly more TKIs.

Pregnancy and CML

Among the AYA cancer population, concerns about fertility preservation and pregnancy constitute an important consideration [30–32]. Currently, no accepted universal guidelines exist for the care of the CML patient during the time of pregnancy as there are limited studies available in this field. One study, by Ault et al. [33], reviewed 19 pregnancies among 18 CML patients at the M.D. Anderson Cancer Center. Ten of these patients were females who became pregnant while receiving imatinib at the time of conception. All of these patients were able to discontinue imatinib therapy immediately upon recognition of the pregnancy with a median estimated time of exposure to imatinib from time of conception to time of imatinib discontinuation of 4 weeks (range 4–9 weeks). One of the female patients had a twin pregnancy. This group had been under imatinib treatment for a median of 8 months (range 1–52 months) for CML (chronic phase, n = 9; accelerated phase, n = 1). In terms of imatinib discontinuation, the median time off imatinib therapy during and after pregnancy was 7 months (range 1–21 months). There were 5 instances of other therapies given during the pregnancy: hydroxyurea (n = 3), interferon α (n = 1) and leukapheresis (n = 1), with 1 resultant complete hematological response. A total of 6 patients had increases in their Philadelphia chromosome-positive metaphases during their pregnancies in the midst of imatinib discontinuation. Two of the women had a spontaneous abortion after discontinuation of imatinib, and 1 patient had an elective abortion. Of the 7 other pregnancies that went to term, 8 babies were born (1 twin birth), with a median weight of 5 lb 13 oz (range from 5 lb 2 oz to 6 lb 13 oz). One of these babies had hypospadias at birth (treated with routine surgical intervention, no complications, otherwise healthy baby). The remaining 7 babies delivered had no complications. Importantly, at the time of the publication, the median age of these children was 17 months (range 3–53 months) with normal development and growth milestones reported. For the female patients (n = 10), all were restarted on imatinib after birth or abortion. With a median follow-up time of 18 months (range 5–48 months), 9 patients achieved complete hematological response; 3 of these patients also achieved a complete cytogenetic response, and none achieved a major molecular response. For the one patient who did not achieve complete hematological response, she went on to transform to CML blast phase and ultimately died 22 months after her delivery. In the male cohort (n = 8), 1 patient conceived a child twice under imatinib therapy. The median time on imatinib was 18 months for this group (range 4 weeks to 48 months) at the time conception was noted. Eight healthy babies were born, 1 spontaneous abortion. With regard to birth defects, 1 baby had mild rotation of the small intestine (routine surgical intervention performed, no complications). The children in this cohort had a median age at the time of the publication of 38 months (range 3–54 months) with no reported growth or development abnormalities. Significantly, none of the male patients had interruption of their imatinib therapy after the conception. Seven of the 8 (88%) male patients achieved complete hematological response, with all of these patients also achieving complete cytogenetic response. The remaining patient ultimately experienced development of clonal evolution and died 42 months after the conception had been noted, in a CML myeloid blast phase.

The second series examining this issue is by Pye et al. [34]. In this report, among 180 female patients who were exposed to imatinib (mostly for the treatment of CML) during pregnancy, the outcome data was reported to the drug manufacturer or to 1 of 2 participating institutions in 125, or 69%, of these patients. Among the patients with known pregnancy outcomes, 28% had elective abortions, while 50% delivered normal infants. Birth defects were reported in 12 babies, 3 of which were considered possible complex malformation syndromes that raised concern, including exomphalos in all 3 of these cases; additionally, both hemivertebrae and kidney abnormalities were noted in 2 of these 3 cases. Data of pregnancy during exposure to other TKIs is much more limited [35]. In contrast, there are also several case reports where babies exposed to TKIs throughout the pregnancy have been born with no detectable abnormalities [36–38]. However, these instances represent mere anecdotes and cannot be considered as evidence of the safety of this approach. Thus, based on the available information and the data from animal studies that suggest that imatinib is teratogenic [39–41], the current recommendation is for female patients to avoid receiving TKIs if they become pregnant.

Another dilemma faced by young AYA patients is the desire to become pregnant while receiving therapy with TKIs. There is currently no formal contraindication for a male patient receiving these drugs to father a baby while under TKI therapy. However, female patients face the challenge of the pregnancy and the need to interrupt therapy if they become pregnant. Two important considerations play against each other in this situation: the need to protect the baby's healthy development, and the need to protect the mother's health and avoid progression of the disease. Whenever possible, patients should be advised to plan for the pregnancy and delay until a deep molecular response is achieved. Treatment should then be interrupted to pursue conception and the patient maintained off therapy for the duration of pregnancy. In our practice we do not intervene with any therapy even if there is loss of molecular, cytogenetic and, in most instances, even hematological response [42]. If treatment is absolutely necessary ideally it can be delayed to the third trimester when it may have the least impact on the baby's growth and development. Interferon and hydroxyurea have been used, and there is anecdotal evidence for both that they can be safely administered in some patients. We prefer hydroxyurea as it is better tolerated and has a faster effect on the white cell count when this is the objective. Whether TKIs can be safely administered in the third trimester remains to be proven but there are anecdotal reports that this is the case. This is unquestionably a clinical setting where studies are necessary to better define the optimal approach.

Adherence to Oral TKI Therapy

The concept of patient adherence to oral medications has been a common concern to providers and patients. This has important implications in settings such as the chronic treatment of infectious disease, such as HIV/AIDS with regard to therapeutic drug-monitoring programs [43] and tuberculosis [44, 45], particularly with regard to directly observed therapy. With the wider use of oral chemotherapy agents, such as TKIs for CML, these concerns have extended to the management of neoplastic diseases.

Regardless of many demographic considerations, including gender, socioeconomic status and education level, the patients' difficulty in adhering to oral oncological agents has been well documented across tumor types, including solid tumors (gastrointestinal stromal tumors) [46], male breast cancer [47, 48], pancreatic neuroendocrine tumors [49], non-small cell lung cancer [50] and renal cell cancer [51], in countries all across the world [52–54]. This has also been documented in hematological malignancies [2] including the whole age spectrum of CML patients: both younger [5] and older age groups [55]. In addition to traditional factors affecting adherence such as financial considerations, presence of adverse events, lack of patient education on the goals of therapy and consequences of lack of adherence, and others, fertility and reproductive health are major concerns among AYA patients with cancer and can affect the AYA patients' ability or willingness to be adherent to their cancer therapies, especially those that require daily, chronic administration [56].

Among patients with CML, patient adherence to oral TKI therapy is the most important factor that determines achievement of a deep molecular response with imatinib therapy [18]. In a study of US veteran patients, 54% of (n = 74) treated with imatinib experienced self-discontinuation or interruption of TKI therapy (median time to discontinuation 395 days, range 31–2,056 days), including patients who ultimately had disease progression, without being switched to other therapies [55]. A retrospective study from Italy compared the ratio between the received daily dose and the prescribed daily dose for CML patients over a 3-year period. This study demonstrated that patient adherence was 83% among patients treated with frontline imatinib, and 85 and 93% with second-generation TKIs (dasatinib, nilotinib, respectively) [17]. With regard to AYA patients, many patients in this age group are for the first time beginning to transition to adult care from their pediatric team and may experience great difficulty in accessing and taking medications regularly without the parent's supervision [11, 57]. The issue of adherence is oftentimes complex for the AYA patient and, especially in the youngest AYAs/teenagers, could pose a major barrier in terms of overall health and cancer care [58]. For CML AYA patients, the group of leukemia patients most specially associated with the necessity to take daily, indefinite, lifelong oral therapy, these hurdles to care are magnified and could decrease the probability of attaining and maintaining optimal responses with the consequential impact on overall survival [2]. A retrospective data set from the M.D. Anderson Center analyzed 61 CML AYA patients (ages 15–29 years) treated with first- and second-generation TKIs. With a median follow-up of 71 months, 24 AYA patients had discontinued therapy, 5 of them due to nonadherence/

becoming lost to follow-up, and 1 additional patient discontinued therapy due to losing health insurance [5]. This is likely an underestimation of the magnitude of this problem as daily adherence to therapy was not prospectively measured. Still, it highlights the fact that many patients, and probably AYAs in particular, are prone to nonadherence, due to a myriad of factors (psychosocial, economic, medical) unique to this subgroup of patients.

Impact of Cost of Care, Insurance and Access to Health Care

Of particular importance to CML patients is the high cost of prescription medications, given that TKIs in general are drugs that must be taken daily, for life. The impact that cost may have on patient care has been highlighted by a world-wide consortium of CML experts [59] and by Kantarjian and Zwelling [60]. The impact of the rising cost of cancer care and cancer drug prices has been noted for cancer patients in general [60], and this important aspect of cancer health care is most importantly noted among the AYA patient subgroup, especially as they transition from pediatric to adult care and may suffer gaps in insurance coverage [61]. In a study performed to evaluate the factors involved with long-term follow-up in the clinic for childhood cancer survivors, a recent study found that 15% of patients did not attend their follow-up appointments, with multiple reasons cited, including among other items lack of patient insurance [62]. This problem is not restricted to CML AYA patients. Historically, AYA patients have been the least represented among all ages in clinical trials, including AYA cancer patients [9]. A recent population-based study by Parsons et al. [20] again demonstrated that AYA patients with cancer had a lower participation in clinical trials than either their younger or older counterparts; furthermore, older AYA patients and those AYAs who did not have insurance demonstrated the lowest likelihood of enrolling in clinical trials. The authors of this analysis concluded that improved access to the health care system and access to clinical trials is urgently needed [20]. Directions for future improvements in this vital area include the focus of cancer patients and advocates on the new developments of health care reform, headlined by the Patient Protection and Affordable Care Act signed by US President Barack Obama in March 2010 [21] and upheld by the US Supreme Court in June 2012 [63] which will allow for adult children to stay on their parents' insurance plans up to the age of 26, encouraging greater awareness and research in this growing field of AYA oncology among providers, researchers and institutions [6], and creating an emphasis on major medical centers and other cancer programs to initiate dedicated AYA oncology programs and multidisciplinary teams at each institution [64].

Conclusions

AYA patients with CML comprise a unique subgroup of hematological malignancy patients. These may have an inferior outcome compared to their counterparts and face specific challenges such as the considerations of fertility and pregnancy. The requirement for lifelong daily therapy, the need for constant adherence to therapy and the frequently limited access to health care represent major aspects of cancer care that will need to be addressed in the AYA subpopulation of CML patients. Since overall, little is known about patient-specific characteristics and outcomes in this group of patients, further studies and clinical trials, particularly focused on AYA patients, will be warranted for a better understanding of the medical, psychosocial and socioeconomic barriers that affect AYA patients with CML.

Acknowledgments

This work was supported in part by the M.D. Anderson Cancer Center Support Grant CA016672.

Disclosure Statement

The authors have no conflicts of interest to disclose with regard to this paper.

References

1 Pui CH, Evans WE: A 50-year journey to cure childhood acute lymphoblastic leukemia. Semin Hematol 2013;50:185–196.
2 Wood WA, Lee SJ: Malignant hematologic diseases in adolescents and young adults. Blood 2011;117:5803–5815.
3 Cortes J, Kantarjian H: How I treat newly diagnosed chronic phase CML. Blood 2012;120:1390–1397.
4 Siegel R, Naishadham D, Jemal A: Cancer statistics, 2013. CA Cancer J Clin 2013;63:11–30.
5 Pemmaraju N, Kantarjian H, Shan J, Jabbour E, Quintas-Cardama A, Verstovsek S, Ravandi F, Wierda W, O'Brien S, Cortes J: Analysis of outcomes in adolescents and young adults with chronic myelogenous leukemia treated with upfront tyrosine kinase inhibitor therapy. Haematologica 2012;97:1029–1035.

6 Thomas DM, Albritton KH, Ferrari A: Adolescent and young adult oncology: an emerging field. J Clin Oncol 2010;28:4781–4782.

7 Pollock BH, Birch JM: Registration and classification of adolescent and young adult cancer cases. Pediatr Blood Cancer 2008;50:1090–1093.

8 Stock W: Adolescents and young adults with acute lymphoblastic leukemia. Hematology Am Soc Hematol Educ Program 2010;2010:21–29.

9 Bleyer A, Budd T, Montello M: Adolescents and young adults with cancer: the scope of the problem and criticality of clinical trials. Cancer 2006;107:1645–1655.

10 Bleyer A, Morgan S, Barr R: Proceedings of a workshop: bridging the gap in care and addressing participation in clinical trials. Cancer 2006;107:1656–1658.

11 Butow P, Palmer S, Pai A, Goodenough B, Luckett T, King M: Review of adherence-related issues in adolescents and young adults with cancer. J Clin Oncol 2010;28:4800–4809.

12 Bleyer A, Viny A, Barr R: Cancer in 15- to 29-year-olds by primary site. Oncologist 2006;11:590–601.

13 Brunner AM, Campigotto F, Sadrzadeh H, Drapkin BJ, Chen YB, Neuberg DS, Fathi AT: Trends in all-cause mortality among patients with chronic myeloid leukemia: a Surveillance, Epidemiology, and End Results database analysis. Cancer 2013;119:2620–2629.

14 Chen Y, Wang H, Kantarjian H, Cortes J: Trends in chronic myeloid leukemia incidence and survival in the United States from 1975 to 2009. Leuk Lymphoma 2013;54:1411–1417.

15 Lakshmaiah KC, Bhise R, Purohit S, Abraham LJ, Lokanatha D, Suresh TM, Appaji L, Arunakumari BS, Govindbabu K: Chronic myeloid leukemia in children and adolescents: results of treatment with imatinib mesylate. Leuk Lymphoma 2012;53:2430–2433.

16 Kalmanti L, Saussele S, Lauseker M, Proetel U, Müller MC, Hanfstein B, Schreiber A, Fabarius A, Pfirrmann M, Schnittger S, Dengler J, Falge C, Kanz L, Neubauer A, Stegelmann F, Pfreundschuh M, Waller CF, Spiekermann K, Krause SW, Heim D, Nerl C, Hossfeld DK, Kolb HJ, Hochhaus A, Hasford J, Hehlmann R; German Chronic Myeloid Leukemia Study Group; Schweizerische Arbeitsgemeinschaft für Klinische Krebsforschung: Younger patients with chronic myeloid leukemia do well in spite of poor prognostic indicators: results from the randomized CML study IV. Ann Hematol 2014;93:71–80.

17 Santoleri F, Sorice P, Lasala R, Rizzo RC, Costantini A: Patient adherence and persistence with imatinib, nilotinib, dasatinib in clinical practice. PLoS One 2013;8:e56813.

18 Marin D, Bazeos A, Mahon FX, Eliasson L, Milojkovic D, Bua M, Apperley JF, Szydlo R, Desai R, Kozlowski K, Paliompeis C, Latham V, Foroni L, Molimard M, Reid A, Rezvani K, de Lavallade H, Guallar C, Goldman J, Khorashad JS: Adherence is the critical factor for achieving molecular responses in patients with chronic myeloid leukemia who achieve complete cytogenetic responses on imatinib. J Clin Oncol 2010;28:2381–2388.

19 Jain N, O'Brien S: The frontline treatment of chronic myeloid leukemia in the chronic phase: current clinical decisions and future prospects for treatment. Expert Rev Hematol 2013;6:575–586.

20 Parsons HM, Harlan LC, Seibel NL, Stevens JL, Keegan TH: Clinical trial participation and time to treatment among adolescents and young adults with cancer: does age at diagnosis or insurance make a difference? J Clin Oncol 2011;29:4045–4053.

21 Moy B, Polite BN, Halpern MT, Stranne SK, Winer EP, Wollins DS, Newman LA: American Society of Clinical Oncology policy statement: opportunities in the patient protection and affordable care act to reduce cancer care disparities. J Clin Oncol 2011;29:3816–3824.

22 O'Brien SG, Guilhot F, Larson RA, Gathmann I, Baccarani M, Cervantes F, Cornelissen JJ, Fischer T, Hochhaus A, Hughes T, Lechner K, Nielsen JL, Rousselot P, Reiffers J, Saglio G, Shepherd J, Simonsson B, Gratwohl A, Goldman JM, Kantarjian H, Taylor K, Verhoef G, Bolton AE, Capdeville R, Druker BJ; IRIS Investigators: Imatinib compared with interferon and low-dose cytarabine for newly diagnosed chronic-phase chronic myeloid leukemia. N Engl J Med 2003;348:994–1004.

23 Kantarjian HM, Shah NP, Cortes JE, Baccarani M, Agarwal MB, Undurraga MS, Wang J, Ipiña JJ, Kim DW, Ogura M, Pavlovsky C, Junghanss C, Milone JH, Nicolini FE, Robak T, Van Droogenbroeck J, Vellenga E, Bradley-Garelik MB, Zhu C, Hochhaus A: Dasatinib or imatinib in newly diagnosed chronic-phase chronic myeloid leukemia: 2-year follow-up from a randomized phase 3 trial (DASISION). Blood 2012;119:1123–1129.

24 Saglio G, Kim DW, Issaragrisil S, le Coutre P, Etienne G, Lobo C, Pasquini R, Clark RE, Hochhaus A, Hughes TP, Gallagher N, Hoenekopp A, Dong M, Haque A, Larson RA, Kantarjian HM; ENESTnd Investigators: Nilotinib versus imatinib for newly diagnosed chronic myeloid leukemia. N Engl J Med 2010;362:2251–2259.

25 Cortes JE, Kantarjian H, Shah NP, Bixby D, Mauro MJ, Flinn I, O'Hare T, Hu S, Narasimhan NI, Rivera VM, Clackson T, Turner CD, Haluska FG, Druker BJ, Deininger MW, Talpaz M: Ponatinib in refractory Philadelphia chromosome-positive leukemias. N Engl J Med 2012;367:2075–2088.

26 Cortes JE, Kantarjian HM, Brümmendorf TH, Kim DW, Turkina AG, Shen ZX, Pasquini R, Khoury HJ, Arkin S, Volkert A, Besson N, Abbas R, Wang J, Leip E, Gambacorti-Passerini C: Safety and efficacy of bosutinib (SKI-606) in chronic phase Philadelphia chromosome-positive chronic myeloid leukemia patients with resistance or intolerance to imatinib. Blood 2011;118:4567–4576.

27 Cortes J, Digumarti R, Parikh PM, Wetzler M, Lipton JH, Hochhaus A, Craig AR, Benichou AC, Nicolini FE, Kantarjian HM; Omacetaxine 203 Study Group: Phase 2 study of subcutaneous omacetaxine mepesuccinate for chronic-phase chronic myeloid leukemia patients resistant to or intolerant of tyrosine kinase inhibitors. Am J Hematol 2013;88:350–354.

28 Saussele S, Lauseker M, Gratwohl A, Beelen DW, Bunjes D, Schwerdtfeger R, Kolb HJ, Ho AD, Falge C, Holler E, Schlimok G, Zander AR, Arnold R, Kanz L, Dengler R, Haferlach C, Schlegelberger B, Pfirrmann M, Müller MC, Schnittger S, Leitner A, Pletsch N, Hochhaus A, Hasford J, Hehlmann R; German CML Study Group: Allogeneic hematopoietic stem cell transplantation (allo SCT) for chronic myeloid leukemia in the imatinib era: evaluation of its impact within a subgroup of the randomized German CML Study IV. Blood 2010;115:1880–1885.

29 Veldman R, El Rassi F, Holloway S, Langston A, Khoury HJ: Advances in hematopoietic stem cell transplantation in chronic myeloid leukemia. Discov Med 2013;16:179–186.

30 Levine J, Canada A, Stern CJ: Fertility preservation in adolescents and young adults with cancer. J Clin Oncol 2010;28:4831–4841.

31 Bresee JM, Nagler HM: Is cryopreservation of sperm effective for preserving fertility in adolescents and young adults with cancer? Nat Clin Pract Urol 2008;5:14–15.

32 Iqbal J, Ali Z, Khan AU, Aziz Z: Pregnancy outcomes in patients with chronic myeloid leukemia treated with imatinib mesylate: short report from a developing country. Leuk Lymphoma, Epub ahead of print.

33 Ault P, Kantarjian H, O'Brien S, Faderl S, Beran M, Rios MB, Koller C, Giles F, Keating M, Talpaz M, Cortes J: Pregnancy among patients with chronic myeloid leukemia treated with imatinib. J Clin Oncol 2006;24:1204–1208.

34 Pye SM, Cortes J, Ault P, Hatfield A, Kantarjian H, Pilot R, Rosti G, Apperley JF: The effects of imatinib on pregnancy outcome. Blood 2008;111:5505–5508.

35 Cortes J, O'Brien S, Ault P, Borthakur G, Jabbour E, Bradley-Garelik B, Debreczeni K, Yang D, Liu D, Kantarjian H: Pregnancy Outcomes among Patients with Chronic Myeloid Leukemia Treated with Dasatinib. ASH Annual Meeting Abstracts 2008;112:3230.

36 Yadav U, Solanki SL, Yadav R: Chronic myeloid leukemia with pregnancy: successful management of pregnancy and delivery with hydroxyurea and imatinib continued till delivery. J Cancer Res Ther 2013;9:484–486.

37 Martin J, Ramesh A, Devadasan L, Palaniappan, Martin JJ: An uneventful pregnancy and delivery, in a case with chronic myeloid leukemia on imatinib. Indian J Med Paediatr Oncol 2011;32:109–111.

38 Meera V, Jijina F, Shrikande M, Madkaikar M, Ghosh K: Twin pregnancy in a patient of chronic myeloid leukemia on imatinib therapy. Leuk Res 2008;32:1620–1622.

39 Pavlovsky C, Giere I, Van Thillo G: Planned pregnancy in a chronic myeloid leukemia patient in molecular remission. Case Rep Hematol 2012;2012:624590.

40 Apperley J: Issues of imatinib and pregnancy outcome. J Natl Compr Canc Netw 2009;7: 1050–1058.

41 Apperley J: CML in pregnancy and childhood. Best Pract Res Clin Haematol 2009;22: 455–474.

42 Cole S, Kantarjian H, Ault P, Cortes JE: Successful completion of pregnancy in a patient with chronic myeloid leukemia without active intervention: a case report and review of the literature. Clin Lymphoma Myeloma 2009;9: 324–327.

43 Babson KA, Heinz AJ, Bonn-Miller MO: HIV medication adherence and HIV symptom severity: the roles of sleep quality and memory. AIDS Patient Care STDS 2013;27:544–552.

44 Uplekar M, Walley J, Newell J: Directly observed treatment for tuberculosis. Lancet 1999;353:145, author reply 7–8.

45 Bayer R, Wilkinson D: Directly observed therapy for tuberculosis: history of an idea. Lancet 1995;345:1545–1548.

46 Saponara M, Pantaleo MA, Nannini M, Biasco G: Chronic therapy in gastrointestinal stromal tumours (GISTs): the big gap between theory and practice. Target Oncol 2012;7:243–246.

47 Pemmaraju N, Munsell MF, Hortobagyi GN, Giordano SH: Retrospective review of male breast cancer patients: analysis of tamoxifen-related side-effects. Ann Oncol 2012;23: 1471–1474.

48 Anelli TF, Anelli A, Tran KN, Lebwohl DE, Borgen PI: Tamoxifen administration is associated with a high rate of treatment-limiting symptoms in male breast cancer patients. Cancer 1994;74:74–77.

49 Cummins M, Pavlakis N: The use of targeted therapies in pancreatic neuroendocrine tumours: patient assessment, treatment administration, and management of adverse events. Ther Adv Med Oncol 2013;5:286–300.

50 Geynisman DM, Wickersham KE: Adherence to targeted oral anticancer medications. Discov Med 2013;15:231–241.

51 Danesi R, Boni JP, Ravaud A: Oral and intravenously administered mTOR inhibitors for metastatic renal cell carcinoma: pharmacokinetic considerations and clinical implications. Cancer Treat Rev 2013;39:784–792.

52 Huiart L, Bardou VJ, Giorgi R: The importance of adherence to oral therapies in the field of oncology: the example of breast cancer. Bull Cancer 2013;100:1007–1015.

53 Chen LC, Chen TC, Huang YB, Chang CS: Disease acceptance and adherence to imatinib in Taiwanese chronic myeloid leukaemia outpatients. Int J Clin Pharm 2014;36:120–127.

54 Conde-Estevez D, Salas E, Albanell J: Survey of oral chemotherapy safety and adherence practices of hospitals in Spain. Int J Clin Pharm 2013;35:1236–1244.

55 Vander Velde N, Chen L, Guo A, Sharma H, Marynchenko M, Wu EQ, Liu J, Yang H, Lizheng S: Study of imatinib treatment patterns and outcomes among US veteran patients with Philadelphia chromosome-positive chronic myeloid leukemia. J Oncol Pract 2013;9:e212–e219.

56 Johnson RH, Kroon L: Optimizing fertility preservation practices for adolescent and young adult cancer patients. J Natl Compr Canc Netw 2013;11:71–77.

57 Morgan S, Davies S, Palmer S, Plaster M: Sex, drugs, and rock 'n' roll: caring for adolescents and young adults with cancer. J Clin Oncol 2010;28:4825–4830.

58 Kondryn HJ, Edmondson CL, Hill J, Eden TO: Treatment non-adherence in teenage and young adult patients with cancer. Lancet Oncol 2011;12:100–108.

59 Experts in Chronic Myeloid Leukemia: The price of drugs for chronic myeloid leukemia (CML) is a reflection of the unsustainable prices of cancer drugs: from the perspective of a large group of CML experts. Blood 2013; 121:4439–4442.

60 Kantarjian H, Zwelling L: Cancer drug prices and the free-market forces. Cancer 2013;119: 3903–3905.

61 Freyer DR: Transition of care for young adult survivors of childhood and adolescent cancer: rationale and approaches. J Clin Oncol 2010; 28:4810–4818.

62 Klosky JL, Cash DK, Buscemi J, Lensing S, Garces-Webb DM, Zhao W, Wiard S, Hudson MM: Factors influencing long-term follow-up clinic attendance among survivors of childhood cancer. J Cancer Surviv 2008;2: 225–232.

63 McDonough JE: The road ahead for the Affordable Care Act. N Engl J Med 2012;367: 199–201.

64 Ferrari A, Thomas D, Franklin AR, Hayes-Lattin BM, Mascarin M, van der Graaf W, Albritton KH: Starting an adolescent and young adult program: some success stories and some obstacles to overcome. J Clin Oncol 2010;28: 4850–4857.

Acta Haematol 2014;132:307–312
DOI: 10.1159/000365117

Published online: September 10, 2014

Acute Promyelocytic Leukemia in Children and Adolescents

Eytan M. Stein[a]   Martin S. Tallman[a, b]

[a]Leukemia Service, Memorial Sloan-Kettering Cancer Center, and [b]Weill Cornell Medical Center, New York, N.Y., USA

Key Words

Acute promyelocytic leukemia · Adolescents · Children

Abstract

Acute promyelocytic leukemia (APL) is a rare subtype of AML characterized by a reciprocal balanced translocation between chromosomes 15 and 17 that fuses the PML gene with the RARα gene and leads to the leukemic phenotype. Although best described in large clinical trials of adults, APL, like other forms of AML, also occurs in children. The positive outcome of children with APL mirrors the dramatic increase in survival seen in adults since the introduction of all-trans retinoic acid (ATRA). In this paper, we review the diagnosis of APL in children as well as large, retrospective, clinical trial data collected on pediatric APL. We also raise management issues and toxicities that are unique to children.

© 2014 S. Karger AG, Basel

Introduction

Acute promyelocytic leukemia (APL) is a unique subtype of acute myeloid leukemia (AML) characterized by a block at the promyelocyte stage of hematopoiesis. The original description and recognition of APL as a unique subtype of AML are credited to Leif Hillestad, a Scandinavian physician who reported 3 patients with rapidly progressive leukemia and a profound coagulopathy [1]. This coagulopathy, similar to disseminated intravascular coagulation, produces a prolonged prothrombin time and partial thromboplastin time and hypofibrinogenemia.

The sine qua non of APL is a recurrent reciprocal translocation between chromosomes 15 and 17. This translocation, first described by Janet Rowley and colleagues, fuses the promyelocytic leukemia gene with the retinoic acid receptor α gene and leads to the promyelocytic leukemia phenotype [2]. In routine practice, this translocation is easily visualized with standard chromosomal analysis. However, cases have been described in the literature of cryptic translocations that fuse promyelocytic leukemia and retinoic acid receptor α genes but are nevertheless not detectable on standard chromosomal analysis.

Until the late 1980s, APL was the most lethal subtype of AML, as a result of the profound hemorrhagic complications seen in the early stages of the disease. The use of all-*trans*-retinoic acid (ATRA) as an effective treatment for APL in adults in the 1980s and 1990s is the major success story in the history of the treatment of acute leukemia in general, and AML specifically. The idea that a single

Eytan M. Stein, MD
Leukemia Service, Memorial Sloan-Kettering Cancer Center
1275 York Avenue
New York, NY 10065 (USA)
E-Mail steine@mskcc.org

oral agent could have such dramatic effects on the outcome of acute leukemia anticipated the advent of targeted therapies more generally in the treatment of solid tumors and hematological malignancies.

APL in the Young

While AML is in general a disease of adults, APL, like AML, also occurs in the young. For the purposes of this review, young patients are defined, somewhat arbitrarily, as those 18 or younger. Because AML is a rare disease and APL is a rare subtype of AML, the numbers of pediatric patients with APL are quite small. However, it does occur and with proper management the outcome of children with APL is as good as that of adults with APL. In this review, we focus our attention on making the initial diagnosis of APL, clinical trials that investigate the optimal treatment of children with APL, outcomes and side effects that are of particular concern in children.

Diagnosis

The diagnostic procedures necessary to diagnose APL in children mirror the diagnosis of APL in adults. For many patients, and especially for children, the most difficult part of the initial evaluation for acute leukemia is a bone marrow aspiration and biopsy. Even with adequate local anesthesia, many experience significant procedural discomfort that leads to subsequent anxiety and, in some cases, refusal of further bone marrow evaluation. The reasons for performing bone marrow biopsy in AML are multiple: assessments of bone marrow blast percentage (which forms the basis for a firm diagnosis of AML), evaluating bone marrow morphology, using immunohistochemical staining to confirm leukemic lineage (lymphoid or myeloid) and obtaining adequate numbers of myeloblasts for cytogenetic and molecular genetic analysis. In AML, the initial bone marrow biopsy is crucial because the results of the cytogenetic and molecular genetic studies form the basis of treatment recommendations in consolidation – specifically whether to proceed to allogeneic stem cell transplantation or consolidate with 3–4 courses of high-dose cytarabine or a similar regimen.

However, APL has unique associations that raise the question as to whether a bone marrow biopsy at diagnosis is actually needed. The morphology of leukemic promyelocytes (if they are present in the peripheral blood) is distinctive and consists of promyelocytes with abundant granules that form bundles resembling collections of sticks (so-called faggot cells). In addition, the presence of the t(15;17) translocation either identified by cytogenetics, fluorescence in situ hybridization (FISH) or molecular genetics is unique to APL and confirms the diagnosis. In many centers, FISH evaluation can be performed within 24 h. Often, review of the peripheral blood in patients with APL reveals the characteristic leukemic promyelocytes and if present, the cytogenetics are also clear. Although additional cytogenetic abnormalities aside from t(15;17) exist in about one third of patients with APL, these have not been consistently associated with disease outcome and are not included in risk stratification. In fact, the prognosis is based solely on peripheral white blood count and age, and as mentioned earlier, treatment strategy is based on risk status and ability to tolerate anthracyclines. For these reasons, it is possible that the diagnosis of APL in children may be obtainable without a bone marrow biopsy.

Minimizing Early Death in Pediatric APL

While the cure rates for APL are remarkable, early death (defined as death within 30 days of diagnosis) continues to be a major cause of treatment failure in adults and children. In large clinical trials performed in adults, the induction death rate ranges between 5 and 9%. In population-based studies (which includes patients that never enrolled on trials), the early death rate ranges between 17 and 30% and is considerably higher in older patients. Indeed, when stratified by 5-year periods, the early death rate has not changed significantly since the introduction of ATRA. The major cause of early death is hemorrhage, usually pulmonary or intracerebral, caused by the characteristic coagulopathy associated with this disease. A review of data in children suggests that, like in adults, hemorrhage remains the major cause of early death.

What accounts for early death? Dedicated pediatric studies are lacking but in a retrospective study in adults, Altman et al. [3] hypothesized that early death could be reduced with the rapid administration of ATRA – without waiting for the results of bone marrow aspiration and confirmation of t(15;17). In a retrospective analysis of 194 adult patients, most (69%) had ATRA administered 2 or more days after presentation [3]. While the early death rate was not increased, the percentage of patients that died due to hemorrhage was markedly increased when ATRA was delayed for more than 2 days. In addition, the

Acta Haematol 2014;132:307–312
DOI: 10.1159/000365117

results of this retrospective analysis confirmed that high-risk patients with APL who received their first dose of ATRA 3 or 4 days after they had been suspected of having APL had an early death rate of 80% compared to a rate of only 18% in those high-risk patients who received ATRA on days 0, 1 or 2.

Clinical Trials

Because of the small numbers of pediatric patients with APL, data come from retrospective analyses of children that enrolled on adult clinical trials with subset analyses of their course, toxicities and outcomes.

Cooperative Group Trials

The first comprehensive retrospective analysis of a cooperative group trial for pediatric APL was published in 2001 by a German-Swiss-Austrian group [4]. Using the BFM-93 trial, where patients with APL were treated with ATRA from 1994 on, they identified 22 pediatric patients. While the initial dose of ATRA used was 45 mg/m^2 as in adults, on account of toxicity seen in the first few children treated that included headache, fever, bone, joint and muscle pain, the dose of ATRA was decreased to 25 mg/m^2. Interestingly, based on this early experience this dose has been used for pediatric APL cases in all subsequent clinical trials with no evidence of decreased efficacy. ATRA was given only in induction, and multiagent chemotherapy was given during induction, consolidation, intensification and maintenance. Of the 22 patients treated with ATRA during induction, 21 achieved a complete remission (CR) with 1 patient dying from hemorrhage. At a median follow-up of 34 months, 20 of the 22 patients were alive. Aside from the early hemorrhagic death, 1 patient died of progressive disease. 50% of the treated patients experienced physiological changes consistent with differentiation syndrome, all of which were treated with steroids and resolved.

The European APL Group conducted the APL93 trial, a randomized trial that asked two fundamental questions. First, whether ATRA needs to be administered concurrently with chemotherapy or whether chemotherapy can be administered sequentially with ATRA and, second, the role of maintenance ATRA and/or chemotherapy in the treatment of APL [5]. Of the 576 patients enrolled on the trial, 31 (5%) of the patients were less than 31 years old and included in the analysis. Of note, ATRA was dosed at

45 mg/m^2 with dose reductions to 25 mg/m^2 in children, when severe headaches or other signs suggesting benign intracranial hypertension were present. Because of the small numbers of pediatric patients in each arm of the trial, the results from each study arm were combined in the final analysis of outcome. Of the 31 patients treated, 30 achieved a CR, and 1 died on day 2 of induction because of central nervous system and pulmonary hemorrhage. The relapse rate at 5 years was 27%, and the 5-year overall survival was 90%. Because of the small numbers of patients assigned to the various maintenance therapies, between-group comparisons between maintenance ATRA, chemotherapy or a combination of ATRA and chemotherapy could not be performed. Toxicities related to therapy included ATRA syndrome in 13% of the children treated, headache in 39% of patients of which 16% had signs and symptoms consistent with benign intracranial hypertension (pseudotumor cerebri).

The results of the European APL93 trial were combined with the European APL2000 trial and updated in 2012 [6]. While the APL93 trial established that combination, rather than sequential, therapy was the preferred treatment paradigm in induction, the APL2000 trial asked whether one could omit cytarabine in consolidation for low- and intermediate-risk patients. Unlike the earlier report, this retrospective look at pediatric patients broke down the analysis between children 12 and under and adolescents who were between 13 and 18 years old. Like the earlier analysis, all pediatric (younger than 18) patients were analyzed together because of the small numbers rather than stratifying based on randomization.

In the final analysis 84 pediatric patients were treated in the APL93 trial – 26 children and 58 adolescents. The CR rate was 92 and 100%, respectively, in children and adolescents. The cumulative incidence of relapse was 28% in children and 20% in adolescents while the 5-year overall survival rate was 80.4% in children and 93.6% in adolescents. Toxicities were similar to those seen in other trials including headache, pseudotumor cerebri and differentiation syndrome.

The PETHEMA group analyzed the results of pediatric patients treated in the single arm LPA96 and LPA99 trials and reported the outcomes in 2005 [7]. Both of these trials had the same induction regimen of idarubicin at a dose of 12 mg/m^2 given on days 2, 4, 6 and 8 and ATRA at a dose of 25 mg/m^2 given twice a day until the achievement of hematological CR or 90 days, whichever came first. Three cycles of consolidation were given on the LPA96 trial: the first with idarubicin, the second with mitoxantrone and the third with idarubicin. ATRA was not given

Acta Haematol 2014;132:307–312
DOI: 10.1159/000365117

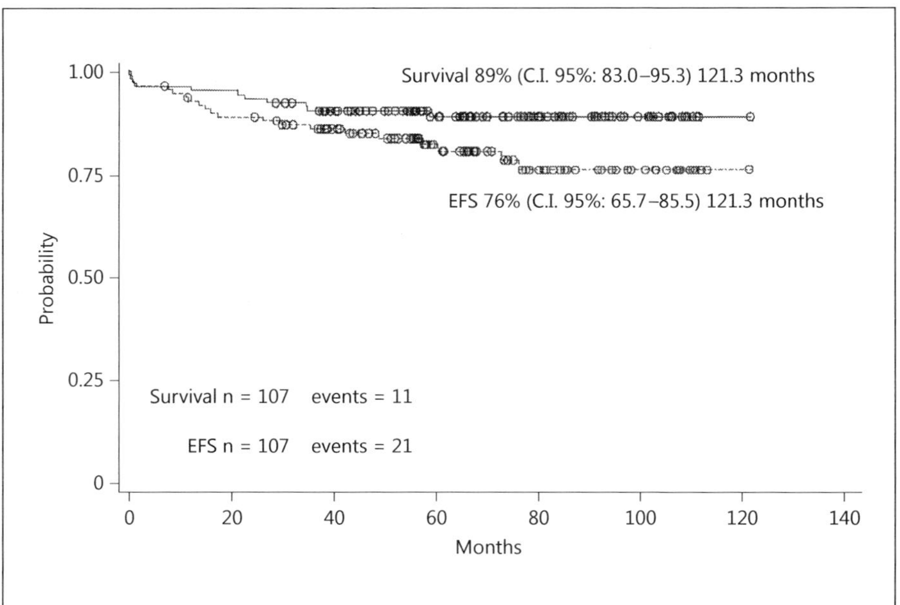

Fig. 1. Overall survival and event-free survival (EFS) probability for the whole cohort of patients. CI = Confidence interval.

in consolidation. In the LPA99 trial, ATRA was given during consolidation at a dose of 25 mg/m^2 as well as chemotherapy with idarubicin for 3 cycles. Maintenance therapy was given in both trials for 15 days every 3 months with 6-mercaptopurine, methotrexate and ATRA. Maintenance was continued for 2 years.

In the combined analysis of both trials, 66 pediatric patients were treated and 61 achieved a CR. Of the 5 patients who did not achieve a CR, 3 died of early hemorrhagic death, and 2 died of differentiation syndrome. Headaches occurred in 30% of the children treated, and pseudotumor cerebri occurred in 6%. Pseudotumor required the discontinuation of ATRA in 2 children and holding – but then restarting – ATRA in 2 other children. The cumulative incidence of relapse when both trials were combined was 17%, 3.5% in children with low- and intermediate-risk disease and 31% in children with high-risk disease. The overall survival at 7 years was 88% for low/intermediate-risk patients and 83% for high-risk patients.

The North American Intergroup conducted a randomized trial of induction chemotherapy with ATRA alone versus standard treatment with chemotherapy [8]. This trial, published in 1997 in the *New England Journal of Medicine*, was one of the first large randomized trials that demonstrated the superiority of ATRA over standard chemotherapy in the treatment of APL. Fifty-three pediatric patients were enrolled on the study and were confirmed by FISH to have a 15;17 translocation. Of these, 27 patients were randomized to receive ATRA monotherapy, and 26 were randomized to chemotherapy alone. The CR rate was 81 and 65%, respectively, for those patients assigned to ATRA or chemotherapy, a result that was not statistically significant. Similar to other studies, the major cause of early death was hemorrhage. Pseudotumor cerebri occurred in 11% of the treated patients.

The Japanese Childhood AML Cooperative Study Group performed a dedicated prospective study of the use of 58 children with de novo APL, between the ages of 11 months and 16 years between 1997 and 2004 [9]. In induction, ATRA at a dose of 45 mg/m^2 was combined with daunorubicin and cytarabine. Consolidation consisted of 3 cycles of multiagent chemotherapy in combination with ATRA, and maintenance consisted of ATRA monotherapy, given for 15 days every 3 months for a year.

Of the 58 patients enrolled on the clinical protocol, 56 achieved a CR and 2 had early hemorrhagic death. The cumulative incidence of relapse was 3.6% and the overall survival at 7 years was 93.1%. Differentiation syndrome, severe headache and pseudotumor cerebri were complications seen with therapy.

In 1993, the GIMEMA (Gruppo Italiano per le Malattie Ematologiche dell'Adulto) designed a study of both adults and children that used daily ATRA at a dose of 25 mg/m^2 in combination with idarubicin on days 2, 4, 6 and 8 for induction, followed by consolidation with 3 cycles of consolidation chemotherapy with chemotherapy alone [10]. In addition, as other groups had done, they asked the question whether maintenance therapy with ATRA alone, chemotherapy, ATRA plus chemotherapy or no maintenance was the preferred approach to maintain a remission and achieve cure. The study was published in 2005.

Of the 107 evaluable patients, 4 died during induction therapy, and 3 of those deaths were from intracerebral hemorrhage. All of the other patients achieved a CR. The overall survival of all evaluable patients was 89% at both 5 and 10 years of follow-up (fig. 1). Ten patients developed pseudotumor cerebri, and 8 patients had definite or possible ATRA syndrome.

Aside from the well-known complications of pseudotumor cerebri and differentiation syndrome seen, there remains a concern about early and late cardiac toxicity in children treated for APL. While there appears to be a very small risk of myocardial injury, the data from the large clinical trials described above do not support any major cardiac risk. In the GIMEMA trial, only 2 children developed transient sinus tachycardia while on study and there have been no episodes of late anthracycline-induced cardiotoxicity [10]. In the combined analysis of the APL93 and APL2000, three children developed heart failure within 2 years of APL diagnosis [6]. The first patient, who received a cumulative anthracycline dose of 495 mg/m^2, recovered his ejection fraction with medical therapy alone. The second patient died from complications related to heart failure, and the third required cardiac transplantation. Of note, both the second and third patients had relapsed APL and received further cardiotoxic chemotherapy as salvage therapy. In the PETHEMA trial, there were no cases of late cardiac toxicity [7].

Arsenic/ATRA without Chemotherapy

The remarkable outcomes demonstrated by Lo-Coco et al. [11] about ATRA/arsenic combination therapy without the use of chemotherapy, recently published in the *New England Journal of Medicine* for low-risk APL patients, has established a new standard of care in the treatment of APL. Whether these results in the adult population treated in this clinical trial can be generalized to pediatric APL patients has not yet been demonstrated in a systematic way. A priori, there is no reason to believe that the efficacy of ATRA/arsenic combination therapy will be worse in children over adults, but there remain concerns about late toxicity that could occur in children including cardiac toxicity and secondary malignancies. Given the low numbers of children diagnosed with APL, an international collaborative effort is necessary to conduct a prospective clinical trial with ATRA in combination with arsenic with monitoring of late toxicities.

Conclusions and Future Directions

A number of themes emerge from the large clinical trials detailed above, of pediatric patients treated for APL. While an increased incidence of the microgranular variant and hyperleukocytosis and diagnosis appears to be increased in pediatric APL, it remains unclear whether this increased incidence translates into poorer outcomes for the children treated in these clinical trials. Indeed, the overall survival of children treated with ATRA rivals that seen in adult studies, even though most of these children were treated with a reduced dose of ATRA. As the standard of care for low-risk APL in adults is rapidly shifting towards ATRA/arsenic alone, without chemotherapy, clinical trials to explore this combination in children are needed as mentioned above. The shift, now, should be towards well-conducted prospective monitoring of late toxicities in pediatric patients that were treated with ATRA and chemotherapy into adulthood with a focus on toxicity, both physical (cardiac, etc.) and emotional.

References

1 Hillestad L: Acute promyelocytic leukemia. Acta Med Scand 1957;159:189–194.
2 Golomb HM, Vardiman J, Rowley JD: Acute nonlymphocytic leukemia in adults: correlations with Q-banded chromosomes. Blood 1976;48:9–21.
3 Altman JK, Rademaker A, Cull E, Weitner BB, Ofran Y, Rosenblat TL, Haidau A, Park JH, Ram SL, Orsini JM Jr, Sandhu S, Catchatourian R, Trifilio SM, Adel NG, Frankfurt O, Stein EM, Mallios G, Deblasio T, Jurcic JG, Nimer S, Peterson LC, Kwaan HC, Rowe JM, Douer D, Tallman MS: Administration of ATRA to newly diagnosed patients with acute promyelocytic leukemia is delayed contributing to early hemorrhagic death. Leuk Res 2013;37:1004–1009.
4 Mann G, Reinhardt D, Ritter J, Hermann J, Schmitt K, Gadner H, Creutzig U: Treatment with all-*trans* retinoic acid in acute promyelocytic leukemia reduces early deaths in children. Ann Hematol 2001;80:417–422.

5 De Botton S, Coiteux V, Chevret S, Rayon C, Vilmer E, Sanz M, de La Serna J, Philippe N, Baruchel A, Leverger G, Robert A, San Miguel J, Conde E, Sotto JJ, Bordessoule D, Fegueux N, Fey M, Parry A, Chomienne C, Degos L, Fenaux P: Outcome of childhood acute promyelocytic leukemia with all-*trans*-retinoic acid and chemotherapy. J Clin Oncol 2004;22: 1404–1412.

6 Bally C, Fadlallah J, Leverger G, Bertrand Y, Robert A, Baruchel A, Guerci A, Recher C, Raffoux E, Thomas X, Leblanc T, Idres N, Cassinat B, Vey N, Chomienne C, Dombret H, Sanz M, Fenaux P, Adès LJ: Outcome of acute promyelocytic leukemia (APL) in children and adolescents: an analysis in two consecutive trials of the European APL Group. J Clin Oncol 2012;30:1641–1646.

7 Ortega JJ, Madero L, Martín G, Verdeguer A, García P, Parody R, Fuster J, Molines A, Novo A, Debén G, Rodríguez A, Conde E, de la Serna J, Allegue MJ, Capote FJ, González JD, Bolufer P, González M, Sanz MA: Treatment with all-trans retinoic acid and anthracycline monochemotherapy for children with acute promyelocytic leukemia: a multicenter study by the PETHEMA Group. J Clin Oncol 2005; 23:7632–7640.

8 Gregory J, Kim H, Alonzo T, Gerbing R, Woods W, Weinstein H, Shepherd L, Schiffer C, Appelbaum F, Willman C, Wiernik P, Rowe J, Tallman M, Feusner J: Treatment of children with acute promyelocytic leukemia: results of the first North American Intergroup trial INT0129. Pediatr Blood Cancer 2009;53: 1005–1010.

9 Imaizumi M, Tawa A, Hanada R, Tsuchida M, Tabuchi K, Kigasawa H, Kobayashi R, Morimoto A, Nakayama H, Hamamoto K, Kudo K, Yabe H, Horibe K, Tsuchiya S, Tsukimoto I: Prospective study of a therapeutic regimen with all-*trans* retinoic acid and anthracyclines in combination of cytarabine in children with acute promyelocytic leukaemia: the Japanese Childhood Acute Myeloid Leukaemia Cooperative Study. Br J Haematol 2010;152:89–98.

10 Testi AM, Biondi A, Lo Coco F, Moleti ML, Giona F, Vignetti M, Menna G, Locatelli F, Pession A, Barisone E, De Rossi G, Diverio D, Micalizzi C, Aricò M, Basso G, Foa R, Mandelli F: GIMEMA-AIEOPAIDA protocol for the treatment of newly diagnosed acute promyelocytic leukemia (APL) in children. Blood 2005;106:447–453.

11 Lo-Coco F, Avvisati G, Vignetti M, Thiede C, Orlando SM, Iacobelli S, Ferrara F, Fazi P, Cicconi L, Di Bona E, Specchia G, Sica S, Divona M, Levis A, Fiedler W, Cerqui E, Breccia M, Fioritoni G, Salih HR, Cazzola M, Melillo L, Carella AM, Brandts CH, Morra E, von Lilienfeld-Toal M, Hertenstein B, Wattad M, et al: Retinoic acid and arsenic trioxide for acute promyelocytic leukemia. N Engl J Med 2013;369:111–121.

Acta Haematol 2014;132:313–325
DOI: 10.1159/000360211

Published online: September 10, 2014

Hematopoietic Stem Cell Transplantation in Adolescents and Young Adults

Priti Tewari[a]   Anna R. Franklin[a]   Nidale Tarek[a]   Martha A. Askins[a]
Scott Mofield[b]   Partow Kebriaei[a]

[a]MD Anderson Cancer Center, Houston, Tex., and [b]Duke University Medical Center, Durham, N.C., USA

Key Words
Adolescents and young adults · Stem cell transplantation

Abstract
Background: Adolescents and young adults (AYAs) are a very unique subset of our population journeying through a dynamic stage of their lives. This age group often remains understudied as a separate entity because they are commonly lumped into either pediatric or adult subgroups. **Methods:** Here we review acute and chronic issues surrounding hematopoietic stem cell transplantation (HSCT) with a focus on the AYA age group. **Results:** HSCT is a commonly used treatment modality for patients with certain types of cancers. AYA patients undergoing HSCT present a very unique perspective, circumstances, medical, psychological and social issues requiring a diligent workup, care and follow-up. **Conclusion:** The medical care of these patients should be approached in a multidisciplinary method involving the patient, caregivers, physicians, psychologists and social workers.

© 2014 S. Karger AG, Basel

Adolescents and young adults (AYAs) are a very unique subset of our population journeying through a dynamic stage of their lives. This age group often remains understudied as a separate entity because they are commonly lumped into either pediatric or adult subgroups. Hematopoietic stem cell transplantation (HSCT) is a commonly used treatment modality for patients with certain types of cancers. AYA patients undergoing HSCT present a very unique perspective, circumstances, medical, psychological and social issues requiring a diligent workup, care and follow-up.

Effects of Stem Cell Source and Conditioning Regimen

Stem Cell Source

In a retrospective analysis of 221 patients (175 between 17 and 40 years old) who received a transplant for acute lymphoblastic leukemia (ALL) in CR1, Kiehl et al. [1] were among the first to report no difference in survival between matched related (45%) and matched unrelated donors (42%). In a later study, Nishiwaki et al. [2] reported that while survival was comparable, treatment-related mortality (TRM) was higher in the unrelated group while relapse was higher in the related group. More recently, umbilical cord blood (UCB) transplants have been compared to matched related and matched unrelated donor SCT. The more immature T-cell repertoire in the UCB graft allows for more human leukocyte antigen mismatch

KARGER

E-Mail karger@karger.com
www.karger.com/aha

© 2014 S. Karger AG, Basel
0001–5792/14/1324–0313$39.50/0

Priti Tewari
1515 Holcombe Blvd, Unit 87
Houston, TX 77040 (USA)
E-Mail ptewari@mdanderson.org

between donor and recipient, and thus more availability of donors. However, UCB transplants are also associated with delayed hematopoietic recovery and increased risk for infection [3, 4]. In a retrospective, multiregistry study, data for 1,525 patients (including 645 with ALL) receiving UCB grafts (n = 165) were compared with 8/8 or 7/8 matched unrelated peripheral blood (n = 888) or bone marrow (n = 472) grafts. Although TRM was higher for UCB grafts, leukemia-free survival was similar among the graft sources [5].

Conditioning Intensity

While the discussion of the intensity of the SCT conditioning therapy is most frequent with very old or very young patients, this discussion may also be appropriate for some adolescent patients with comorbidities often sustained from extensive prior therapy for their ALL. The conditioning regimen broadly serves three goals: (1) to treat the disease burden to a minimal level, (2) to create 'space' within the marrow microenvironment to allow engraftment of hematopoietic stem cells and (3) to provide sufficient host immunosuppression to prevent graft rejection and allow for donor engraftment. Until the last decade, all patients received myeloablative conditioning (MAC) regimens, defined as a regimen which contained a combination of agents expected to produce profound and irreversible pancytopenia and myeloablation within 1–3 weeks from administration, and required hematopoietic stem cells to restore hematopoiesis. The continued understanding of the curative potential of the immune-mediated graft-versus-tumor effect has led to increasing use of reduced intensity conditioning (RIC) regimens, which rely more on the graft-versus-tumor effect, rather than myeloablation, to treat the patient. These regimens are associated with lower toxicities and thus can be safely performed in patients in whom SCT would have been previously contraindicated. Although broadly classified as RIC regimens, there are significant differences in the relative degree of immunosuppression and myelosuppression involved, and the regimens can be further divided into the truly nonmyeloablative (NMA) and RIC regimens [6, 7]. NMA regimens are defined as regimens associated with minimal cytopenia that do not require stem cell support. In NMA regimens, the conditioning regimen is mainly for immunosuppression to allow stem cell engraftment and depends mainly on the graft-versus-tumor effect for disease control.

Due to the rapid growth kinetics of ALL blasts, the standard approach to SCT conditioning is to use a MAC regimen, and thus there are few published reports of RIC and NMA conditioning in ALL, and the majority are in older adults with ALL [8–11]. However, for younger patients with comorbidities, a RIC or NMA regimen may need to be considered. The Pediatric Blood and Marrow Transplant Consortium study ONC0313 was one of the earliest studies to look at the role of RIC SCT specifically in children [12]. Forty-seven patients with a median age of 11 years (range 2–20 years) receiving SCT for a variety of cancers including ALL beyond first remission (n = 35) were evaluated following conditioning with intravenous busulfan (Bu), fludarabine and antithymocyte globulin. At 2 years, the TRM rate was very favorable at 11%, although the overall survival (OS) was only 45% due to the high relapse rate of 43%. Not surprisingly, patients with detectable disease at the time of SCT had a significantly worse OS compared with those in remission (0 vs. 63%, p = 0.01).

The role of RIC regimens specifically in patients with ALL was evaluated and reported in a retrospective study from the Center for International Blood and Marrow Transplant Research (CIBMTR) [13]. Patients with a median age of 12 years (range 1–18, 25 patients >11 years) received RIC SCT for ALL in CR1 (n = 5), CR2 or higher (n = 23) or active disease (n = 8). In contrast to the study by Pulsipher et al. [12], the 3-year TRM was reported to be 40%, although relapse and OS were similar at 37 and 36%. The difference in TRM may be related to the difference in patient population and treatment regimens. Although both of these studies report a fairly high relapse rate, the OS of an estimated 35–45% is not dissimilar to survival rates for MAC regimens in advanced ALL [14–16]. Indeed, a retrospective analysis of transplants for ALL in CR1 or CR2 reported to the CIBMTR failed to show an impact for SCT conditioning intensity on age-adjusted survival (RIC 38% vs. MAC 43%, p = 0.39) [17]. The study group was comprised of 1,428 patients who received a MAC regimen and 93 who received RIC; 38 of the RIC patients were between 16 and 39 years of age, and among this group 61% had at least 1 significant adverse clinical factor. The TRM rate was similar for the two groups despite the more infirm patients in the RIC group. Finally, the results of an NMA regimen were reported by Ram et al. [18] in 51 patients with a median age of 56 years (range 8–69 years, 6 patients <18 years) who received SCT following conditioning with fludarabine/total body irradiation (TBI) of 2 Gy for ALL in CR1 (n = 32) or more advanced remission (n = 19). At 3 years, OS, relapse and TRM were 34, 40 and 28%, respectively. Not surprisingly, survival was higher for patients in CR1 (52 vs. 8% for Philadelphia-negative patients), and highest for patients with

Acta Haematol 2014;132:313–325
DOI: 10.1159/000360211

Tewari/Franklin/Tarek/Askins/Mofield/
Kebriaei

Philadelphia-positive disease who received post-SCT imatinib (65%). In conclusion, as these studies illustrate, RIC regimens are an acceptable approach for patients who cannot tolerate a MAC regimen.

While the standard MAC regimen consists of TBI combined with a second alkylating agent such as cyclophosphamide (Cy) or etoposide, alternative MAC regimens without TBI continue to be investigated, due to the long-term toxicities of radiation, which include impaired growth and cognitive function [19, 20], increased incidence without plateau in secondary malignancies and increased incidence of the cardiometabolic trait, leading to diabetes and accelerated atherosclerotic cardiovascular disease [21, 22]. Early studies compared the combination of oral with Cy with TBI/Cy and found increased TRM, including fatal veno-occlusive disease, for the Bu/Cy combination, and consequently worse outcome with Bu/Cy [23]. However, more recent studies, using intravenous Bu combined with Cy [24], fludarabine [25, 26] or clofarabine [27], yield equivalent or superior outcomes to TBI-based regimens.

Fertility

A unique issue facing AYAs undergoing HSCT is fertility. Just as the potential adverse effects of graft failure, graft-versus-host disease (GVHD) and organ dysfunction are discussed during the consent process and documented in the medical record, so should the high risk of infertility. However, frank discussion of infertility rarely occurs for multiple reasons [28].

Oncologists are trained to treat the life-threatening cancer and prioritize the prompt initiation of treatment. Most oncologists report they lack adequate knowledge to have a discussion about infertility including options for fertility preservation [29, 30]. Patients can and should be promptly referred to a fertility specialist for a detailed discussion, just as a cardiologist would be consulted for a patient with heart disease [31, 32].

Other barriers to the fertility preservation discussion include our discomfort with a sensitive topic, failure to recognize the importance of the issue to the patient, costs which may be perceived as prohibitive and concerns about the possible delay in starting treatment. As medicine shifts to being more patient centered, patients should be given the opportunity to make well-informed decisions based on their own morals, values, religion, culture and finances. Social workers and psychologists are often helpful in facilitating the decision-making process. Current evidence demonstrates such a discussion about infertility decreases patient distress and improves their quality of life.

Unfortunately, the data on the risk of infertility from transplantation is less robust. Gonadotoxicity of chemotherapy is difficult to study as agents are almost exclusively used in combination. Also, many studies of women used resumption of menses as a surrogate marker for fertility, which we now know is unreliable. Current data shows HSCT portends a greater than 90% risk of infertility with TBI and high doses of alkylating agents being the main culprits of sterility. Novel preparative regimens have not been adequately studied, specifically regimens including antimetabolites, such as fludarabine and clofarabine, monoclonal antibodies and NMA regimens [33].

Fertility Preservation

Ideally, patients who desire fertility preservation will have the opportunity to do so prior to receiving any cytotoxic chemotherapy. However, treatment must begin urgently in many cases of hematological malignancies. Also, the recommendation for a transplant or other treatment causing infertility may not have been known at the time of initial diagnosis and treatment initiation. For example, a patient with early favorable Hodgkin's lymphoma may receive 4 cycles of ABVD (Adriamycin, bleomycin, vinblastine, dacarbazine), which has a low risk of infertility. However, a relapse may be treated with ifosfamide, carboplatin and etoposide followed by an autologous HSCT, significantly increasing the risk of infertility. Patients with aplastic anemia and other nonmalignant disorders that may require HSCT do not receive cytotoxic therapy prior to transplantation, and time constraints are rare. As such, these patients should have the opportunity to preserve their fertility before proceeding to transplantation.

For men, cryopreservation of sperm is the only established fertility preservation method [33]. The patient provides a semen specimen via masturbation. A semen analysis is performed prior to cryopreservation to ensure the quality of the specimen. The cost of banking sperm varies by provider and geographic location. Upfront charges of USD 500–700 include the semen analysis and the first year of storage. Annual storage fees of about USD 500 are an ongoing cost. Often, these costs are not covered by insurance. Financial assistance may be available through the clinic or philanthropic and advocacy organizations.

Ideally 2–3 specimens are collected, but a single specimen is adequate when treatment needs to be started emergently. With today's assisted reproduction techniques, very few sperm are required to create embryos. Intracytoplasmic sperm injection is the injection of a single sperm into an oocyte to directly fertilize the egg. The number of sperm cryopreserved and the number of desired children will guide the choice of technique in creating a pregnancy. Sperm can be safely cryopreserved for decades.

For many years cryopreservation of embryos was the only established method of fertility preservation for women [33]. As of October 2012, the American Society of Reproductive Medicine considers oocyte cryopreservation as a standard procedure due to improvements in techniques resulting in similar rates of live birth compared with embryo cryopreservation [34]. The time constraints are now decreased from the previous 4–6 weeks as the timing is no longer dependent on the menstrual cycle. Currently, only 2–4 weeks are required for ovarian stimulation and oocyte harvesting. The typical cost ranges from USD 10,000 to 15,000. Again, many of these costs are not covered by insurance; however, financial assistance may be available from the clinic. Several pharmaceutical companies will donate the hormone injections (USD 2,500–4,000) to cancer patients undergoing fertility preservation [31].

Investigational methods of fertility preservation include cryopreservation of ovarian and testicular tissue. Insufficient evidence exists to recommend ovarian suppression with gonadotropin-releasing hormone analogues to preserve fertility. However, such agents induce menstrual suppression preventing menorrhagia in the transplant setting [31, 33].

Late Effects

Fortunately with improving technology and supportive care within the SCT field, we have increasing numbers of long-term survivors, and this certainly entails survivors within our AYA cohort. Aside from acute SCT issues, this age group provides a unique series of late and long-term effects. Much awareness and attention have been drawn to this topic with both European and international working groups to survey and evaluate late effects following SCT [35–38]. The National Comprehensive Cancer Network provides very comprehensive guidelines and recommendations regarding AYA oncology patients (nccn.org) [39]. While many late effects within our AYA SCT population overlap those of the AYA oncology population, this is and should be a major area of focus when managing survivors. Late effects can appear many years following SCT and require lifelong follow-up and screening. The AYA population, similar to the pediatric populations is unique in that they have decades of life ahead of them. Surviving patients require appropriate care, follow-up and screening programs focused on late effects following SCT to recognize and manage new and chronic health issues. These evaluations should entail knowledge of SCT conditioning regimens, acute toxicities and posttransplantation complications.

Secondary Malignancies

SCT patients are often exposed to therapies that predispose them to secondary malignancies. When stratifying these risks and evaluating for an appropriate follow-up, both therapy prior to transplantation and agents used for conditioning need to be assessed. Table 1 summarizes secondary tumor types by primary risk and contributing factors. Treatment with epipodophyllotoxins and alkylators predisposes to an increased risk of secondary acute myeloid leukemia and myelodysplastic syndrome [40–42]. Aside from chemotherapeutic agents causing secondary malignancy, radiation in the forms of focal, cranial irradiation or TBI predispose patients to a unique subset of solid and cutaneous malignancies. Oeffinger and Hudson [43] describe the various late effects as stratified by radiation type ranging from cataracts to gonadal dysfunction. A wide-range of secondary malignancies can occur as a result of late-effects of radiation and generally entailing solid tumors within radiation fields. Any radiation predisposes to secondary tumors within or near the radiation field, and aside from traditional solid tumors this includes skin cancer such as basal cell or squamous cell carcinoma and melanomas. With TBI often the traditional treatment of choice for transplant conditioning, these patients in particular need to be monitored closely for secondary malignancies, including skin cancers. Chest radiation, which is often used in the treatment of patients with Hodgkin's and non-Hodgkin's lymphoma, increases risks of breast and thyroid cancers. Monitoring for these solid tumors is imperative in the AYA HSCT patients.

Endocrine Effects

One major area requiring screening and focus is endocrine effects. These survivors are at an increased risk for thyroid dysfunction, gonadal dysfunction, growth impairments and bony abnormalities [44–48]. As highlighted earlier, gonadal dysfunction occurs in both males and females exposed to chemotherapy and/or radiation, and with this particular age group this is an important area of

Acta Haematol 2014;132:313–325
DOI: 10.1159/000360211

Tewari/Franklin/Tarek/Askins/Mofield/
Kebriaei

Table 1. Secondary malignancies with causative agents following HSCI [38, 85–96]

Secondary malignancies	Causative agents	Predisposing risk factors	Median onset, cumulative incident rate
Solid tumors	TBI-based conditioning regimen GVHD Immunosuppression following SCT	History of radiation therapy prior to SCT Younger age at TBI exposure Genetic predisposition: Fanconi anemia, underlying immunodeficiency	6–8 years 1–4% at 10 years
Skin cancer Cancers of the oral cavity		Light skin Chronic lichenoid lesions of the oral mucosa, history of smoking, HPV	
Breast cancer Lung cancer CNS tumors Thyroid cancer Bone and soft tissue sarcomas Liver cancer Gastrointestinal cancers Genitourinary cancers		Disruption of ovarian function by chemotherapy History of smoking	
MDS/acute leukemia	TBI-based conditioning regimen Alkylating agents	Exposure to melphalan or etoposide prior to SCT	17 months 4% at 10 years
Posttransplant lymphoproliferative disease	Epstein-Barr virus infection	T-cell depletion of the graft In vivo T-cell depletion (ATG, alemtuzumab) GVHD Immunosuppression following SCT	6–12 months 1–2% at 10 years

ATG = Antithymocyte globulin; CNS = central nervous system; HPV = human papillomavirus; MDS = myelodysplastic syndrome.

focus. Although younger patients are at times spared, in the AYA population transplant conditioning regimens often result in gonadal dysfunction with the highest risk following the use of TBI and alkylating agents for transplant conditioning [49–51]. Many RIC and NMA regimens are being explored and may spare patients from these effects.

The frequency of thyroid dysfunction following transplantation is high, and although this is traditionally thought to result from TBI-containing regimens, this late effect is not limited to radiation exposure [52, 53]. Although thyroid dysfunction usually occurs within a few years following HSCT, Sanders et al. [52] observed thyroid dysfunction as late as 28 years after TBI and 10 years following Bu/Cy preparative regimens. In this review of 791 patients over a 30-year time period, the most significant risk is associated with HSCT preparative regimens using TBI and Bu. When the risk of thyroid dysfunction is stratified by primary malignancy type, the highest risk is with Hodgkin's lymphoma followed by hematological malignancies. Multivariate analysis of thyroid function following HSCT resulted in 73% of Hodgkin's lymphoma survivors with thyroid dysfunction, as compared to 35 and 33% for myeloid and lymphoid malignancies, respectively. With Hodgkin's lymphoma, a malignancy that often targets the AYA age group, thyroid function is very important to monitor in the long term.

Although more of a focus for pediatric age patients proceeding to transplantation, it is important to recognize that some younger AYA HSCT patients are still undergoing physical growth and development. Receiving cytotoxic therapies during this period can have detrimental effects on both growth and bone development [44, 54, 55]. Aside from not achieving the projected adult height [56, 57], decreased bone density can play a role in the development of osteonecrosis and avascular necrosis, leading to high morbidity in adulthood [58–61]. Kaste et al. [62] evaluated 48 allogeneic HSCT recipients aged 21 years and younger for bone mineral density and osteonecrosis in these survivors reporting the cumulative incidence of osteopenia and osteonecrosis in childhood survivors 10 years after transplantation to be 47.7 and 44%, respectively. In a retrospective review of 100 patients after HSCT, 12% of patients developed avascular necrosis following allogeneic trans-

Acta Haematol 2014;132:313–325
DOI: 10.1159/000360211

plantation and 4% following autologous transplantation with 15 different affected joints [63]. This highlights the importance of evaluating bone density and thorough musculoskeletal examinations on follow-up [62, 64].

Chronic Organ Dysfunction

In HSCT recipients, chronic organ dysfunction can result from both pretransplantation- and transplantation-related therapies. When compared to sibling controls, survivors of HSCT are more likely to have chronic health conditions [65]. This can include extensive pretransplantation therapies to attain remission, GVHD, severe or chronic infections. Table 2 summarizes risk factors associated with various chronic organ dysfunctions. In particular, the focus needs to be on pulmonary, renal and cardiovascular sequelae. In the review of 155 pediatric HSCT survivors by Leung et al. [54], at least 1 parameter of the pulmonary function tests was abnormal in 77 patients, with a cumulative incidence of abnormalities at 10 years of 63.2%. Renal sequelae include hypertension and chronic renal insufficiency, and cardiovascular sequelae include hypertension, abnormal electrocardiograms and decreased cardiac function. While these risks are certainly not exclusive to the AYA population, the survivors from this age group have decades of life ahead of them, and diligent attention needs to be focused on maintaining adequate health and appropriately managing chronic health issues.

Chronic GVHD

Chronic GVHD is one of the most common late complications of SCT that can result in high morbidity and mortality. This can have effects on all organs potentially resulting in extensive damage and dysfunction [54, 66–68]. Depending on graft source the incidence of chronic GVHD can range between 40 and 70% [69, 70]. While we have limited data and publications with a specific focus on the AYA populations, certainly this is a group at risk with a possibly higher morbidity due to the fragile stage of their lives that they are in. Chronic GVHD can be especially daunting to the AYA population, where their lives are initially interrupted during their cancer diagnosis, and now, after surviving cancer and their transplantation, their quality of life and function are impaired due to chronic GVHD.

Counseling Transplant Survivors about Family-Building Options

As highlighted earlier, infertility is a prevalent late effect following HSCT. Survivors should be counseled that the high risk of infertility should not be used as a form of birth control, as evidenced by multiple case reports of transplant survivors having children naturally. Adequate measures to protect against sexually transmitted diseases are critical in this immunosuppressed patient population. HSCT survivors have an increased risk of cervical dysplasia [71, 72] and, as such, a theoretical risk of human papillomavirus-related malignancies of the oral cavity and skin.

Most experts recommend waiting at least 1 year after transplantation before assessing residual fertility. For men, a semen analysis is performed. The average cost is USD 100. The urologist or reproductive endocrinologist can counsel the man or couple as to what their options are based on these results. If no sperm are in the semen analysis, testicular sperm extraction may be offered. Needle biopsies of the testicle are examined for the presence of sperm. Sperm can be extracted under direct visualization and cryopreserved for future use [31, 33].

The assessment of ovarian reserve utilizes serum anti-müllerian hormone level and antral follicle count on transvaginal ultrasound. Luteinizing hormone and follicle-stimulating hormone are no longer used as they are surrogate markers and need to be measured on day 3 of a menstrual cycle in the absence of exogenous hormones (i.e. oral contraceptives, estrogen) [73]. Based on the results of these tests, an obstetrician/gynecologist or reproductive endocrinologist can discuss the available options.

Transplant survivors who are unable to have a biological child naturally have several other family-building options. Donor oocytes, sperm and embryos are available. A woman surviving transplantation may desire to become pregnant with an embryo created with her partner's sperm or with a donor embryo. Donor sperm would allow a female partner of a transplant survivor to have a biological child and carry the pregnancy.

Gestational surrogates would not typically be needed in transplant survivors as the infertility is caused by iatrogenic oocyte destruction. However, cardiomyopathy and other organ dysfunction may classify the pregnancy as high risk or not recommended [74].

Adoption is another option but can be challenging. Some domestic adoption agencies exclude cancer survivors as candidates, as do some countries. Other agencies and countries limit the options of cancer survivors; for example, currently China will only allow adoption of special needs children to cancer survivors. Being a foster parent is an avenue to adoption.

All family-building options for cancer and transplant survivors are expensive. As such, survivors should be counseled to create a savings plan in advance of their desire to start a family.

Table 2. Summary of potential chronic health issues following HSCT with risk factors and screening recommendations [39, 97, 98]

Tissues/organs	Risk factors	Screening recommendations
Immune system	GVHD and immunosuppressive therapy, T-cell depletion	CD4 count and immunoglobulin levels as clinically indicated
Oral	GVHD, radiation therapy	Clinical evaluation at 6 months, 1 year and yearly, dental assessment yearly
Endocrine		
Thyroid problems	TBI, radiation involving the thyroid gland	TSH, free T_4 and neck examination yearly
Gonadal dysfunction	TBI, cranial irradiation, high-dose alkylating agents, testicular irradiation (male), abdominal/pelvic irradiation (female)	Male: FSH, LH, testosterone, semen analysis, as clinically indicated Female: FSH, LH, estradiol, at 1 year, then as clinically indicated
Central adrenal insufficiency	TBI, cranial irradiation, corticosteroids	8 a.m. serum cortisol level yearly
Diabetes	Corticosteroids	Fasting glucose and HbA_{1c} yearly
Neurocognitive	TBI, cranial irradiation	Neuropsychological evaluation as clinically indicated
Cardiovascular	TBI, mediastinal/chest/abdominal irradiation	
Vascular disease	Calcineurin inhibitors, corticosteroids	Blood pressure and BMI yearly, fasting glucose and lipid profile every 2 years
Ischemic coronary artery disease	Anthracycline >300/m^2	Clinical assessment yearly, cardiology consult as clinically indicated
Cardiomyopathy		EKG, echocardiogram (or MUGA scan) every 1–2 years
Respiratory	TBI, bleomycin >400 U/m^2, Bu >500 mg, carmustine >600 mg/m^2, history of chest irradiation, infections, GVHD	Clinical assessment at 6 months, 1 year and yearly; chest X-ray and pulmonary function tests at end of treatment, then as clinically indicated
Kidney	Radiation therapy, nephrotoxic chemotherapy and other medications	BUN, creatinine, electrolytes, urinalysis, urine microalbumin and blood pressure at 6 months, 1 year and then yearly
Bladder	Pelvic irradiation, Cy >3 g/m^2	Urinalysis yearly
Liver	GVHD, infections, drug-related injuries, blood transfusions	Liver function tests every 3–6 months for the first year, then yearly, ferritin at 1 year, then as clinically indicated, viral testing as clinically indicated
Central nervous system	TBI, cranial irradiation, intrathecal chemotherapy	Clinical evaluation yearly
Bones	Corticosteroids, TBI, gonadal insufficiency	Vitamin D, bone densitometry at 1 year
Muscles	GVHD, corticosteroids	Clinical screen and physical therapy, consult as clinically indicated
Eyes	TBI, GVHD, corticosteroids	Clinical evaluation at 6 months, 1 year and yearly, ophthalmology evaluation with Schirmer test and intraocular pressure measurement at 1 year
Ears	Cisplatin >360 mg/m^2, radiation involving the ear	Audiology testing at end of treatment, then as clinically indicated

TSH = Thyroid-stimulating hormone; T_4 = thyroxine; FSH = follicle-stimulating hormone; LH = luteinizing hormone; HbA_{1c} = glycosylated hemoglobin A_{1c}; BMI = body mass index; EKG = electrocardiogram; MUGA = multigated acquisition; BUN = blood urea nitrogen.

Psychosocial Considerations

Cancer and its treatment can have both negative and positive psychological effects on teens and young adults. SCT is inherently an intensive process with many physical, social and psychological challenges [75]. Physically, patients often experience nausea, malaise and decreased energy during the time of hospitalization. In addition, changes in appearance can result from alopecia, weight gain or loss, edema and GVHD of the skin. Socially, AYAs have to deal with separation from their peers and usual community activities. Moreover, they find themselves necessarily depending on their parents at a time they would otherwise be developing increased autonomy. Psychologically, AYAs may experience a sense of loss of control as well as uncertainty about the future. These themes have emerged in studies specifically examining AYAs who have undergone hematopoietic cell transplantation [76]. Depending on one's coping skills and the intensity of challenges faced during stem cell transplantation and recovery, it is possible for patients to develop brief symptoms of depression and anxiety, such as is seen with the psychiatric diagnoses of adjustment disorders. For a small minority of children undergoing SCT, and depending on a complex set of treatment and health-related factors, psychological symptoms may persist and merit ongoing psychological care [77].

Developmentally Appropriate Care

It is helpful to conceptualize adolescence as a maturation process during which youth achieve a number of important psychosocial tasks, including: (1) adjusting to a physically maturing body, (2) achieving more mature relationships with peers of both genders, (3) achieving emotional independence from parents and other adults, (4) acquiring a set of values that will serve as an ethical guide to behavior, (5) completing educational requirements and preparing for a career and (6) preparing for the possibility of marriage and family in the future. With the support of their families, adolescents mature as they participate in social activities, make decisions/solve problems and manage responsibilities well. Success with these opportunities engenders feelings of self-efficacy and autonomy, which in turn give the adolescent the confidence he or she needs to launch from home. Whereas being away from home, school, organized activities, e.g. sports, and one's friends can limit typical opportunities for adolescent growth, there are many aspects of going through cancer treatment that actually promote a positive development, especially when medical care providers take the time to engage AYAs in active discussions about their care.

Cancer centers often provide educational, social and recreational programs and spaces tailored for AYAs that promote peer interaction and support. Most children's cancer centers provide academic support and are opportunities for vocational and career guidance [78]. Designated spaces in the clinic and hospital reserved for teens and young adults are enjoyable and afford a measure of autonomy. Summer camps, adventure trips and retreats sponsored by national cancer support organizations (e.g. Sunshine Kids, Planet Cancer, First Descents) and the treatment centers themselves can provide excellent settings in which to build friendship networks [79]. In these venues, teens and young adults casually discuss commonalities in their cancer experience, but also affirm appreciation for one another's individuality and personality, experiences that foster positive psychosocial development.

Medical Compliance Issues

Adolescence can be an exhilarating time – teens have tremendous energy and creativity. As they are developing their sense of judgment regarding safety in the environment, they engage in both positive and risky behaviors. Adolescents are naturally inclined towards greater impulsivity than adults, because their brains are still maturing, including the areas of the frontal lobe responsible for attention and control. The brain does not reach its full development until the young adult years [80]. Teens sometimes rebel against rules or medical advice in an effort to establish a sense of independence. Other reasons for medical noncompliance include a lack of appreciation for the benefits of treatment, forgetfulness and discomfort with side effects such as malaise or changes in physical appearance. And for some AYAs, finances may present a limiting factor. Therefore, it is not surprising that medication noncompliance rates among adolescents have been estimated to range from 27 to 60%, with openness of family relationships and support predicting adherence [81]. Noncompliance with medications during cancer treatment presents a significant problem, because it may not only have deleterious consequences for a person's physical well-being and survival but can even negatively skew the results of clinical trials. Windebank and Spinetta [82] provide a thoughtful review of our contemporary knowledge of compliance in adolescents with cancer and propose moving from a 'compliance' model to a 'concordance' model. Importantly, they recommend an increase in doctor/patient/family discussions that are characterized by openness, honesty and thoroughness with a focus on building positive relationships and trust. More research is merited to study the subject of adolescent compliance with cancer treatment, especially in the area of stem cell therapy, as rigorous treatment and follow-up regimens are required to help ensure engraftment and survivor health.

Promoting Positive Coping

AYAs typically feel invincible. Developmentally, this sense of strength and safety gives them the confidence to try new endeavors and to aspire to reach their goals. The

Acta Haematol 2014;132:313–325
DOI: 10.1159/000360211

Tewari/Franklin/Tarek/Askins/Mofield/
Kebriaei

sudden diagnosis of cancer, a life-threatening illness, creates cognitive dissonance, requiring the young person to assimilate this new information and to begin actively coping with cancer and cancer treatment. Zebrack and Isaacson [83] have identified 5 domains of stress and coping for AYAs undergoing cancer treatment that include informational, practical, emotional, interpersonal and existential issues. The authors note that coping occurs throughout the continuum of care, beginning at diagnosis, progressing through treatment and ultimately continuing through transitions to survivorship or end of life. These domains provide a useful framework from which health care providers can work to promote positive coping among teens and young adults with cancer. For example, with regard to informational issues, health care providers are encouraged to ask AYAs directly (and regularly) about how much information they want and to whom it should be communicated. This strategy conveys respect for the young person's autonomy and proactively involves him or her in decision-making. Technology-based information and supports are also effective in conveying information to AYAs. Modeling problem-solving, e.g. sharing examples of what other AYAs have done in similar situations, and providing positive reinforcement for coping efforts constitute other important ways how positive coping can be fostered. Overall, AYAs manage the challenges of cancer treatment and stem cell therapy well; however, they benefit greatly from age-appropriate information and support services in the health care setting [84].

Society's Role

For AYA patients proceeding to HSCT, their primary focus and concern is inevitably their own health and survival. While many have undoubtedly been exposed to some 'real-life' or practical issues, it is rare that they would have the depth of experience at the level required to manage the expense of their health care along with all the psychosocial constraints they endure. These patients are often asked to mirror the expectations and requirements of their peers, and to do so in an acute life or death circumstance.

As these patients try to make these adjustments before proceeding to HSCT and during their treatment, the corresponding challenge for survivors comes with their adjustment back into society. Many of society's 'normal' structures, which prepare and educate AYAs on responsibility and independence, have been absent for a signifi-

Table 3. Multidisciplinary approach to AYA HSCT patients

Pretransplantation workup	HSCT physicians Fertility/reproductive specialists
Medical care and decision-making	HSCT physicians Nurses Mid-level providers
Social support	Parents Spouse Caregivers AYA life specialists
Behavioral health care	Psychologists Social workers Teachers/educators AYA life specialists Chaplains Art/music therapists
Rehabilitation	Physical therapists Occupational therapists
Transition after HSCT	Teachers/educators Career/life counselors Financial counselors
Long-term care	Late-effects/survivorship clinics Fertility specialist

The approach to care for AYA patients undergoing HSCT should involve multidisciplinary teams with the patient central to this care.

cant period of time. As a reference while AYA patients are making tough treatment decisions and striving to survive, most commonly peers face the stress of choosing a college or first job.

Often during their course of treatment patients are counseled to develop goals for the time after transplantation, and naturally many of these for older AYA patients revolve around higher education and jobs. The challenges that these present, however, are many as there are formal processes (cost, school/job applications, financial aid, etc.) creating variables out of the patient's control.

While there has to be an understanding from the patients and their families that they have responsibility for their lives, perhaps some support from society is appropriate. Cancer and HSCT introduce significant psychological and financial stresses that few peers experience. Support from society can include assistance in helping pay medical bills, educational support, career training programs targeted for these survivors, and certainly the financial ability for survivors to have continued medical

Acta Haematol 2014;132:313–325
DOI: 10.1159/000360211

care and follow-up including appropriate psychosocial support [79, 83].

Psychology and social work represent key behavioral health services standard to most HSCT centers. These professionals not only provide emotional and problem-solving support, but ideally advocate for AYA HSCT patients as well. An even more robust and appropriate approach should involve school teachers, life counselors, financial counselors and career specialists. Table 3 summarizes a comprehensive approach to care for AYA patients undergoing HSCT. Incorporating a language of survival and life planning as the patient progresses through transplantation is important to establish, and medical staff should be prepared to provide these cues for the patient support for planning posttransplantation life.

References

1 Kiehl MG, Kraut L, Schwerdtfeger R, Hertenstein B, Remberger M, Kroeger N, Stelljes M, Bornhaeuser M, Martin H, Scheid C, Ganser A, Zander AR, Kienast J, Ehninger G, Hoelzer D, Diehl V, Fauser AA, Ringden O: Outcome of allogeneic hematopoietic stem-cell transplantation in adult patients with acute lymphoblastic leukemia: no difference in related compared with unrelated transplant in first complete remission. J Clin Oncol 2004;22:2816–2825.

2 Nishiwaki S, Inamoto Y, Sakamaki H, Kurokawa M, Iida H, Ogawa H, Fukuda T, Ozawa Y, Kobayashi N, Kasai M, Mori T, Iwato K, Yoshida T, Onizuka M, Kawa K, Morishima Y, Suzuki R, Atsuta Y, Miyamura K: Allogeneic stem cell transplantation for adult Philadelphia chromosome-negative acute lymphocytic leukemia: comparable survival rates but different risk factors between related and unrelated transplantation in first complete remission. Blood 2010;116:4368–4375.

3 Laughlin MJ, Eapen M, Rubinstein P, Wagner JE, Zhang MJ, Champlin RE, Stevens C, Barker JN, Gale RP, Lazarus HM, Marks DI, van Rood JJ, Scaradavou A, Horowitz MM: Outcomes after transplantation of cord blood or bone marrow from unrelated donors in adults with leukemia. N Engl J Med 2004;351:2265–2275.

4 Rocha V, Labopin M, Sanz G, Arcese W, Schwerdtfeger R, Bosi A, Jacobsen N, Ruutu T, de Lima M, Finke J, Frassoni F, Gluckman E: Transplants of umbilical-cord blood or bone marrow from unrelated donors in adults with acute leukemia. N Engl J Med 2004;351:2276–2285.

5 Eapen M, Rocha V, Sanz G, Scaradavou A, Zhang MJ, Arcese W, Sirvent A, Champlin RE, Chao N, Gee AP, Isola L, Laughlin MJ, Marks DI, Nabhan S, Ruggeri A, Soiffer R, Horowitz MM, Gluckman E, Wagner JE: Effect of graft source on unrelated donor haemopoietic stem-cell transplantation in adults with acute leukaemia: a retrospective analysis. Lancet Oncol 2010;11:653–660.

6 Bacigalupo A, Ballen K, Rizzo D, Giralt S, Lazarus H, Ho V, Apperley J, Slavin S, Pasquini M, Sandmaier BM, Barrett J, Blaise D, Lowski R, Horowitz M: Defining the intensity of conditioning regimens: working definitions. Biol Blood Marrow Transplant 2009;15:1628–1633.

7 Giralt S: Reduced-intensity conditioning regimens for hematologic malignancies: what have we learned over the last 10 years? Hematol Am Soc Hematol Educ Program 2005, pp 384–389.

8 Martino R, Giralt S, Caballero MD, Mackinnon S, Corradini P, Fernandez-Aviles F, San Miguel J, Sierra J: Allogeneic hematopoietic stem cell transplantation with reduced-intensity conditioning in acute lymphoblastic leukemia: a feasibility study. Haematologica 2003;88:555–560.

9 Hamaki T, Kami M, Kanda Y, Yuji K, Inamoto Y, Kishi Y, Nakai K, Nakayama I, Murashige N, Abe Y, Ueda Y, Hino M, Inoue T, Ago H, Hidaka M, Hayashi T, Yamane T, Uoshima N, Miyakoshi S, Taniguchi S: Reduced-intensity stem-cell transplantation for adult acute lymphoblastic leukemia: a retrospective study of 33 patients. Bone Marrow Transplant 2005;35:549–556.

10 Mohty M, Labopin M, Tabrizzi R, Theorin N, Fauser AA, Rambaldi A, Maertens J, Slavin S, Majolino I, Nagler A, Blaise D, Rocha V: Reduced intensity conditioning allogeneic stem cell transplantation for adult patients with acute lymphoblastic leukemia: a retrospective study from the European Group for Blood and Marrow Transplantation. Haematologica 2008;93:303–306.

11 Stein AS, Palmer JM, O'Donnell MR, Kogut NM, Spielberger RT, Slovak ML, Tsai NC, Senitzer D, Snyder DS, Thomas SH, Forman SJ: Reduced-intensity conditioning followed by peripheral blood stem cell transplantation for adult patients with high-risk acute lymphoblastic leukemia. Biol Blood Marrow Transplant 2009;15:1407–1414.

12 Pulsipher MA, Boucher KM, Wall D, Frangoul H, Duval M, Goyal RK, Shaw PJ, Haight AE, Grimley M, Grupp SA, Kletzel M, Kadota R: Reduced-intensity allogeneic transplantation in pediatric patients ineligible for myeloablative therapy: results of the Pediatric Blood and Marrow Transplant Consortium Study ONC0313. Blood 2009;114:1429–1436.

13 Verneris MR, Eapen M, Duerst R, Carpenter PA, Burke MJ, Afanasyev BV, Cowan MJ, He W, Krance R, Li CK, Tan PL, Wagner JE, Davies SM: Reduced-intensity conditioning regimens for allogeneic transplantation in children with acute lymphoblastic leukemia. Biol Blood Marrow Transplant 2010;16:1237–1244.

14 Forman SJ, Rowe JM: The myth of the second remission of acute leukemia in the adult. Blood 2013;121:1077–1082.

15 Fielding AK, Richards SM, Chopra R, Lazarus HM, Litzow MR, Buck G, Durrant IJ, Luger SM, Marks DI, Franklin IM, McMillan AK, Tallman MS, Rowe JM, Goldstone AH: Outcome of 609 adults after relapse of acute lymphoblastic leukemia (ALL): an MRC UKALL12/ECOG 2993 study. Blood 2007;109:944–950.

16 Kebriaei P, Poon LM: The role of allogeneic hematopoietic stem cell transplantation in the therapy of patients with acute lymphoblastic leukemia. Curr Hematol Malig Rep 2012;7:144–152.

17 Marks DI, Wang T, Perez WS, Antin JH, Copelan E, Gale RP, George B, Gupta V, Halter J, Khoury HJ, Klumpp TR, Lazarus HM, Lewis VA, McCarthy P, Rizzieri DA, Sabloff M, Szer J, Tallman MS, Weisdorf DJ: The outcome of full-intensity and reduced-intensity conditioning matched sibling or unrelated donor transplantation in adults with Philadelphia chromosome-negative acute lymphoblastic leukemia in first and second complete remission. Blood 2010;116:366–374.

18 Ram R, Storb R, Sandmaier BM, Maloney DG, Woolfrey A, Flowers ME, Maris MB, Laport GG, Chauncey TR, Lange T, Langston AA, Storer B, Georges GE: Non-myeloablative conditioning with allogeneic hematopoietic cell transplantation for the treatment of high-risk acute lymphoblastic leukemia. Haematologica 2011;96:1113–1120.

19 Bushhouse S, Ramsay NK, Pescovitz OH, Kim T, Robison LL: Growth in children following irradiation for bone marrow transplantation. Am J Pediatr Hematol Oncol 1989;11:134–140.

20 Sanders JE: The impact of marrow transplant preparative regimens on subsequent growth and development. The Seattle Marrow Transplant Team. Semin Hematol 1991;28:244–249.

Acta Haematol 2014;132:313–325
DOI: 10.1159/000360211

21 Chow EJ, Simmons JH, Roth CL, Baker KS, Hoffmeister PA, Sanders JE, Friedman DL: Increased cardiometabolic traits in pediatric survivors of acute lymphoblastic leukemia treated with total body irradiation. Biol Blood Marrow Transplant 2010;16:1674–1681.

22 Baker KS, Ness KK, Steinberger J, Carter A, Francisco L, Burns LJ, Sklar C, Forman S, Weisdorf D, Gurney JG, Bhatia S: Diabetes, hypertension, and cardiovascular events in survivors of hematopoietic cell transplantation: a report from the Bone Marrow Transplantation Survivor Study. Blood 2007;109:1765–1772.

23 Davies SM, Ramsay NK, Klein JP, Weisdorf DJ, Bolwell B, Cahn JY, Camitta BM, Gale RP, Giralt S, Heilmann C, Henslee-Downey PJ, Herzig RH, Hutchinson R, Keating A, Lazarus HM, Milone GA, Neudorf S, Perez WS, Powles RL, Prentice HG, Schiller G, Socie G, Vowels M, Wiley J, Yeager A, Horowitz MM: Comparison of preparative regimens in transplants for children with acute lymphoblastic leukemia. J Clin Oncol 2000;18:340–347.

24 Tang W, Wang L, Zhao WL, Chen YB, Shen ZX, Hu J: Intravenous busulfan-cyclophosphamide as a preparative regimen before allogeneic hematopoietic stem cell transplantation for adult patients with acute lymphoblastic leukemia. Biol Blood Marrow Transplant 2011;17:1555–1561.

25 Russell JA, Savoie ML, Balogh A, Turner AR, Larratt L, Chaudhry MA, Storek J, Bahlis NJ, Brown CB, Quinlan D, Geddes M, Stewart DA: Allogeneic transplantation for adult acute leukemia in first and second remission with a novel regimen incorporating daily intravenous busulfan, fludarabine, 400 cGy total-body irradiation, and thymoglobulin. Biol Blood Marrow Transplant 2007;13:814–821.

26 Santarone S, Pidala J, Di Nicola M, Field T, Alsina M, Ayala E, Janssen W, Kharfan-Dabaja MA, Ochoa L, Perez L, Perkins J, Raychaudhuri J, Fernandez H, Anasetti C: Fludarabine and pharmacokinetic-targeted busulfan before allografting for adults with acute lymphoid leukemia. Biol Blood Marrow Transplant 2011;17:1505–1511.

27 Kebriaei P, Basset R, Ledesma C, Ciurea S, Parmar S, Shpall EJ, Hosing C, Khouri I, Qazilbash M, Popat U, Alousi A, Nieto Y, Jones RB, de Lima M, Champlin RE, Andersson BS: Clofarabine combined with busulfan provides excellent disease control in adult patients with acute lymphoblastic leukemia undergoing allogeneic hematopoietic stem cell transplantation. Biol Blood Marrow Transplant 2012;18:1819–1826.

28 Neuss MN, Malin JL, Chan S, Kadlubek PJ, Adams JL, Jacobson JO, Blayney DW, Simone JV: Measuring the improving quality of outpatient care in medical oncology practices in the United States. J Clin Oncol 2013;31:1471–1477.

29 Quinn GP, Vadaparampil ST, Bell-Ellison BA, Gwede CK, Albrecht TL: Patient-physician communication barriers regarding fertility preservation among newly diagnosed cancer patients. Soc Sci Med 2008;66:784–789.

30 Loren AW, Brazauskas R, Chow EJ, Gilleece M, Halter J, Jacobsohn DA, Joshi S, Pidala J, Quinn GP, Wang Z, Apperley JF, Burns LJ, Hale GA, Hayes-Lattin BM, Kamble R, Lazarus H, McCarthy PL, Reddy V, Warwick AB, Bolwell BJ, Duncan C, Socie G, Sorror ML, Wingard JR, Majhail NS: Physician perceptions and practice patterns regarding fertility preservation in hematopoietic cell transplant recipients. Bone Marrow Transplant 2013;48:1091–1097.

31 Loren AW, Mangu PB, Beck LN, Brennan L, Magdalinski AJ, Partridge AH, Quinn G, Wallace WH, Oktay K: Fertility preservation for patients with cancer: American Society of Clinical Oncology clinical practice guideline update. J Clin Oncol 2013;31:2500–2510.

32 Coccia PF, Altman J, Bhatia S, Borinstein SC, Flynn J, George S, Goldsby R, Hayashi R, Huang MS, Johnson RH, Beaupin LK, Link MP, Oeffinger KC, Orr KM, Pappo AS, Reed D, Spraker HL, Thomas DA, von Mehren M, Wechsler DS, Whelan KF, Zebrack BJ, Sundar H, Shead DA: Adolescent and young adult oncology. Clinical practice guidelines in oncology. J Natl Compr Canc Netw 2012;10:1112–1150.

33 Levine J, Canada A, Stern CJ: Fertility preservation in adolescents and young adults with cancer. J Clin Oncol 2010;28:4831–4841.

34 Practice Committees of the American Society for Reproductive Medicine and Society for Assisted Reproductive Technology: Mature oocyte cryopreservation: a guideline. Fertil Steril 2013;99:37–43.

35 Bhatia S, Davies SM, Scott Baker K, Pulsipher MA, Hansen JA: NCI, NHLBI first international consensus conference on late effects after pediatric hematopoietic cell transplantation: etiology and pathogenesis of late effects after HCT performed in childhood – methodologic challenges. Biol Blood Marrow Transplant 2011;17:1428–1435.

36 Tichelli A, Labopin M, Rovo A, Badoglio M, Arat M, van Lint MT, Lawitschka A, Schwarze CP, Passweg J, Socie G: Increase of suicide and accidental death after hematopoietic stem cell transplantation: a cohort study on behalf of the Late Effects Working Party of the European Group for Blood and Marrow Transplantation (EBMT). Cancer 2013;119:2012–2021.

37 Tichelli A, Passweg J, Wojcik D, Rovo A, Harousseau JL, Masszi T, Zander A, Bekassy A, Crawley C, Arat M, Sica S, Lutz P, Socie G: Late cardiovascular events after allogeneic hematopoietic stem cell transplantation: a retrospective multicenter study of the Late Effects Working Party of the European Group for Blood and Marrow Transplantation. Haematologica 2008;93:1203–1210.

38 Cohen A, Rovelli A, Merlo DF, van Lint MT, Lanino E, Bresters D, Ceppi M, Bocchini V, Tichelli A, Socie G: Risk for secondary thyroid carcinoma after hematopoietic stem-cell transplantation: an EBMT Late Effects Working Party Study. J Clin Oncol 2007;25:2449–2454.

39 National Comprehensive Cancer Network. www.nccn.org.

40 Hijiya N, Ness KK, Ribeiro RC, Hudson MM: Acute leukemia as a secondary malignancy in children and adolescents: current findings and issues. Cancer 2009;115:23–35.

41 Smith MA, Rubinstein L, Ungerleider RS: Therapy-related acute myeloid leukemia following treatment with epipodophyllotoxins: estimating the risks. Med Pediatr Oncol 1994;23:86–98.

42 Pui CH, Ribeiro RC, Hancock ML, Rivera GK, Evans WE, Raimondi SC, Head DR, Behm FG, Mahmoud MH, Sandlund JT, Crist WM: Acute myeloid leukemia in children treated with epipodophyllotoxins for acute lymphoblastic leukemia. N Engl J Med 1991;325:1682–1687.

43 Oeffinger KC, Hudson MM: Long-term complications following childhood and adolescent cancer: foundations for providing risk-based health care for survivors. CA Cancer J Clin 2004;54:208–236.

44 Dvorak CC, Gracia CR, Sanders JE, Cheng EY, Baker KS, Pulsipher MA, Petryk A: NCI, NHLBI/PBMTC first international conference on late effects after pediatric hematopoietic cell transplantation: endocrine challenges-thyroid dysfunction, growth impairment, bone health, and reproductive risks. Biol Blood Marrow Transplant 2011;17:1725–1738.

45 Sanchez-Ortega I, Canals C, Peralta T, Parody R, Clapes V, de Sevilla AF, Duarte RF: Thyroid dysfunction in adult patients late after autologous and allogeneic blood and marrow transplantation. Bone Marrow Transplant 2012;47:296–298.

46 Ishiguro H, Yasuda Y, Tomita Y, Shinagawa T, Shimizu T, Morimoto T, Hattori K, Matsumoto M, Inoue H, Yabe H, Yabe M, Shinohara O, Kato S: Long-term follow-up of thyroid function in patients who received bone marrow transplantation during childhood and adolescence. J Clin Endocrinol Metab 2004;89:5981–5986.

47 Bakker B, Oostdijk W, Bresters D, Walenkamp MJ, Vossen JM, Wit JM: Disturbances of growth and endocrine function after busulphan-based conditioning for haematopoietic stem cell transplantation during infancy and childhood. Bone Marrow Transplant 2004;33:1049–1056.

48 Ghavamzadeh A, Larijani B, Jahani M, Khoshniat M, Bahar B, Tabatabaei O: Thyroid, parathyroid, gonadal, and pancreatic beta-cell function after bone marrow transplantation with chemotherapy-only conditioning. Transplant Proc 2003;35:3101–3104.

49 Shalet SM: Effects of cancer chemotherapy on gonadal function of patients. Cancer Treat Rev 1980;7:141–152.

50 Barton C, Waxman J: Effects of chemotherapy on fertility. Blood Rev 1990;4:187–195.

51 Shalet SM: Gonadal function following radiation and cytotoxic chemotherapy in childhood. Ergeb Inn Med Kinderheilkd 1989;58:1–21.

52 Sanders JE, Hoffmeister PA, Woolfrey AE, Carpenter PA, Storer BE, Storb RF, Appelbaum FR: Thyroid function following hematopoietic cell transplantation in children: 30 years' experience. Blood 2009;113:306–308.

53 Slatter MA, Gennery AR, Cheetham TD, Bhattacharya A, Crooks BN, Flood TJ, Cant AJ, Abinun M: Thyroid dysfunction after bone marrow transplantation for primary immunodeficiency without the use of total body irradiation in conditioning. Bone Marrow Transplant 2004;33:949–953.

54 Leung W, Ahn H, Rose SR, Phipps S, Smith T, Gan K, O'Connor M, Hale GA, Kasow KA, Barfield RC, Madden RM, Pui CH: A prospective cohort study of late sequelae of pediatric allogeneic hematopoietic stem cell transplantation. Medicine (Baltimore) 2007;86:215–224.

55 McDonald L, Luke J, Jude V, Chan K, Cuellar N: Development of an evidence-based clinical guideline for age-appropriate screening, prevention, and management of bone abnormalities in children post-hematopoietic stem cell transplant. J Pediatr Oncol Nurs 2013;30:78–89.

56 Bernard F, Bordigoni P, Simeoni MC, Barlogis V, Contet A, Loundou A, Thuret I, Leheup B, Chambost H, Play B, Auquier P, Michel G: Height growth during adolescence and final height after haematopoietic SCT for childhood acute leukaemia: the impact of a conditioning regimen with BU or TBI. Bone Marrow Transplant 2009;43:637–642.

57 Sanders JE: Growth and development after hematopoietic cell transplant in children. Bone Marrow Transplant 2008;41:223–227.

58 McClune BL, Polgreen LE, Burmeister LA, Blaes AH, Mulrooney DA, Burns LJ, Majhail NS: Screening, prevention and management of osteoporosis and bone loss in adult and pediatric hematopoietic cell transplant recipients. Bone Marrow Transplant 2011;46:1–9.

59 Kulak CA, Borba VZ, Kulak Junior J, Campos DJ, Shane E: Post-transplantation osteoporosis. Arq Bras Endocrinol Metabol 2010;54:143–149.

60 Ruble K, Hayat MJ, Stewart KJ, Chen AR: Bone mineral density after bone marrow transplantation in childhood: measurement and associations. Biol Blood Marrow Transplant 2010;16:1451–1457.

61 Stein E, Ebeling P, Shane E: Post-transplantation osteoporosis. Endocrinol Metab Clin North Am 2007;36:937–963, viii.

62 Kaste SC, Shidler TJ, Tong X, Srivastava DK, Rochester R, Hudson MM, Shearer PD, Hale GA: Bone mineral density and osteonecrosis in survivors of childhood allogeneic bone marrow transplantation. Bone Marrow Transplant 2004;33:435–441.

63 Serio B, Pezzullo L, Fontana R, Annunziata S, Rosamilio R, Sessa M, Giudice V, Ferrara I, Rocco M, De Rosa G, Ricci P, Tauchmanova L, Montuori N, Selleri C: Accelerated bone mass senescence after hematopoietic stem cell transplantation. Transl Med UniSa 2013;5:7–13.

64 Carpenter PA, Hoffmeister P, Chesnut CH 3rd, Storer B, Charuhas PM, Woolfrey AE, Sanders JE: Bisphosphonate therapy for reduced bone mineral density in children with chronic graft-versus-host disease. Biol Blood Marrow Transplant 2007;13:683–690.

65 Armenian SH, Sun CL, Kawashima T, Arora M, Leisenring W, Sklar CA, Baker KS, Francisco L, Teh JB, Mills G, Wong FL, Rosenthal J, Diller LR, Hudson MM, Oeffinger KC, Forman SJ, Robison LL, Bhatia S: Long-term health-related outcomes in survivors of childhood cancer treated with HSCT versus conventional therapy: a report from the Bone Marrow Transplant Survivor Study (BMTSS) and Childhood Cancer Survivor Study (CCSS). Blood 2011;118:1413–1420.

66 Shikari H, Antin JH, Dana R: Ocular graft-versus-host disease: a review. Surv Ophthalmol 2013;58:233–251.

67 Bacigalupo A, Chien J, Barisione G, Pavletic S: Late pulmonary complications after allogeneic hematopoietic stem cell transplantation: diagnosis, monitoring, prevention, and treatment. Semin Hematol 2012;49:15–24.

68 Arai S, Jagasia M, Storer B, Chai X, Pidala J, Cutler C, Arora M, Weisdorf DJ, Flowers ME, Martin PJ, Palmer J, Jacobsohn D, Pavletic SZ, Vogelsang GB, Lee SJ: Global and organ-specific chronic graft-versus-host disease severity according to the 2005 NIH Consensus Criteria. Blood 2011;118:4242–4249.

69 Sullivan KM, Agura E, Anasetti C, Appelbaum F, Badger C, Bearman S, Erickson K, Flowers M, Hansen J, Loughran T, Martin P, Matthews D, Petersdorf E, Radich J, Riddell S, Rovira D, Sanders J, Schuenig F, Siadak M, Storb R, Witherspoon RP: Chronic graft-versus-host disease and other late complications of bone marrow transplantation. Semin Hematol 1991;28:250–259.

70 Vogelsang GB: How I treat chronic graft-versus-host disease. Blood 2001;97:1196–1201.

71 Savani BN, Stratton P, Shenoy A, Kozanas E, Goodman S, Barrett AJ: Increased risk of cervical dysplasia in long-term survivors of allogeneic stem cell transplantation – implications for screening and HPV vaccination. Biol Blood Marrow Transplant 2008;14:1072–1075.

72 Wang Y, Brinch L, Jebsen P, Tanbo T, Kirschner R: A clinical study of cervical dysplasia in long-term survivors of allogeneic stem cell transplantation. Biol Blood Marrow Transplant 2012;18:747–753.

73 Su HI: Measuring ovarian function in young cancer survivors. Minerva Endocrinol 2010;35:259–270.

74 Loren AW, Chow E, Jacobsohn DA, Gilleece M, Halter J, Joshi S, Wang Z, Sobocinski KA, Gupta V, Hale GA, Marks DI, Stadtmauer EA, Apperley J, Cahn JY, Schouten HC, Lazarus HM, Savani BN, McCarthy PL, Jakubowski AA, Kamani NR, Hayes-Lattin B, Maziarz RT, Warwick AB, Sorror ML, Bolwell BJ, Socie G, Wingard JR, Rizzo JD, Majhail NS: Pregnancy after hematopoietic cell transplantation: a report from the late effects working committee of the Center for International Blood and Marrow Transplant Research (CIBMTR). Biol Blood Marrow Transplant 2011;17:157–166.

75 Haase JE, Phillips CR: The adolescent/young adult experience. J Pediatr Oncol Nurs 2004;21:145–149.

76 Cooke L, Chung C, Grant M: Psychosocial care for adolescent and young adult hematopoietic cell transplant patients. J Psychosoc Oncol 2011;29:394–414.

77 Barrera M, Atenafu E, Pinto J: Behavioral, social, and educational outcomes after pediatric stem cell transplantation and related factors. Cancer 2009;115:880–889.

78 Butler RW, Sahler OJ, Askins MA, Alderfer MA, Katz ER, Phipps S, Noll RB: Interventions to improve neuropsychological functioning in childhood cancer survivors. Dev Disabil Res Rev 2008;14:251–258.

79 D'Agostino NM, Penney A, Zebrack B: Providing developmentally appropriate psychosocial care to adolescent and young adult cancer survivors. Cancer 2011;117(suppl):2329–2334.

80 Sowell ER, Thompson PM, Holmes CJ, Jernigan TL, Toga AW: In vivo evidence for post-adolescent brain maturation in frontal and striatal regions. Nat Neurosci 1999;2:859–861.

81 Butow P, Palmer S, Pai A, Goodenough B, Luckett T, King M: Review of adherence-related issues in adolescents and young adults with cancer. J Clin Oncol 2010;28:4800–4809.

82 Windebank KP, Spinetta JJ: Do as I say or die: compliance in adolescents with cancer. Pediatr Blood Cancer 2008;50(suppl):1099–1100.

83 Zebrack B, Isaacson S: Psychosocial care of adolescent and young adult patients with cancer and survivors. J Clin Oncol 2012;30:1221–1226.

84 Zebrack B, Mathews-Bradshaw B, Siegel S: Quality cancer care for adolescents and young adults: a position statement. J Clin Oncol 2010;28:4862–4867.

85 Curtis RE, Rowlings PA, Deeg HJ, Shriner DA, Socie G, Travis LB, Horowitz MM, Witherspoon RP, Hoover RN, Sobocinski KA, Fraumeni JF Jr, Boice JD Jr: Solid cancers after bone marrow transplantation. N Engl J Med 1997;336:897–904.

86 Straathof KC, Savoldo B, Heslop HE, Rooney CM: Immunotherapy for post-transplant lymphoproliferative disease. Br J Haematol 2002;118:728–740.

Acta Haematol 2014;132:313–325
DOI: 10.1159/000360211

87 Metayer C, Curtis RE, Vose J, Sobocinski KA, Horowitz MM, Bhatia S, Fay JW, Freytes CO, Goldstein SC, Herzig RH, Keating A, Miller CB, Nevill TJ, Pecora AL, Rizzo JD, Williams SF, Li CY, Travis LB, Weisdorf DJ: Myelodysplastic syndrome and acute myeloid leukemia after autotransplantation for lymphoma: a multicenter case-control study. Blood 2003; 101:2015–2023.

88 Hertenstein B, Hambach L, Bacigalupo A, Schmitz N, McCann S, Slavin S, Gratwohl A, Ferrant A, Elmaagacli A, Schwertfeger R, Locasciulli A, Zander A, Bornhauser M, Niederwieser D, Ruutu T: Development of leukemia in donor cells after allogeneic stem cell transplantation – a survey of the European Group for Blood and Marrow Transplantation (EBMT). Haematologica 2005;90:969–975.

89 Leisenring W, Friedman DL, Flowers ME, Schwartz JL, Deeg HJ: Nonmelanoma skin and mucosal cancers after hematopoietic cell transplantation. J Clin Oncol 2006;24:1119–1126.

90 Gallagher G, Forrest DL: Second solid cancers after allogeneic hematopoietic stem cell transplantation. Cancer 2007;109:84–92.

91 Friedman DL, Rovo A, Leisenring W, Locasciulli A, Flowers ME, Tichelli A, Sanders JE, Deeg HJ, Socie G: Increased risk of breast cancer among survivors of allogeneic hematopoietic cell transplantation: a report from the FHCRC and the EBMT-Late Effect Working Party. Blood 2008;111:939–944.

92 Rizzo JD, Curtis RE, Socie G, Sobocinski KA, Gilbert E, Landgren O, Travis LB, Travis WD, Flowers ME, Friedman DL, Horowitz MM, Wingard JR, Deeg HJ: Solid cancers after allogeneic hematopoietic cell transplantation. Blood 2009;113:1175–1183.

93 Landgren O, Gilbert ES, Rizzo JD, Socie G, Banks PM, Sobocinski KA, Horowitz MM, Jaffe ES, Kingma DW, Travis LB, Flowers ME, Martin PJ, Deeg HJ, Curtis RE: Risk factors for lymphoproliferative disorders after allogeneic hematopoietic cell transplantation. Blood 2009;113:4992–5001.

94 Tarella C, Passera R, Magni M, Benedetti F, Rossi A, Gueli A, Patti C, Parvis G, Ciceri F, Gallamini A, Cortelazzo S, Zoli V, Corradini P, Carobbio A, Mule A, Bosa M, Barbui A, Di Nicola M, Sorio M, Caracciolo D, Gianni AM, Rambaldi A: Risk factors for the development of secondary malignancy after high-dose chemotherapy and autograft, with or without rituximab: a 20-year retrospective follow-up study in patients with lymphoma. J Clin Oncol 2011;29:814–824.

95 Majhail NS, Brazauskas R, Rizzo JD, Sobecks RM, Wang Z, Horowitz MM, Bolwell B, Wingard JR, Socie G: Secondary solid cancers after allogeneic hematopoietic cell transplantation using busulfan-cyclophosphamide conditioning. Blood 2011;117:316–322.

96 Curtis RE, Metayer C, Rizzo JD, Socie G, Sobocinski KA, Flowers ME, Travis WD, Travis LB, Horowitz MM, Deeg HJ: Impact of chronic GVHD therapy on the development of squamous-cell cancers after hematopoietic stem-cell transplantation: an international case-control study. Blood 2005;105:3802–3811.

97 Rizzo JD, Wingard JR, Tichelli A, Lee SJ, Van Lint MT, Burns LJ, Davies SM, Ferrara JL, Socie G: Recommended screening and preventive practices for long-term survivors after hematopoietic cell transplantation: joint recommendations of the European Group for Blood and Marrow Transplantation, the Center for International Blood and Marrow Transplant Research, and the American Society of Blood and Marrow Transplantation. Biol Blood Marrow Transplant 2006;12:138–151.

98 Majhail NS, Rizzo JD, Lee SJ, Aljurf M, Atsuta Y, Bonfim C, Burns LJ, Chaudhri N, Davies S, Okamoto S, Seber A, Socie G, Szer J, Van Lint MT, Wingard JR, Tichelli A: Recommended screening and preventive practices for long-term survivors after hematopoietic cell transplantation. Biol Blood Marrow Transplant 2012;18:348–371.

Acta Haematol 2014;132:326–330
DOI: 10.1159/000360237

Published online: September 10, 2014

Challenging Aspects of Managing Hemostasis in Adolescents

Ulrike Nowak-Göttl[a, b]   Gili Kenet[c, d]

Department of Coagulation and Haemostasis, Institute of Clinical Chemistry, University Hospital Schleswig-Holstein at [a]Campus Kiel, Kiel, and [b]Campus Lübeck, Lübeck, Germany; [c]Thrombosis Unit and Israel National Hemophilia Center, Sheba Medical Center, Tel Hashomer, [d]Sackler School of Medicine, Tel Aviv University, Tel Aviv, Israel

Key Words

Adolescents · Menorrhagia · Thrombophilia · Venous thromboembolism · Von Willebrand disease

Abstract

The prevalence of symptomatic childhood venous thromboembolism increases among adolescents. The occurrence of nonhereditary prothrombotic risk factors, e.g. oral contraceptive pills, often prescribed to adolescent females for various indications, such as tobacco use, obesity and hypertension may trigger symptomatic thrombosis, especially in carriers of genetic thrombophilia traits. On the other hand, heavy menstrual bleeding is a common clinical problem of young adolescent women. A proper diagnostic workup of these women may enable physicians to detect and treat congenital bleeding disorders, e.g. von Willebrand disease, presenting with menorrhagia. The challenges of diagnosis and treatment of either thrombosis or bleeding disorders in young adults will be discussed in this review.

© 2014 S. Karger AG, Basel

Venous Thromboembolism in Adolescents and Young Adults: Unique Epidemiological Concerns

Over the last decades venous thromboembolism (VTE) has been increasingly recognized as an important clinical entity in children and young adults [1, 2].

Within the entire childhood population, neonates are at the greatest risk for VTE (5.1/100,000 live births per year in Caucasian children) [1–3], with a second peak in incidence during puberty and adolescence (fig. 1). The annual incidence of venous events was estimated to be 0.07–0.14/10,000 children, or 5.3/10,000 hospital admissions of children younger than 18 years.

Thrombosis mostly occurs as a secondary complication of primary underlying diseases such as sepsis, cancer, congenital heart disease or after therapeutic interventions such as central venous lines [4, 5].

VTE is a severe disease, associated with mortality and significant morbidity including lack of thrombus resolution in 50% of cases, risk for recurrence, loss of venous access and development of postthrombotic syndrome [6, 7].

Some unique risk factors may be associated with the increased prothrombotic risk among adolescents. A re-

Prof. Gili Kenet
Thrombosis Unit, National Hemophilia Center
Sheba Medical Center
Tel Hashomer 52621 (Israel)
E-Mail gili.kenet@sheba.health.gov.il

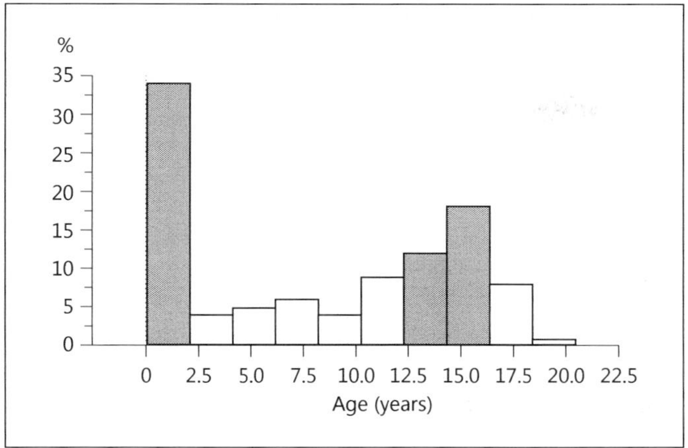

Fig. 1. Age distribution of symptomatic VTE onset in children.

cent study that analyzed population-based data of 7,084 community schoolchildren and adolescents showed that school level peer smoking was positively related to adolescent smoking, irrespective of socioeconomic status and background variables of responders [8]. Furthermore, in another study of 5,141 adolescents, an association was demonstrated between adolescence substance abuse and obesity (body mass index above 30) in young adulthood [9]. Growing concern about elevated blood pressure associated with obesity in young adults should be aimed at prevention of adult cardiovascular disease by healthy lifestyle counseling at early ages, as well as avoidance of other preventable risk factors (e.g. smoking, hormonal therapy) that may lead to thrombosis.

As VTE may be associated with hormonal contraception use, special awareness should be referred to this issue. In adults, an increased VTE rate among contraception users is associated with age above 35 years, tobacco use and high-dose estrogen [10, 11]. Thrombosis risk is associated with high estrogen content, causing increased resistance to activated protein C and promoting coagulation activation while decreasing inhibition of the coagulation cascade [12]. As oral contraceptive pills are often prescribed to adolescent females, either for contraception or to treat heavy menstrual bleeding, dysmenorrhea or acne, the risk for VTE, especially among obese, smoking, young females, should be considered. In a small population of adolescents presenting to a children's hospital with contraception-related VTE, the majority of patients had multiple risk factors, among which obesity prevailed [13]. According to Centers for Disease Control reports in the USA, about 60% of sexually active adolescents aged

15–19 years used some type of hormonal contraception [14]. On the other hand, two thirds of adolescents presenting to emergency rooms reported high-risk behaviors, including early onset of nonprotected sexual intercourse that may lead to teen pregnancy [15], increasing, among other risks, the rate of potential thrombotic complications.

Role of Inherited Thrombophilias in Adolescent VTE

In 3 recent systematic reviews and meta-analyses of observational studies including observational studies in pediatric patients aged 0–18 years with deep VTE and cerebrovascular occlusion (cerebral venous thrombosis and stroke), more than 70% of patients had at least 1 clinical risk factor [16–18]. The pooled odds ratios (ORs) showed statistically significant associations between factor V G1691A, factor II G20210A, protein C, protein S or antithrombin deficiency, elevated lipoprotein (a), combined thrombophilic risk factors and the presence of lupus anticoagulants/antiphospholipid antibodies and VTE onset. For second VTE events, statistically significant associations with recurrence were found for protein S or antithrombin deficiency, the factor II variant and combined thrombophilia [16]. The pooled OR for VTE onset ranged from 2.4 for the factor II G20210A mutation (cerebrovascular occlusion) to 9.4 in children with antithrombin deficiency (VTE). The factor II G20210A mutation (OR: 2.1), protein C (OR: 2.4), S (OR: 3.1) and antithrombin deficiency (OR: 3.0) played a significant role in the recurrence of VTE.

As recurrence rates of up to 21% for idiopathic VTE have been reported [6, 7], it is important to screen all adolescent index cases for thrombophilia in order to provide individually tailored prophylactic regimens for future high-risk situations.

Treatment Modalities

In adolescents, included and reported among pediatric VTE patients, randomized therapeutic trials are missing, and treatment guidelines are mainly adapted from adult protocols [19, 20]. Until results from randomized trials are available for anticoagulant treatment and duration of symptomatic index patients, children with clinically and imaging-proven VTE are treated according to recommendations based on small-scale studies.

Notably, whereas in children the consideration of an increased bleeding risk (due to intense physical activity) may dictate the need for individualized therapy protocols, among adolescents and young adults therapy compliance may become a significant issue, affecting the risk of recurrence or postthrombotic complications.

Unfractionated heparin, low-molecular-weight heparins and vitamin K antagonists are commonly used as antithrombotic drugs, whereas newly developed antithrombotic agents such as argatroban, bivalirudin, fondaparinux or new oral anticoagulants are under discussion, the latter still within phase 1–2 clinical trials for patients younger than 18 years [19–22]. Keeping in mind the low level of evidence for treatment-related recommendations, along with the presence of unique acquired risk factors in this age group as previously described, it has to be pointed out here that each patient with an early VTE manifestation should receive secondary anticoagulant prophylaxis in future clinical risk situations prone to thromboembolism. Nonetheless, as treatment trials for adolescents are lacking, the doses and durations of secondary anticoagulation should be individually adapted to the patient's risk.

Bleeding in Adolescents and Young Adult Women

Heavy menstrual bleeding is a common clinical problem, and menorrhagia may be the symptom leading to diagnosis of congenital bleeding disorders. As reproductive tract bleeding in women naturally occurs during menstruation or childbirth, congenital bleeding disorders may be first diagnosed at adolescence [23]. Although menstrual problems are not life threatening, they can pose a significant burden on the quality of life of young teenagers and women. In a recent study of health-related quality of life among 184 adolescents, 34% complained of heavy bleeding [24]. Population-based studies estimate that 10–35% of women report heavy menstrual bleeding, and physicians, including hematologists and gynecologists, may often be consulted regarding the etiology and the proper treatment of this symptom [25–27]. Objectively, heavy menstrual bleeding is defined as prolonged (over 7 days) and yields above 80 ml blood loss per menstrual cycle [27]. A detailed history and careful physical examination evaluating any skin signs of easy bruising, petechiae, purpura, dental or mucosal bleeds as well as a detailed family history regarding bleeding complications may lead to the diagnosis of inherited bleeding disorders [25]. As the validity and reproducibility of bleeding classification according to mucocutaneous bleeding questionnaires has not been fully elucidated for children and adolescents [28], efforts should be made to quantify bleeding and further assess laboratory parameters in order to accurately establish the diagnosis.

The prevalence of menorrhagia in women with a bleeding disorder ranges from 32 to 100% in patients with von Willebrand's disease (VWD), from 5 to 98% in patients with thrombocytopenia or platelet dysfunction and from 35 to 70% in women with rare factor deficiencies or rare disorders of fibrinolysis [26, 27, 29]. Women are more likely to present in early adulthood with bleeding disorders, and they are also more likely to be diagnosed with other gynecological manifestations (e.g. corpus luteum bleeding, bleeding of ovarian cysts and last but not least postpartum hemorrhage) due to their underlying hemostatic disorders [26]. The first case of VWD, the commonest bleeding disorder, was described in a 13-year-old adolescent girl by Eric von Willebrand in 1926 [30]. The girl suffered heavy menstrual bleeding and subsequently bled to death. Her maternal grandmother had died of postpartum hemorrhage following her first delivery [30]. Increased awareness among clinicians currently improves the chances of proper diagnosis and therapy for such cases. In a recent US study of gynecologists, 77% considered the diagnosis of VWD among adolescents with heavy menstrual bleeding [31].

Consequently, any adolescent presenting with heavy menses, especially if there is a history of easy bruising and/or mucocutaneous bleeds on other occasions, a family history of bleeding symptoms or a known bleeding disorder, presence of anemia and iron deficiency, should be referred to an expert hematologist for further laboratory diagnosis. Initial laboratory testing should include a complete blood cell count, prothrombin time, partial thromboplastin time, levels of factor VIII (FVIII), von Willebrand factor (VWF) antigen, ristocetin cofactor and platelet function tests. Evaluation of multimers and detailed factor assays for rare bleeding disorders may be performed later, at the hematologist's discretion [25, 29, 32]. Naturally, laboratory assessments should be made at the time of menstrual bleeding in order to capture the nadir of the lowest documented levels of VWF antigen [27]. Notably, the presence of blood group 0 may be a strong modifier, lowering VWF ristocetin cofactor below the normal reference range. However, in a recent study of young women, no strict VWD diagnosis could be established among women with bleeding symptoms and blood group 0 despite a higher frequency of a low VWF:ristocetin cofactor ratio [33].

Acta Haematol 2014;132:326–330
DOI: 10.1159/000360237

Treatment of Menorrhagia and Heavy Bleeding in Young Women

The optimal management of acute menorrhagia in young women without a diagnosed bleeding disorder includes first-line therapy with antifibrinolytics and hormonal agents. This combined attitude is sufficient for most cases. However, for cases of acute, severe menorrhagia, local surgical interventions may follow (e.g. blood tamponade, dilatation and curettage, endometrial ablation – if there is no desire for future fertility preservation, up to uterine artery embolization – as a lifesaving procedure in acute fulminant postpartum hemorrhage) and even the off-label use of procoagulant drugs, such as recombinant activated factor VII (rFVIIa) in extreme cases [29, 32]. Treatment options for VWD include antifibrinolytics, combined hormonal oral contraceptives, use of desmopressin that may be applied to treat type 1 VWD, and for some severe cases transfusion of plasma-derived factor concentrates that contain FVIII with VWF [27]. Specific coagulation factor concentrates (e.g. FVII or rFVIIa for severe FVII deficiency, FVIII/FIX for hemophilia A/B carriers with very low plasma factor activity, respectively, platelets for patients with Glanzmann thrombasthenia, fibrinogen for afibrinogenemia, etc.) may be applied in cases of severe bleeding once a specific rare coagulopathy has been diagnosed [29, 32]. The choice of combined oral contraception, used for maintenance therapy in many young women with heavy menstrual bleeding, should be individualized, bearing in mind the potential increased risk for VTE, as previously discussed.

Conclusion

Treatment of adolescents and young adults presents hemostatic challenges. On one hand, in this age group risk factors for early onset of venous thrombosis manifest themselves; on the other hand, bleeding disorders may also present at this age, especially among young women diagnosed due to heavy menstrual bleeding. Increased physician's awareness and referral for proper diagnostic testing would lead to an optimal individualized treatment of these conditions.

References

1 Andrew M, David M, Adams M, Ali K, Anderson R, Barnard D, Bernstein M, Brisson L, Cairney B, DeSai D: Venous thromboembolic complications (VTE) in children: first analyses of the Canadian Registry of VTE. Blood 1994;83:1251–1257.

2 Van Ommen CH, Heijboer H, Büller HR, Hirasing RA, Heijmans HS, Peters M: Venous thromboembolism in childhood: a prospective two-year registry in the Netherlands. J Pediatr 2001;139:676–681.

3 Schmidt B, Andrew M: Neonatal thrombosis: report of a prospective Canadian and international registry. Pediatrics 1995;96:939–943.

4 Journeycake JM, Buchanan GR: Thrombotic complications of central venous catheters in children. Curr Opin Hematol 2003;10:369–374.

5 Revel-Vilk S: Central venous line-related thrombosis in children. Acta Haematol 2006;115:201–206.

6 Goldenberg NA: Long-term outcomes of venous thrombosis in children. Curr Opin Hematol 2005;12:370–376.

7 Goldenberg NA, Donadini MP, Kahn SR, Crowther M, Kenet G, Nowak-Gottl U, Manco-Johnson MJ: Post-thrombotic syndrome in children: a systematic review of frequency of occurrence, validity of outcome measures, and prognostic factors. Haematologica 2010;95:1952–1959.

8 Kristjansson AL, Sigfusdottir ID, Allegrante JP: Adolescent substance use and peer use: a multilevel analysis of cross-sectional population data. Subst Abuse Treat Prev Policy 2013;8:27.

9 Huang DY, Lanza HI, Anglin MD: Assocation between adolescent substance use and obesity in young adulthood: a group-based dual trajectory analysis. Addict Behav 2013;38:2653–2660.

10 Gomes MP, Deitcher SR: Risk of venous thromboembolic disease associated with hormonal contraceptives and hormone replacement therapy: a clinical review. Arch Intern Med 2004;164:1965.

11 Farmer RD, Lawrenson RA, Thompson CR, Kennedy JG, Hambleton IR: Population-based study of risk of venous thromboembolism associated with various oral contraceptives. Lancet 1997;349:83.

12 Tans G, Bouma BN, Buller HE, Rosing J: Changes of hemostatic variables during oral contraceptive use. Semin Vasc Med 2003;3:61.

13 Pillai P, Bonny AE, O'Brien SH: Contraception-related venous thromboembolism in a pediatric institution. J Pediatr Adolesc Gynecol 2013;26:186–188.

14 Centers for Disease Control and Prevention: Sexual experience and contraceptive use among female teens – United States, 1995, 2002, and 2006–2010. MMWR Morb Mortal Wkly Rep 2012;61:297–301.

15 Miller MK, Pickett M, Leisner K, Sherman AK, Humiston SG: Sexual health behaviors, preferences for care, and use of health services among adolescents in pediatric emergency departments. Pediatr Emerg Care 2013;29:907–911.

16 Young G, Albisetti M, Bonduel M, Brandao L, Chan A, Friedrichs F, Goldenberg NA, Grabowski E, Heller C, Journeycake J, Kenet G, Krumpel A, Kurnik K, Lubetsky A, Male C, Manco-Johnson M, Mathew P, Monagle P, Van Ommen H, Simioni P, Svirin P, Tormene D, Nowak-Gottl U: Impact of inherited thrombophilia on venous thromboembolism in children: a systematic review and meta-analysis of observational studies. Circulation 2008;118:1373–1382.

17 Kenet G, Lutkhoff LK, Albisetti M, Bernard T, Bonduel M, Brandao L, Chabrier S, Chan A, De Veber G, Fiedler B, Fullerton HJ, Goldenberg NA, Grabowski E, Gunther G, Heller C, Holzhauer S, Iorio A, Journeycake J, Junker R, Kirkham FJ, Jurnik K, Lynch JK, Male C, Manco-Johnson M, Mesters R, Monagle P, van Ommen CH, Raffini L, Rostasy K, Simioni P, Strater RD, Young G, Nowak-Gottle U: Impact of inherited thrombophilia on arterial ischemic stroke and cerebral sinovenous thrombosis in children: a systematic review and meta-analysis of observational studies. Circulation 2010;121:1838–1847.

Acta Haematol 2014;132:326–330
DOI: 10.1159/000360237

18 Kenet G, Aronis S, Berkun Y, Bonduel M, Chan A, Goldenberg NA, Holzhauer S, Iorio A, Journeycake J, Junker R, Male C, Manco-Hohnson M, Massicotte P, Mesters R, Monagle P, van Ommen H, Rafini L, Simioni P, Young G, Nowak-Gottle U: Impact of persistent antiphospholipid antibodies on symptomatic thromboembolism in children: a systematic review and meta-analysis (observational studies). Semin Thromb Haemost 2011;37:802–809.

19 Monagle P, Chalmers E, Chan A, De Veber G, Kirkham F, Massicotte P, Michelson AD; American College of Chest Physicians: Antithrombotic therapy in neonates and children: American College of Chest Physicians Evidence-Based Clinical Practice Guidelines (8th ed). Chest 2008;133:887S–968S.

20 Bidlingmaier C, Kenet G, Kurnik K, Mathew P, Manner D, Mitchell L, Krumpel A, Nowak-Gottle U: Safety and efficacy of low molecular weight heparin in children: a systematic review of the literature and meta-analysis of single arm studies. Semin Thromb Haemost 2011;37:814–825.

21 Nowak-Gottl U, Dietrich K, Schaffranek D, Eldin NS, Yasui Y, Geisen C, Mitchell G: In pediatric patients, age has more impact on dosing of vitamin K antagonists than VKORC1 or CYP2C9 genotypes. Blood 2010; 116:5789–5790.

22 Young G: New anticoagulants in children: a review of recent studies and a look to the future. Thromb Res 2011;127:70–74.

23 James AH, Kouides PA, Abdul-Kadir R, Edlund M, Federici AB, Halimeh S, Kamphuisen PW, Konkle BA, Martinez-Perez O, McLintock C, Peyvandi F, Winikoff R: Von Willebrand disease and other bleeding disorders in women: consensus on diagnosis and management from an international expert panel. Am J Obst Gynecol 2009;201:12.e1–e8.

24 Nur Azura AG, Sanci L, Moore E, Grover S: The quality of life of adolescents with menstrual problems. J Pediatr Adolesc Gynecol 2013;26:102–108.

25 Pai M, Chan A, Barr R: How I manage heavy menstrual bleeding. Br J Haematol 2013;162: 721–729.

26 Ahuja SP, Hetweck SP: Overview of bleeding disorders in adolescent females with menorrhagia. J Ped Adolesc Gynecol 2010; 23(suppl):S15–S21.

27 Halimeh S: Menorrhagia and bleeding disorders in adolescent females. Hemostaseologie 2012;32:45–50.

28 Hedlund Treutiger I, Ravel Vilk S, Blanchette VS, Curtin JA, Lilicrap D, Rand ML: Reliability and reproducibility of classification of children as 'bleeders' versus 'non-bleeders' using a questionnaire for significant mucocutaneous bleeding. J Pediatr Hematol Oncol 2004;26:488–491.

29 Kadir RA, Davies J: Hemostatic disorders in women. J Thromb Haemost 2013;11(suppl 1):170–179.

30 Von Willebrand E: Hereditary pseudohemophilia. Finska Läkarsällskapets Handl 1926; 67:7–112.

31 Byams VR, Anderson BL, Grant AM, Atrash H, Schulkin J: Evaluation of bleeding disorders in women with menorrhagia: a survey of obstetrician-gynecologists. J Obstet Gynecol 2012;207:269.e1–e5.

32 James AH, Kouides PA, Abdul-Kadir RA, Dietrich JE, Edlund M, Federici AB, Halimeh S, Kamphuisen PW, Lee CA, Martinez-Perez O, McLintock O, Peyvandi F, Philipp C, Wilkinson J, Winikoff R: Evaluation and management of acute menorrhagia in women with and without underlying bleeding disorders: consensus from an international expert panel. Eur J Obstet Gynecol 2011;158:124–134.

33 Lethagen S, Hillarp A, Ekolm C, Mattson E, Halden C, Friberg B: Distribution of von Willebrand factor levels in young women with and without bleeding symptoms. Influence of ABO blood group and promoter haplotypes. Thromb Haemost 2008;99:1013–1018.

Acta Haematol 2014;132:331–339
DOI: 10.1159/000360209

Published online: September 10, 2014

Aplastic Anemia in Adolescents and Young Adults

Amy E. DeZern[a]   Eva C. Guinan[b]

[a] Johns Hopkins University School of Medicine, Baltimore, Md., and [b] Harvard Medical School, Boston, Mass., USA

Key Words

Aplastic anemia · Bone marrow failure · Adolescent · Hematopoietic cell transplant · Immunosuppressive therapy

Abstract

Adolescent and young adult patient presentations of aplastic anemia require a particular perspective on both diagnosis and treatment. This unique age group necessitates a thorough diagnostic evaluation to ensure the etiology, acquired or inherited, is sufficiently determined. The treatment options include human leukocyte antigen-identical sibling hematopoietic cell transplantation or immunosuppressive therapy, and both require attention to the specific medical and social needs of these adolescents and young adults. Longitudinal surveillance throughout life for the development of late complications of the disease and treatment is mandatory.

© 2014 S. Karger AG, Basel

Introduction

Aplastic anemia (AA) is a diagnosis that can present in any age group. Adolescent and young adult patients (up to the age of 30 years) with severe aplastic anemia (SAA) can have unique presentations of marrow failure in comparison to older adults. As a younger cohort may exhibit different proportions of inherited and acquired conditions, the differential diagnosis is broad and requires a more comprehensive workup. Accurate diagnosis is critical, as etiology and age at diagnosis may dictate therapeutic decisions.

Once alternative diagnoses have been eliminated, appropriate therapy for SAA should be initiated promptly. Although considerable debate continues over the upper age limit at which either hematopoietic cell transplantation (HCT) or immunosuppressive therapy (IST) should be used as the first-line approach for idiopathic SAA, the definitive treatment for a younger patient with a human leukocyte antigen (HLA)-identical sibling is an HCT. The cure rate for this younger cohort now approaches 90%, primarily due to advances in supportive care and standardization of conditioning regimens. In the absence of an HLA-identical sibling, IST is the most common alternative first-line approach to treatment.

Irrespective of the treatment method, longitudinal surveillance throughout life for development of late complications of marrow failure and its treatment is mandatory in these adolescents and young adults. This review serves to cover the presentation, treatment options and survivorship care in this unique age range.

Pathophysiology

AA can be inherited or acquired. Inherited forms may result from DNA repair defects (Fanconi anemia, FA), abnormal telomere physiology (dyskeratosis congenita,

Amy E. DeZern, MD, MHS
Assistant Professor of Oncology and Medicine
Cancer Research Building I, Room 3M87
1650 Orleans Street, Baltimore, MD 21287-0013 (USA)
E-Mail adezern1 @ jhmi.edu

DKC) or abnormalities of ribosomal biogenesis (Shwachman-Diamond syndrome). With rare exceptions, the pathophysiology of acquired AA in adolescents and young adults is not distinct from that of other populations. Acquired forms of AA are believed to be the result of an autoimmune attack directed at hematopoietic progenitor cells. The immune attack is primarily directed by cytotoxic T cells that target hematopoietic stem cells and cause apoptosis leading to hematopoietic failure. It remains unclear which antigens the T cells are targeting.

Presentation and Diagnosis

AA is defined as a clinical syndrome characterized by pancytopenia with a hypocellular bone marrow in the absence of abnormal infiltration or increased reticulin [1]. The clinical presentation is directly linked to the severity of the underlying cytopenias as well as the etiology. In this physically active age group, diagnosis may be delayed as fatigue, infection or bruising can be attributed to other causes. Cardiac reserve in younger patients may also delay appreciation of anemia as the cause of systemic symptoms. It is also possible that young adults suffer delays in diagnosis due to less frequent interactions with the medical system, related to overall good health or to social issues such as lack of insurance or increased geographic mobility.

The considerations applied to any patient with pancytopenia pertain equally to this age group. However, additional considerations may have more weight. For example, particular attention should be paid to history and findings suggestive of an inherited bone marrow failure syndrome (IBMFS). Some patients may have overt manifestations (e.g. short stature, hyperpigmentation, triphalangeal thumbs) that had been overlooked previously whereas the findings in some disorders (e.g. hair graying and reticulate pigmentation in DKC, premature menopause in FA) can become more obvious with age. Previous reports have suggested that a significant number of patients present with FA (9%) or DKC (46%) over the age of 16 [2]. With improved testing and a higher index of suspicion, it is becoming evident that these numbers are likely an underestimate. Table 1 reviews the differential diagnosis in this age group. Other etiologies of marrow failure, while in and of themselves infrequent, may also be more common in this age group. Aplasia secondary to anorexia nervosa is a pertinent example.

As in any age group, a thorough history and physical examination are imperative for diagnosis. For adolescents, it may be difficult for the patient to be forthcoming in the presence of parents. It may be easier to get an adequate history of relevant issues such as eating disorders, recreational drug use or an unplanned pregnancy without parents present. Family history may contribute significantly to the diagnosis of IBMFS (e.g. short stature, abnormal pigmentation, pulmonary failure). Physical examination should include a search for subtle findings associated with IBMFS. The etiology of any surgical scars should be determined with certainty as adolescents and young adults may not know why they have a scar, yet a history of orthopedic, cardiac, renal or gastrointestinal repairs may raise suspicion of an IBMFS. For young adults, we suggest special attention to the items in table 2.

The diagnostic workup must be thorough. Bone marrow evaluations including an aspirate and a biopsy are obligatory. Traditionally, in older adults conscious sedation is not necessary for the procedure but should be considered (as it is in pediatrics) in this age group. Once diagnosed with marrow hypocellularity, table 3 reviews how to classify AA severity [3]. The natural history of SAA is continued progression of the cytopenias, with minimal chance of spontaneous remission. Clinical outcomes do correlate with severity at presentation – with a worse prognosis for very SAA [4]. Moderate AA may spontaneously remit and may not require treatment [5].

It is important to realize that cytogenetic studies, including fluorescence in situ hybridization for common abnormalities, are an essential component of testing for

Table 1. Differential diagnosis of pancytopenia in young adults

	Diagnosis
Infection	Epstein-Barr virus, cytomegalovirus, human herpesvirus 6 Hepatitis B, C Human immunodeficiency virus Parvovirus
Environmental exposures	Recreational drugs Prescription drugs Toxic exposures
Clonal disorders	Leukemia Paroxysmal nocturnal hemoglobinuria Histiocytic disorders
Bone marrow failure syndromes	DKC FA Shwachman-Diamond syndrome Diamond-Blackfan anemia
Other	Pregnancy

Table 2. Initial evaluation of adolescents and young adults presenting with cytopenias

Patient history	Duration of cytopenias (are pediatric records available?) Medications (prescribed and over-the-counter supplements) Immunization records Exposures Transfusions
Family history	Constitutional abnormalities Malignancies
Physical examination	Height (in context of mean parental height) Limb abnormalities Skin and nail abnormalities (café-au-lait spots, nail dystrophy, pale patches)

Laboratory	Peripheral blood
	    β-Human chorionic gonadotropin (consider even if intercourse is not explicitly stated)
	    Complete blood count with differential
	    Reticulocyte counts
	    Chemistries
	    Transaminases and bilirubin
	    Hepatitis serologies
	    Fluorescent aerolysin assay for paroxysmal nocturnal hemoglobinuria
	    Chromosome breakage tests
	    Telomere length and mutational analysis (if DKC suspected)
	Bone marrow
	    Aspirate and biopsy
	    Flow cytometry (including quantitative CD34)
	    Cytogenetics

Table 3. Diagnostic criteria for the classification of AA

Peripheral blood cytopenias	Nonsevere (moderate) AA (not meeting criteria for severe disease)	SAA (any 2 of 3)	Very SAA (meeting criteria for severe disease and absolute neutrophils <200)
Bone marrow cellularity	<25%	<25%	<25%
Absolute neutrophil count		<500/µl	<200/µl
Platelet count		<20,000/µl	
Reticulocyte count		<1.0% corrected or <60,000/µl	

any patient with SAA regardless of age. Myelodysplasia (MDS) can occur in younger as well as older patients. As hypocellular MDS can be exceedingly difficult to differentiate from SAA, chromosomal studies may be critical to diagnosing MDS. Clinical paroxysmal nocturnal hemoglobinuria (PNH, e.g. accompanied by hemolysis) is less frequent in younger patients but not unknown. Moreover, evidence of a PNH clone may suggest both acquired AA and greater responsiveness to IST [6]. While not every patient requires an extensive laboratory evaluation for

IBMFS, chromosomal breakage studies are almost always warranted to exclude FA as FA patients may present without any obvious physical manifestations of the disease. Given that they would be unlikely to respond to IST, can respond to androgens and would require a reduced intensity conditioning regimen for HCT, making this diagnosis is critical [7]. Likewise, in a patient with a family history (pulmonary fibrosis, early graying, liver disease) or physical findings (nail dystrophy, mucosal leukoplakia) suggestive of DKC, telomere length studies or gene muta-

Acta Haematol 2014;132:331–339
DOI: 10.1159/000360209

tion testing should be considered as these patients are also often androgen responsive and extremely sensitive to myeloablative conditioning regimens [8]. The ramifications of making an IBMFS diagnosis extend beyond the patient to the family – from ascertaining appropriate HCT donors to providing genetic counseling.

Treatment

Hematopoietic Cell Transplantation

Adolescents and young adults (age of <30 years) with SAA who have an HLA-matched sibling donor should proceed directly to HCT as this is potentially curative (fig. 1). Results of HCT for SAA have improved over the last few decades, particularly in regard to use of donors other than matched family members. A report from the European Group for Blood and Marrow Transplantation (EBMT) of over 1,500 patients transplanted from 1991 to 2002 confirmed that predictors of survival following HCT included matched sibling donor, recipient age of less than 16 years, early HCT (time from diagnosis to HCT of less than 83 days) and a nonradiation conditioning regimen [9]. An advantage of HCT over standard IST is a marked reduction in the risk of relapse and abrogation of the risk for late clonal disorders such as MDS and PNH. The risks of acute and chronic graft-versus-host disease (GVHD) remain a challenge after HCT. The EBMT and the Center for International Blood and Marrow Transplant Research (CIBMTR) reviewed outcomes in nearly 700 patients with SAA receiving transplants from HLA-matched siblings. Their results showed that day-100 probabilities of acute grade 2–4 GVHD in younger patients were 10 and 14%, after bone marrow (BM) and peripheral blood progenitor cell (PBPC) HCT, respectively. Chronic GVHD rates were higher after PBPC (27%) than after BM HCT (12%) in patients less than 20 years old [10].

Graft rejection rates have fallen in past decades, but early and late graft failures with persistent or recurrent pancytopenia may occur. In the context of immunosuppression for GVHD prophylaxis, most patients achieve full donor chimerism after HCT. It is imperative to have detailed and regular conversations with the younger patients, who may be in more fluid and less regimented social settings, to ensure compliance with the full HCT immunosuppressive regimen. Failure to adhere to regular medication dosing may predispose to graft rejection. Patients with the greatest risk of late graft failure are those with a progressive increase in recipient cells (>5%), especially around the time of withdrawal of IST [11].

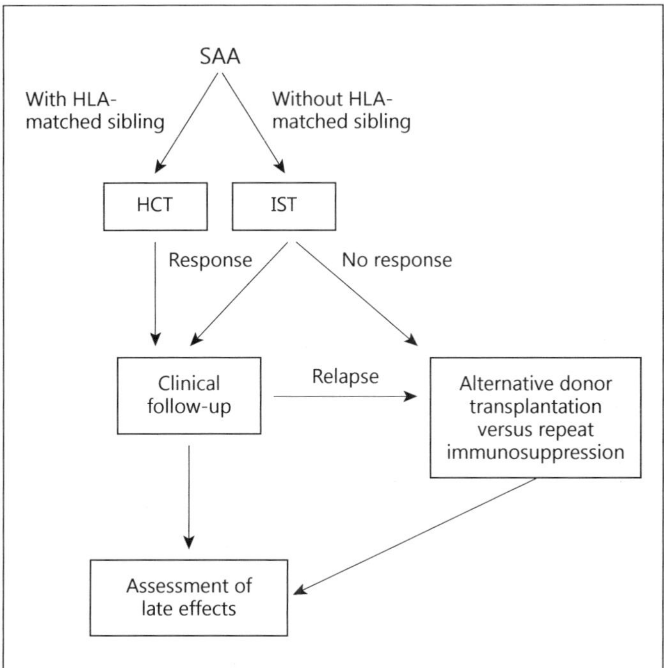

Fig. 1. Treatment schema for SAA.

Improving HCT outcomes in adolescents and young adults is an area of active research, including choice of donor as well as source of stem cells. As above from the EBMT and CIBMTR, in patients younger than 20 years of age, rates of chronic GVHD (relative risk 2.82; p = 0.002) and overall mortality (relative risk 2.04; p = 0.024) were higher after transplantation of PBPC grafts than after BM HCT. In younger patients, the 5-year survival was 85% after BM HCT but only 73% after PBPC HCT. These data suggest that BM grafts are preferable in this age group [10]. Further development of alternative donor options is under evaluation. None have moved to first-line therapy as of yet given historically poor survival rates, but there are promising results in haploidentical, [12, 13] unrelated donor, and cord blood HCT [14, 15]. These options are currently considered in the relapsed and refractory settings only.

Frontline IST

Another highly effective therapy for SAA is antithymocyte globulin (ATG) and cyclosporine (CsA) IST. This is generally the first-line therapy for adolescent and young adult SAA patients who lack matched sibling donors [16]. The hematopoietic response rate after ATG/CsA is 60–70%, and the probability of survival at 5 years ranges from

60 to 85% [9]. However, up to 40% of patients eventually relapse, a significant concern in this age group with long life expectancy. In a recent meta-analysis outcomes study from the EBMT of 2,479 patients with SAA, actuarial survival analyses were performed according to whether the patient's first-line treatment was HCT or IST. At 10 years, the survival was 73% in HCT recipients and 68% in those treated with IST (p = 0.002). The rates of secondary malignancy were tenfold higher in the patients who received IST alone (1.2%) compared with those who received HCT (0.1%) [17].

Other Immunosuppressive Options

Considering the rates of relapse and secondary clonal disease following ATG/CsA, a need for better nontransplant approaches persists, perhaps even more so in the young adult patient population. In hopes of decreasing rates of relapse and progression to secondary clonal conditions, additional IST, including mycophenolate, tacrolimus and alemtuzumab, have been added to the ATG/CsA platform, but no improvement in outcome has been observed [18–20]. While excess relative toxicity has been reported [21], high-dose cyclophosphamide has been utilized in younger populations with durable complete remissions [22] and may provide an alternative for some adolescent and young adult patients without a matched sibling donor.

Late Effects after Treatment

Clonal outgrowth with secondary hematological malignancies and impaired fertility are among the most profound late effects of IST and HCT, respectively, for adolescents and young adults treated for AA. Patients treated with IST should be told that there is a 1–5% chance of secondary hematological malignancies with clonal evolution to MDS or clinical PNH [17, 23]. Routine monitoring (generally annual) should be performed. Fear of infertility should not be considered a reason to withhold an HCT in a young patient. Both female and male survivors of matched sibling HCT for SAA have demonstrated fertility. The majority with successful reproduction after HCT received nonmyeloablative matched-sibling HCT with ATG/cyclophosphamide [24]. While transient ovarian and testicular dysfunction are common after cyclophosphamide-based HCT preparative regimens for SAA, fertility can return over the longer term [25]. In those who receive myeloablative preparatory regimens, preserved fertility is much less likely [23]. Fertility preservation techniques such as semen, egg or embryo cryopreservation should be attempted where possible and desired.

Such attempts must weigh the planned conditioning regimen, the rapidity with which the move to HCT is anticipated and any procedural complications due to risks of infection or bleeding. While they may or may not be at an age where this is a current concern, fertility issues should be discussed at length as limited options could later have significant social consequences. Monitoring for fertility after transplantation can be done as part of a survivorship program in consultation with reproductive endocrinologists.

Finally bone health and overall endocrine function must also be monitored over the long term [26]. After IST or HCT, hip or other persistent joint pain should prompt imaging to evaluate for avascular necrosis and appropriate orthopedic or physical therapy referral. Monitoring for osteopenia may be appropriate if steroid use and/or inactivity have been prolonged or if there is endocrine dysfunction. Serial thyroid monitoring should be implemented because as many as 10% of patients may have hypothyroidism after HCT.

Plans for long-term monitoring should also reflect other regimen-related toxicities. Rates of both melanoma and nonmelanoma skin cancer are increased after IST and HCT. Renal dysfunction and hypertension have also emerged as treatment-related issues. Evaluation for metabolic syndrome, which can be considered as a late treatment effect, is often not part of routine medical screening in this age group and may be missed. To this end, additional guidance from the National Comprehensive Cancer Network guidelines for adolescent and young adult oncology patient long-term follow-up after HCT can be reviewed and applied to the AA survivor population.

Supportive Care

Vascular Access

Placement of a central venous catheter should be strongly considered for all patients with AA, given the frequency of phlebotomy, transfusions and administration of therapeutic medications. Adolescents and young adults may need coaxing to agree to this as it is an obvious manifestation of illness that may be socially undesirable to them. The specific type of catheter (peripherally inserted central catheter, central insertion or subcutaneously located port) should be selected after discussion with the patient to ensure they will respect its physical limitations and maintain the device's care. While peripherally inserted central catheters may limit arm mobility and be more obvious, their weekly flush schedule could

Acta Haematol 2014;132:331–339
DOI: 10.1159/000360209

be an advantage to a young adult who does not want to come to the clinic more frequently or is unwilling to flush a catheter daily at home.

Blood Transfusions

Patients with severe cytopenias require frequent and sometimes urgent support with blood products. Blood products should be irradiated to prevent transfusion-associated GVHD [27] and leukofiltered to reduce the incidence of viral infections and prevent alloimmunization [28]. Parents and other family members often offer to be the source of transfusions, but this should be avoided to decrease sensitization to potential HCT donors. The initial goal of transfusion therapy for anemia should be to correct or avoid cardiopulmonary complications. Most adolescent and young adult patients without significant comorbidities should be transfused with packed red blood cells when symptomatic. A restrictive transfusion policy may be judiciously applied as long as a hemoglobin ≥6 g/dl is maintained. The goal of platelet transfusion is to maintain a high enough platelet count to prevent spontaneous bleeding. For most patients, platelet transfusions are indicated when platelet levels are below 10,000/µl or if the patient is experiencing bleeding. The young patient who feels well enough to continue day-to-day activities should be cautioned that there is an increased risk for bleeding with activities such as contact sports. Granulocyte transfusions remain controversial in SAA and should be used judiciously. Granulocyte transfusions may have an adjunctive role in patients with SAA and severe infections such as invasive bacterial and fungal infections unresponsive to maximal antibiotic and/or antifungal therapy [29].

Growth Factors

Hematopoietic growth factors (HGFs) may provide clinical benefit in some circumstances but do not induce disease remissions. The use of HGFs to support blood counts is of limited value in SAA, as predicted by both in vitro studies and the markedly elevated endogenous serum levels of HGFs. There may be a limited role for granulocyte colony-stimulating factor administration in an attempt to stimulate a neutrophil response to a severe infection, although there have been no prospective randomized studies in SAA that show a survival benefit with granulocyte colony-stimulating factor [30, 31]. These data suggest that granulocyte colony-stimulating factor support with IST might be used for patients with SAA as it may enhance neutrophil recovery, but it must be recognized that it does not modify the overall response and survival [32]. There are also some data suggesting that

HGFs may be linked to earlier presentations of MDS or leukemia [33].

Infections

Fungal and bacterial infections are a major cause of death in patients with SAA. Data from children suggest that mortality from fungal infections is higher in patients with SAA than in patients with acute myelogenous or lymphoblastic leukemia [34]. However, an active fungal infection should not delay a more definitive therapy such as IST or HCT [35]. It has been recognized that there may be a possible role for tobacco and/or marijuana smoking in increased risk for aspergillus exposure and infection [36]. Thus, young patients should be discouraged from these activities, especially in the setting of SAA.

There is no standardized approach to antibiotic therapy in AA at any age group. Vigilance and proactive prescription of prophylactic antibiotics (when deemed clinically appropriate), antivirals and antifungals in this patient population is imperative [37]. Where possible, it is prudent to avoid agents associated with high rates of marrow suppression, but therapy should be directed as dictated by the requirements of supportive care or as indicated by positive cultures. IST may render patients susceptible to viral infections, particularly community-acquired respiratory viruses and members of the Herpesviridae family. There is also an association between the viral hepatitides and SAA, such that patients may have ongoing or resolving hepatitis at the time of diagnosis.

Iron Overload

Iron overload may result from prolonged red blood cell transfusion support which is a reason to target lower hemoglobin levels in this population if tolerated. If ignored, iron overload can potentially produce irreversible organ damage, in particular to the liver and heart but also to endocrine organs, which may be of particular importance in younger patients. Chelation schedules vary significantly, but most often chelation therapy with deferoxamine is instituted if the patient's serum ferritin level is greater than 1,000–2,000 µg/l [16]. Data on alternative chelating agents in SAA is increasingly available [38, 39].

Menstrual Suppression/Pregnancy/Contraceptive Options

This is an area of importance in this age group, who may have irregular cycles (postmenarchal) or are premenarchal. Menstrual bleeding can be a source of significant blood loss, especially with profound thrombocytopenia and can be difficult to stop. Increased platelet transfusion goals to greater than 30,000 may be required until bleeding ceases. The method of menstrual suppression with the greatest likelihood of inducing amenorrhea should be chosen to protect against blood loss as well as possible gonadal and fertility protection. The most frequently reported method in females in HCT is a gonadotropin-releasing hormone agonist such as leuprolide. Given the bleeding and potential infection concerns of injection in neutropenic, thrombocytopenic patients, hormonal contraceptive pills are a reasonable alternative. This can be difficult to discuss with adolescents if parents are present, particularly as family members may be unaware or unrealistic about the current sexual activities or the fertility goals of the patient. Patients should be strongly discouraged from conception during this time period.

Rarely, AA can develop in pregnancy. Spontaneous remission can occur in 25–30% of patients, often upon birth or termination of the pregnancy. If termination is either not desired or medically appropriate, patients can be followed with stringent supportive care. CsA may be a safe drug antenatally in such patients. Complications appear to be more likely in pregnant patients with low platelet counts and associated PNH [40].

Social Issues and Survivorship

Patients in this age category have unique health issues and health care insurance coverage requirements. Efforts to address these issues are critical to assure support for a smooth transition into adulthood with a disease such as AA. There is an unfortunate lack of social, financial and standardized health care delivery to young adults. Individuals aged 19–29 are the group most likely to be uninsured in the USA. The same concerns extend to their social milieu. They may be living in communal settings, such as dormitories or military barracks, which make adherence to medical requirements very difficult. They may also be alone with minimal social support and nascent careers, making it difficult for them to care for themselves in times of increased medical need. As their peer cohort is equivalently likely to have less command of resources, including workplace flexibility, their peer community may be particularly limited in its ability for support and practical assistance.

At diagnosis, careful consideration should be given to topics that may be ambiguous yet critical for individuals of this age with significant illness. Such issues range from autonomy, support structure, information sharing, alternative decision makers (for advanced directives, for example) to the primary holder of insurance coverage. As AA is a rare disease, a detailed discussion at the time of diagnosis surrounding the nature of the disease, treatment, prognostic and social impact is imperative for the patients as well as their families. The treating doctor should provide a comprehensive explanation regarding all possible situations that may occur during the treatment, with emphasis on the chronic nature and the potentially slow response of the disease. Younger patients may have life plans, such as secondary education or employment endeavors, that make being tolerant with the pace of recovery challenging. As cytopenias will persist in a significant proportion of patients, it is useful to address quality of life with treatment as well as the goal of curing the disease. For young individuals, just starting life out on their own, overt discussion of guidelines for maintaining their social life are helpful – especially in patients with persistent neutropenia. The goal is to avoid excessive limitations on acceptable social outlets. Similarly, direct discussions about sexual function in relation to cytopenias and their treatment are essential. A life, as normal as possible, in most patients is a vital adjunct for psychological health. As the diagnosis of AA is a life-changing experience, some patients, especially in this age group, may want to consider professional psychological support. As their physicians, we should be proactive in destigmatizing this need and make referrals early. For some individuals, it may be helpful to contact other patients through marrow failure organizations. Details of patient support groups should be provided and encouraged.

Transition to Adult Care Providers
When a diagnosis of this magnitude is made in adolescence and even in young adults, the parents and other family members may be involved in treatment discussions. Once the treatments have been provided and outcomes completed, a longitudinal follow-up with adult providers is important. With adolescents, it is important to address why they may not want to leave their current pediatric provider, and review why medically this will be of benefit to them [41, 42]. Even after HCT when cure may be assumed, the patient will benefit from long-term follow-up with appropriate physicians, either in a defined survivorship program or with adult hematologists to follow for late effects and potential relapse. Survivorship clinics after HCT are often available at larger institutions.

Conclusions

Adolescent and young adult patients diagnosed with AA are a unique patient population that requires added attention to both diagnosis and treatment. The treatment of choice remains an HLA-identical sibling HCT if available. IST is an option in those patients who do not have an HLA-identical sibling. Regardless of the treatment method in these adolescents and young adults, long-term follow-up for the development of late complications of the disease and treatment is mandatory.

References

1 Brodsky RA, Jones RJ: Aplastic anaemia. Lancet 2005;365:1647–1656.
2 Alter BP: Diagnosis, genetics, and management of inherited bone marrow failure syndromes. Hematology Am Soc Hematol Educ Program 2007, pp 29–39.
3 Rozman C, Nomdedeu B, Marin P, Montserrat E: Criteria for severe aplastic-anemia. Lancet 1987;2:955–957.
4 Marsh JC, Hows JM, Bryett KA, Al-Hashimi S, Fairhead SM, Gordon-Smith EC: Survival after antilymphocyte globulin therapy for aplastic anemia depends on disease severity. Blood 1987;70:1046–1052.
5 Brock K, Goldenberg N, Graham DK, Liang X, Hays T: Moderate aplastic anemia in children: Preliminary outcomes for treatment versus observation from a single-institutional experience. J Pediatr Hematol Oncol 2013;35: 148–152.
6 Sugimori C, Chuhjo T, Feng X, Yamazaki H, Takami A, Teramura M, Mizoguchi H, Omine M, Nakao S: Minor population of CD55-CD59- blood cells predicts response to immunosuppressive therapy and prognosis in patients with aplastic anemia. Blood 2006; 107:1308–1314.
7 Socie G, Devergie A, Girinski T, Piel G, Ribaud P, Esperou H, Parquet N, Maarek O, Noguera MH, Richard P, Brison O, Gluckman E: Transplantation for Fanconi's anaemia: long-term follow-up of fifty patients transplanted from a sibling donor after low-dose cyclophosphamide and thoraco-abdominal irradiation for conditioning. Br J Haematol 1998;103:249–255.
8 Rocha V, Devergie A, Socie G, Ribaud P, Esperou H, Parquet N, Gluckman E: Unusual complications after bone marrow transplantation for dyskeratosis congenita. Br J Haematol 1998;103:243–248.
9 Locasciulli A, Oneto R, Bacigalupo A, Socie G, Korthof E, Bekassy A, Schrezenmeier H, Passweg J, Fuhrer M: Outcome of patients with acquired aplastic anemia given first line bone marrow transplantation or immunosuppressive treatment in the last decade: a report from the European Group for Blood and Marrow Transplantation (EBMT). Haematologica 2007;92:11–18.
10 Schrezenmeier H, Passweg JR, Marsh JC, Bacigalupo A, Bredeson CN, Bullorsky E, Camitta BM, Champlin RE, Gale RP, Fuhrer M, Klein JP, Locasciulli A, Oneto R, Schattenberg AV, Socie G, Eapen M: Worse outcome and more chronic GVHD with peripheral blood progenitor cells than bone marrow in HLA-matched sibling donor transplants for young patients with severe acquired aplastic anemia. Blood 2007;110:1397–1400.
11 Lawler M, McCann SR, Marsh JC, Ljungman P, Hows J, Vandenberghe E, O'Riordan J, Locasciulli A, Socie G, Kelly A, Schrezenmeier H, Marin P, Tichelli A, Passweg JR, Dickenson A, Ryan J, Bacigalupo A: Serial chimerism analyses indicate that mixed haemopoietic chimerism influences the probability of graft rejection and disease recurrence following allogeneic stem cell transplantation (SCT) for severe aplastic anaemia (SAA): indication for routine assessment of chimerism post SCT for SAA. Br J Haematol 2009;144:933–945.
12 Im HJ, Koh KN, Choi ES, Jang S, Kwon SW, Park CJ, Chi HS, Seo JJ: Excellent outcome of haploidentical hematopoietic stem cell transplantation in children and adolescents with acquired severe aplastic anemia. Biol Blood Marrow Transplant 2013;19:754–759.
13 Xu LP, Liu KY, Liu DH, Han W, Chen H, Chen YH, Zhang XH, Wang Y, Wang FR, Wang JZ, Huang XJ: A novel protocol for haploidentical hematopoietic SCT without in vitro T-cell depletion in the treatment of severe acquired aplastic anemia. Bone Marrow Transplant 2012;47:1507–1512.
14 Yamamoto H, Kato D, Uchida N, Ishiwata K, Araoka H, Takagi S, Nakano N, Tsuji M, Asano-Mori Y, Matsuno N, Masuoka K, Izutsu K, Wake A, Yoneyama A, Makino S, Taniguchi S: Successful sustained engraftment after reduced-intensity umbilical cord blood transplantation for adult patients with severe aplastic anemia. Blood 2011;117:3240–3242.
15 Peffault de Latour R, Rocha V, Socie G: Cord blood transplantation in aplastic anemia. Bone Marrow Transplant 2013;48:201–202.
16 Marsh JC, Ball SE, Cavenagh J, Darbyshire P, Dokal I, Gordon-Smith EC, Keidan J, Laurie A, Martin A, Mercieca J, Killick SB, Stewart R, Yin JA: Guidelines for the diagnosis and management of aplastic anaemia. Br J Haematol 2009;147:43–70.
17 Gafter-Gvili A, Ram R, Gurion R, Paul M, Yeshurun M, Raanani P, Shpilberg O: ATG plus cyclosporine reduces all-cause mortality in patients with severe aplastic anemia – systematic review and meta-analysis. Acta Haematol 2008;120:237–243.
18 Scheinberg P, Nunez O, Weinstein B, Scheinberg P, Wu CO, Young NS: Activity of alemtuzumab monotherapy in treatment-naive, relapsed, and refractory severe acquired aplastic anemia. Blood 2012;119:345–354.
19 Scheinberg P, Nunez O, Wu C, Young NS: Treatment of severe aplastic anaemia with combined immunosuppression: anti-thymocyte globulin, ciclosporin and mycophenolate mofetil. Br J Haematol 2006;133:606–611.
20 Alsultan A, Goldenberg NA, Kaiser N, Graham DK, Hays T: Tacrolimus as an alternative to cyclosporine in the maintenance phase of immunosuppressive therapy for severe aplastic anemia in children. Pediatr Blood Cancer 2009;52:626–630.
21 Tisdale JF, Dunn DE, Geller N, Plante M, Nunez O, Dunbar CE, Barrett AJ, Walsh TJ, Rosenfeld SJ, Young NS: High-dose cyclophosphamide in severe aplastic anaemia: a randomised trial. Lancet 2000;356:1554–1559.
22 Brodsky RA, Chen AR, Dorr D, Fuchs EJ, Huff CA, Luznik L, Smith BD, Matsui WH, Goodman SN, Ambinder RF, Jones RJ: High-dose cyclophosphamide for severe aplastic anemia: long-term follow-up. Blood 2010; 115:2136–2141.
23 Eapen M, Ramsay NK, Mertens AC, Robison LL, DeFor T, Davies SM: Late outcomes after bone marrow transplant for aplastic anaemia. Br J Haematol 2000;111:754–760.
24 Loren AW, Chow E, Jacobsohn DA, Gilleece M, Halter J, Joshi S, Wang Z, Sobocinski KA, Gupta V, Hale GA, Marks DI, Stadtmauer EA, Apperley J, Cahn JY, Schouten HC, Lazarus HM, Savani BN, McCarthy PL, Jakubowski AA, Kamani NR, Hayes-Lattin B, Maziarz RT, Warwick AB, Sorror ML, Bolwell BJ, Socie G, Wingard JR, Rizzo JD, Majhail NS: Pregnancy after hematopoietic cell transplantation: a report from the late effects working committee of the center for international blood and marrow transplant research (CIBMTR). Biol Blood Marrow Transplant 2011;17:157–166.
25 Sanders JE: The impact of marrow transplant preparative regimens on subsequent growth and development. The Seattle Marrow Transplant Team. Semin Hematol 1991;28:244–249.

26 Konopacki J, Porcher R, Robin M, Bieri S, Cayuela JM, Larghero J, Xhaard A, Andreoli AL, Dhedin N, Petropoulou A, Rodriguez-Otero P, Ribaud P, Moins-Teisserenc H, Carmagnat M, Toubert A, Chalandon Y, Socie G, Peffault de Latour R: Long-term follow up after allogeneic stem cell transplantation in patients with severe aplastic anemia after cyclophosphamide plus antithymocyte globulin conditioning. Haematologica 2012;97:710–716.

27 Laundy GJ, Bradley BA, Rees BM, Younie M, Hows JM: Incidence and specificity of HLA antibodies in multitransfused patients with acquired aplastic anemia. Transfusion 2004; 44:814–825.

28 Marsh J, Socie G, Tichelli A, Schrezenmeier H, Hochsmann B, Risitano AM, Fuehrer M, Bekassy AN, Korthof ET, Locasciulli A, Ljungman P, Bacigalupo A, Camitta B, Young NS, Passweg J: Should irradiated blood products be given routinely to all patients with aplastic anaemia undergoing immunosuppressive therapy with antithymocyte globulin (ATG)? A survey from the European Group for Blood and Marrow Transplantation severe aplastic anaemia working party. Br J Haematol 2010;150:377–379.

29 Quillen K, Wong E, Scheinberg P, Young NS, Walsh TJ, Wu CO, Leitman SF: Granulocyte transfusions in severe aplastic anemia: An eleven-year experience. Haematologica 2009; 94:1661–1668.

30 Marsh JC, Ganser A, Stadler M: Hematopoietic growth factors in the treatment of acquired bone marrow failure states. Semin Hematol 2007;44:138–147.

31 Tichelli A, Schrezenmeier H, Socie G, Marsh J, Bacigalupo A, Duhrsen U, Franzke A, Hallek M, Thiel E, Wilhelm M, Hochsmann B, Barrois A, Champion K, Passweg JR: A randomized controlled study in patients with newly diagnosed severe aplastic anemia receiving antithymocyte globulin (ATG), cyclosporine, with or without G-CSF: a study of the SAA working party of the European Group for Blood and Marrow Transplantation. Blood 2011;117:4434–4441.

32 Gluckman E, Rokicka-Milewska R, Hann I, Nikiforakis E, Tavakoli F, Cohen-Scali S, Bacigalupo A: Results and follow-up of a phase III randomized study of recombinant human-granulocyte stimulating factor as support for immunosuppressive therapy in patients with severe aplastic anaemia. Br J Haematol 2002; 119:1075–1082.

33 Socie G, Mary JY, Schrezenmeier H, Marsh J, Bacigalupo A, Locasciulli A, Fuehrer M, Bekassy A, Tichelli A, Passweg J: Granulocyte-stimulating factor and severe aplastic anemia: a survey by the European Group for Blood and Marrow Transplantation (EBMT). Blood 2007;109:2794–2796.

34 Aytac S, Yildirim I, Ceyhan M, Cetin M, Tuncer M, Kara A, Cengiz AB, Secmeer G, Yetgin S: Risks and outcome of fungal infection in neutropenic children with hematologic diseases. Turk J Pediatr 2010;52:121–125.

35 Aki ZS, Sucak GT, Yegin ZA, Guzel O, Erbas G, Senol E: Hematopoietic stem cell transplantation in patients with active fungal infection: not a contraindication for transplantation. Transplant Proc 2008;40:1579–1585.

36 Verweij PE, Kerremans JJ, Voss A, Meis JF: Fungal contamination of tobacco and marijuana. JAMA 2000;284:2875.

37 Valdez JM, Scheinberg P, Nunez O, Wu CO, Young NS, Walsh TJ: Decreased infection-related mortality and improved survival in severe aplastic anemia in the past two decades. Clin Infect Dis 2011;52:726–735.

38 Cappellini MD, Porter J, El-Beshlawy A, Li CK, Seymour JF, Elalfy M, Gattermann N, Giraudier S, Lee JW, Chan LL, Lin KH, Rose C, Taher A, Thein SL, Viprakasit V, Habr D, Domokos G, Roubert B, Kattamis A, Investigators ES: Tailoring iron chelation by iron intake and serum ferritin: the prospective EPIC study of deferasirox in 1,744 patients with transfusion-dependent anemias. Haematologica 2010;95:557–566.

39 Lee JW, Yoon SS, Shen ZX, Ganser A, Hsu HC, El-Ali A, Habr D, Martin N, Porter J: Hematologic responses in patients with aplastic anemia treated with deferasirox: a post-hoc analysis from the EPIC study. Haematologica 2013;98:1045–1048.

40 Tichelli A, Socie G, Marsh J, Barge R, Frickhofen N, McCann S, Bacigalupo A, Hows J, Marin P, Nachbaur D, Symeonidis A, Passweg J, Schrezenmeier H: Outcome of pregnancy and disease course among women with aplastic anemia treated with immunosuppression. Ann Intern Med 2002;137:164–172.

41 Van Staa A, van der Stege HA, Jedeloo S, Moll HA, Hilberink SR: Readiness to transfer to adult care of adolescents with chronic conditions: exploration of associated factors. J Adolesc Health 2011;48:295–302.

42 Bryant R, Young A, Cesario S, Binder B: Transition of chronically ill youth to adult health care: experience of youth with hemoglobinopathy. J Pediatr Health Care 2011;25:275–283.

Acta Haematol 2014;132:340–347

DOI: 10.1159/000360235

Published online: September 10, 2014

Thalassemia Major and Sickle Cell Disease in Adolescents and Young Adults

Joanne Yacobovich[a, b]   Hannah Tamary[a, b]

[a] Department of Pediatric Hematology-Oncology, Schneider Children's Medical Center of Israel, Petah Tikva, and
[b] Sackler Faculty of Medicine, Tel Aviv University, Tel Aviv, Israel

Key Words

Adolescence · Care transition · Sickle cell anemia · Thalassemia major · Young adults

Abstract

The increased longevity of patients with thalassemia and sickle cell disease (SCD) introduces new clinical challenges due to the accumulation of disease-related morbidity, psychosocial issues and health care adjustments. Patients with thalassemia major now live into adulthood without suffering heart failure but must confront delayed puberty, impaired fertility and progressive bone disease. The increased survival in SCD brings to the front previously unrecognized complications including pulmonary hypertension, silent cerebral infarcts and also reproductive dysfunction. Adolescents and young adults (AYAs) have age-related psychosocial needs in their transition from the pediatric health care environment to the adult system. In this review we present the uniquely age-related medical issues facing the AYA thalassemia and SCD cohort in their transition into adulthood.

© 2014 S. Karger AG, Basel

Introduction

Adolescents and young adults (AYAs) with thalassemia major (TM) and sickle cell disease (SCD) pose unique challenges in their medical treatment. Improved availability of medical services, growing knowledge of the pathogenesis of disease symptoms, novel pharmaceutics and advancing technology are all responsible for the longevity of patients with the hereditary hemoglobinopathies. In Italy 60% of the patients with TM in 2009 were above 30 years of age [1], while in Greece the probability of survival was 65% at the age of 50 years [2]. Similarly, in SCD the survival has greatly improved; in 1994 the median survival for males with sickle cell anemia was 42 years and for females 48 years [3], while one decade later the Dallas cohort reported 85.6% overall survival [4]. Children with thalassemia require regular blood transfusions and have to adhere to iron chelation protocols in order to minimize iron overload complications leading to cardiac and endocrine toxicity. As AYAs they often face problems of delayed puberty and infertility as well as osteopenic/osteoporotic bone disease. Similarly, sickle cell AYA patients continue to experience the complications that manifest in childhood such as vaso-occlusive crises, and additionally suffer the accumulating effects of lung

Hannah Tamary, MD
Head of Hematology Unit, Schneider Children's Medical Center of Israel
14 Kaplan Street
Petah Tikva 49202 (Israel)
E-Mail htamary@post.tau.ac.il

disease, neurocognitive impairment and also reproductive dysfunction. In addition to the medical aspects of being AYAs with a chronic disease, these patients are faced with the challenges of the transition to adult treatment facilities, becoming independent individuals, considering family planning and a productive future. In this review we will address the issues uniquely facing the AYA patients with β-TM and SCD.

Thalassemia Major

Regular red cell transfusion effectively prevented classical complications of thalassemia, including facial malformations and high-output heart failure. Unfortunately iron overload complications leading to cardiac, endocrine and hepatic dysfunction have become a major cause of morbidity and mortality. In recent years however, the development of oral, parenteral and combination iron chelation therapy and access to noninvasive measures of iron burden by various MRI techniques have improved the survival of thalassemia patients [5]. Therefore there is an increasing AYA population that faces age-related endocrine complications including delayed puberty and reduced fertility. In addition, the development of bone disease [6–10], a major problem affecting a large proportion of adult patients with β-TM, starts manifesting in AYAs.

Delayed Puberty

Hypogonadotropic hypogonadism (HH) is the commonest endocrinopathy in thalassemic patients affecting 70–80% of patients and causing sexual infantilism, poor growth, infertility and osteoporosis [11–13]. Since quality of life and not merely preservation of life is a major issue for thalassemia patients today, the morbidity related to sexual infantilism is significant. Clinical signs of HH appear early in the second decade of life with failure of initiation of puberty, failure of progression of puberty and primary or secondary amenorrhea [14]. High serum ferritin levels have been associated with delayed puberty implicating poor chelation in the clinical signs of HH [15, 16]. Since it is known that iron loading precedes clinical signs of toxic damage in the heart and pancreas [17, 18], it is logical to assume that the same is relevant for the pituitary. Wood et al. [19] found decreased pituitary volume in thalassemic patients using T2 MRI which was accentuated with iron accumulation. This study showed that pituitary iron loading occurs commonly in children below the age of 10 years and as young as 4 years [19]. A susceptibility to develop HH was associated with severity of the thalassemic genotype. Patients with severe defects have increased red cell requirements, thus greater iron loading, and may also have a greater vulnerability to free radical damage. Endocrine tissue, similarly to cardiac tissue, takes up circulating labile iron species not bound by transferring, thereby suffering its more toxic effects [14].

Iron accumulation in the gonadotrope cells is not the sole cause of HH in thalassemic patients. Adipose tissue also suffers from iron loading, and in turn leptin synthesis is impaired. Leptin is a hormone produced in fat cells and has a physiological role in sexual maturation and fertility, most probably as a permissive signal for the process of puberty. The decreased levels of leptin in thalassemia seem to correlate with transferring receptor levels, indicating a relationship with iron toxicity [14].

Pituitary function must be monitored from an early age to guide chelation therapy. It was shown that intensive combination therapy can reverse existing HH and prevent new-onset hypogonadism [20]. Once diagnosed early, the treatment of delayed puberty with gonadotropin-releasing hormone can induce sexual maturation in up to 80% of cases [14]. If irreversible damage has already occurred, sex steroid replacement therapy is indicated. The timely treatment of HH is critical as it can prevent sexual infantilism and stunted growth as well as improve reproductive potential and minimize bone disease.

Fertility

Fertility is a growing issue and point of concern for the thalassemic AYA. Young women with thalassemia have impaired fertility mainly due to HH. Iron loading of the pituitary begins as early as at the age of 4 years with marked volume loss in the second decade of life [19]. The effect of iron overload on the ovary is less clear. Recently, use of antimüllerian hormone as a biomarker for the assessment of ovarian reserve has shown that fertility is preserved in the majority of thalassemic women younger than 30–35 years [21]. Over 400 pregnancies have been reported, more than half of them in women with amenorrhea, requiring ovulation induction [22]. Despite these optimistic data, infertility still disrupts family planning for the patients stressing the importance of early stringent chelation, active assessment of reproductive capacity and specialized fertility counseling. Pregnancies in thalassemic women bear a high risk, for the mother and fetus. Underlying cardiac and glucose metabolism impairments are more pronounced, and blood requirements increase [23]. A close follow-up is necessary with the cooperation of maternal-fetal clinics and hematologists familiar with the complications of pregnancies in thalassemia.

There is a paucity of literature on the effects of thalassemia on male fertility. One study found that in addition to the hormonal disturbances due to hypothalamic/pituitary axis failure, thalassemic males have a decreased sperm count, sperm motility and proportion of sperm with normal morphology. A comprehensive assessment is required to determine the source of male infertility in order to compile the appropriate fertility therapy [24].

Intensive combined chelation with deferiprone and deferoxamine was shown to prevent progression of subclinical endocrinopathies and even reverse hypothalamic dysfunction due to iron overload toxicity [20]. Recognizing this possibility should provide the incentive for the AYA thalassemic population to aggressively chelate with the goal of normalizing the iron status.

Bone Disease

Osteoporosis is another complication that becomes problematic in the AYA population [25]. The pathogenesis of bone disease is multifactorial being affected by delayed sexual maturation, endocrine dysfunction, extramedullary hematopoiesis, iron toxicity and chelator therapy [26]. Normally, bone mineral density rises throughout childhood until the age of 12 years and then accelerates during the onset of puberty paralleling the growth spurt. Thalassemic youth, often suffering from absent or delayed puberty due to HH, may fail to proceed with the proper bone mineralization and not achieve peak bone mass [27–30]. Thalassemic patients also continue later on to have an increased bone resorption secondary to hypogonadism [31]. Genotype differences including β^0/β^+ compound heterozygotes and additional α-thalassemia mutations mediate red cell consumption, iron loading and thereby the rate of endocrine complications. When patients were grouped according to thalassemia genotype, gonadal function was found to be the only factor associated with decreased bone mineral density [32, 33]. Additionally, polymorphisms known to affect bone mineral density can identify patients at greater risk for osteoporosis and fractures [34]. Growth hormone secretory dysfunction has been described in thalassemia as well as diminished levels of insulin-like growth factor-1 [35, 36]; these may also directly contribute to demineralization of the femoral head [37]. Additional factors that affect the tendency for osteoporosis include vitamin D deficiency and depletion of trace elements by poor nutrition combined with chelation therapy [38–41]. The best way to treat osteoporosis in thalassemics is prevention. Regular transfusions, adequate diet and correction of nutritional deficiencies with supplementation are essential, especially during childhood and puberty. Induction of puberty and further hormone replacement therapy are important in the prevention of bone disease [42, 43]. If osteoporosis is diagnosed, the use of biphosphonates has shown short-term success in improving bone mass Z score [44]. Specifically, monthly infusions of pamidronate were shown to significantly improve bone volume in thalassemic men and women [45], while neridronate, a third-generation bisphosphonate, significantly reduced bone resorption, increased bone density and reduced back pain [46]. Implementation of hormone replacement, dietary supplementation and bisphosphonate therapy should lead to improved quality of life and better daily functioning.

Sickle Cell Disease

The clinical complications of SCD begin from early childhood and continue to accumulate through the AYA age group into later adulthood. With contemporary care the survival of these patients has also greatly increased. The major vaso-occlusive events such as pain crises, acute chest syndrome and stroke that contribute to significant morbidity from the pediatric age range have been extensively documented [47, 48], while pulmonary hypertension (PH), silent cerebral infarcts and fertility difficulties are increasingly related to a significant handicap in the AYA age group. Research into age-related trends has shown poorer outcome and increased mortality during the period of transition of patients from pediatric to adult care [3, 49, 50]. By recognizing the specific health needs of the AYA sickle cell anemia population, it will be possible to focus on improving their care and outcome.

Pulmonary Disease

Acute chest syndrome (ACS) is the leading cause of premature death and the second most common reason for admission among patients with SCD [3]. The major causes of ACS include pneumonia, bone marrow/fat embolism and in situ sickling/pulmonary infarct [51]. This complication is most common in children, however severer in adults [52]. In adults often ACS follows pain crises, supposedly secondary to hypoventilation due to splinting with chest wall pain or immobilization due to lower limb pain [53]. Additionally is has been recognized that secretory phospholipase A_2 can induce inflammatory lung injury by converting bone marrow fat into free fatty acids and may predict the onset of ACS [54]. In a study of 14 adolescents, secretory phospholipase A_2 was used as a

Acta Haematol 2014;132:340–347
DOI: 10.1159/000360235

biomarker for ACS in patients hospitalized for vaso-occlusive crises. Early red blood cell transfusion prevented the development of ACS in these patients [55].

PH is recognized as a significant contributor to morbidity and mortality in older SCD patients. Right heart catheterization showing mean pulmonary artery pressure ≥25 mm Hg is the gold standard to define PH; however, many studies are based on the use of tricuspid valve regurgitant jet velocity (TRJV) in transthoracic echocardiography as a surrogate marker of PH. Increased TRJV has been associated with early mortality [56]; however, 2 recent studies demonstrate that the positive predictive value for PH is only 25–32% and that the true prevalence of PH is only 2.9–3.8% in adults [57, 58]. It appears that PH may develop in children and adolescents [51, 59]. The risk factors in the younger age group vary from those in adults [60]. In children, history of ACS and history of sepsis or bacteremia strongly associate with the development of PH, while in adults severity of hemolysis, age and end organ disease are the major risk factors [60, 61]. Studies investigating the correlation of TRJV to PH in the AYA age group have yet to be performed. It seems clear today that an increased TRJV should direct further investigation by cardiac catheterization to most accurately diagnose PH; nevertheless, it also defines a high-risk group that requires a closer clinical follow-up.

Neurological/Cognitive Complications

Cerebral and/or neurocognitive insult due to multiple factors is of growing concern in the treatment of SCD as it limits the functioning potential of the developing child and young adult. Silent cerebral infarct (SCI) is the most common neurological injury in SCD and occurs in about one third of children before their 14th birthday [62]. The definition of SCI is challenging requiring investigation of the previous history of any neurological complaints (seizure, focal weakness, ataxia, dizziness), specific requirements upon MRI and strict guidelines to rule out mimickers of SCI [63]. The Silent Cerebral Infarct Trial included 814 children with SCI-like lesions who were examined by a pediatric neurologist to rule out the presence of focal deficits that were explained by the radiological findings. It was found that hemoglobin <7.6 g/dl, systolic blood pressure in the highest quartile and male sex were significantly associated with an increased risk for SCI [64]. The outcome of SCIs has been studied depicting deficits specifically in executive functions and related poor academic achievements [65].

More recently the entity of acute silent cerebral ischemic events has been distinguished [66]. These events were originally detected in patients during acute illnesses with anemia exacerbation. A second study found evidence of acute silent cerebral ischemic events among asymptomatic patients undergoing prescheduled, study-related MRIs. In the follow-up, not all acute events led to permanent neuroradiological findings [67]. This provides evidence that supports the hypothesis that chronic, intermittent ischemia occurs in the brain as in other organs in SCD patients. The significance of these events must be researched but may manifest as the neurocognitive impairment that is invisible in imaging studies. Evidence of neuropsychological dysfunction is found in patients that appear neurologically intact. Mean nonverbal function as well as global cognitive function, working memory, processing speed and executive function were found to be significantly lower in adult SCD patients than in community-matched controls [68]. Similar deficits were found in a pediatric-adolescent population including decreased general cognitive functions, subtle deficits in executive function and impaired visuomotor abilities. One third of the children in this study had a full-scale IQ below 75, defining learning disability with definite negative consequences on academic functioning [69]. The study of long-term effects of acute silent cerebral ischemic events and the effectiveness of interventional therapy in AYAs diagnosed with neurocognitive deficits could significantly influence their productive potential and future quality of life.

Fertility

Reports analyzing reproductive functioning in SCD patients are rare in the literature; the majority of articles discussing fertility in males were published approximately 30 years ago. A single recent publication presents the evaluation of sperm parameters and fertility of men with SCD and the potential deleterious impact of hydroxyurea therapy. Among measurements of spermatozoal concentration per volume and per ejaculate 40% were below normal. Two thirds of the cases had abnormal sperm morphology. Overall, at least 1 sperm parameter was abnormal in 91% of patients prior to treatment. Hydroxyurea treatment had a further negative effect on all semen samples collected under therapy and this occurred within 6 months of initiation. In the 4 cases with semen analysis before and after hydroxyurea therapy 3 had altered sperm production after cessation of treatment, 1 with azospermia [70]. This study recommends consideration of sperm cryopreservation prior to initiating therapy with hydroxyurea.

Fertility difficulties in women with SCD are not well documented; however, the use of hydroxyurea is not recommended from 3 months prior to conception since it was found teratogenic in animal models [71]. Pregnancy complications for the mother and fetus have been described. Villers et al. [72] evaluated nearly 18,000 deliveries to SCD mothers compared to controls. They found that infectious sequelae (sepsis, urinary tract infections and pneumonia) and thrombotic complications (cerebral vein and deep venous thrombosis) were significantly more frequent in pregnant SCD women. SCD females were more prone to pregnancy-specific complications, and rates of maternal mortality were significantly higher [72]. Intensive specialized support is necessary for SCD mothers prior to, during pregnancy and postpartum in order to minimize complications and maximally promote proper fetal development.

Transition from Pediatric to Adult Medicine

Beyond the age-related medical complications of their disease, psychosocial issues are of paramount importance to the AYA patients with both hemoglobinopathies as they transition from childhood to adulthood. The critical issues include academic achievement, financial independence, career, family and health care. These issues come to a head during the process of transition from pediatric to adult medical care. The transitioning of AYAs from pediatric health care settings to adult systems is a growing issue of interest in many pediatric subspecialties as up to 90% of adolescents with previously lethal diseases will reach adulthood today [73]. Among patients with hemoglobinopathies, an Italian survey found that 95.8% of TM patients born between 1975 and 1979 survived 20 years and 99% of the 1980–1984 cohort survived 15 years [74], whereas an American study in Dallas, Tex., found that 98.4% of SCD patients survived to the age of 18 years [49]. The greatly improved survival necessitates a transition to adult medical services, a process that was unexplored when the majority of patients did not reach adulthood. The transfer of care, as described by the Society for Adolescent Medicine, is the 'purposeful, planned and timely transition from child and family-centered pediatric health care to patient-centered adult-oriented health care' [75]. This must be a process and not a step or a leap. The issues to be addressed are many, including assessment of the psychocognitive readiness of the patients, identification of appropriate adult treatment centers, education of the patient in his/her personal health care needs, facilitation of the transfer of information to the adult caretakers and physical transfer of the patient to the new medical facilities.

The readiness of patients developmentally depends on maturity, ethnic and environmental influences as well as the preparation provided by the pediatric health providers. The actual timing of transition is often dictated by the health insurance providers and not dependent on the patients' needs or health care professionals' recommendations. Transition readiness of SCD patients was assessed in a recent study [76] using a survey compiling five components: amount of thought given to the transition, knowledge of the steps in transition of care, interest in learning about the process, anticipated difficulty, perceived importance of continuance of care. The results showed that the patients found the transition to be 'extremely important'; however, the score of 'knowledge of the steps of transition' ranked lowest in the assessment. The 17- to 20-year-old cohort demonstrated significantly more interest and knowledge than the 14- to 16-year-olds. A main concern expressed in numerous studies on transition among patients with various chronic diseases involves the fear of unfamiliar caretakers and surroundings; as one patient explained, 'it's like losing a part of my family' [76–79]. In order to be ready for the moment, the process of transition should in essence begin from the onset of care at the facility. Creating a trusting relationship, encouraging participation of the family in decision-making processes and teaching the child about his illness and health care needs from a young age is paramount in the success of transition in the future [80] as is the establishment of transition programs with dedicated support staff [81].

There are significant differences in the specific process of transfer to adult care among TM and SCD patients. Transfusion-dependent thalassemics are inherently connected to specialized comprehensive care centers for blood transfusion, chelation management and periodic multidisciplinary workups. In contrast, SCD patients are largely managed by primary care physicians with consultations in subspecialty care [81]. For thalassemics the transition occurs in the hospital setting, while for SCD patients the care must be handed over to an adult community care service as well as a specialized consulting center. The lack of knowledge that adult hematologists have in the treatment of TM often creates the major barrier to transition, the receiver must be ready to receive [80, 82]. More adult specialty centers are being established enabling the treatment of adult thalassemics in a comprehensive manner. For SCD patients the education

Acta Haematol 2014;132:340–347
DOI: 10.1159/000360235

must focus on community primary care physicians as well as adult hematology experts. The responsibilities of the patients in their own health care must be taught in a step-wise manner over time leading up to independence. Thalassemia patients must understand the importance of compliance with chelation therapy and regular periodic end organ assessment. SCD patients in turn must be aware of the importance of seeking prompt medical attention for acute vaso-occlusive events as well as planning appropriate outpatient treatment schemes for mild pain crises [81, 83]. Compliance with maintenance therapy such as hydroxyurea or transfusion regimens is also essential to the prevention of sequelae.

The transfer of information between staff is central to the success of the adult caretakers in maintaining a continuum of care. Proper medical and psychosocial summaries and collaborative meetings will enable this process. Patients have expressed the desire for joint transfer meetings in order to ease the process, reduce the uncertainty and relieve anxiety. Since there is documentation that the period of transition can be associated with increased morbidity, poorer compliance and even mortality, more attention is required to assure that the transfer to the adult team be straightforward, organized and welcoming [81, 84, 85]. Most adolescents cling on to the familiarity of the pediatric clinic and fear the supposed 'coldness' of the adult clinical setting. Personal 'hand-off' sessions with the adult physicians soften this passage and can improve the chances for future compliance with the new system.

The AYA period is associated with the transition from childhood to adulthood beyond just the health care setting. AYA patients are concerned with the process of becoming mature independent individuals. Due to the nature of their chronic disease, patients have become dependent on parents and the medical staff. They must be encouraged to seek education and employment to further financial independence and to learn to take responsibility for their health needs. These processes are challenging for their healthy counterparts and even more so for AYAs with TM or SCD. According to a study by Compagno [82], adult TM patients spend 271 h per month on health care-related tasks. This burden interferes with studies and work opportunities. Intensive efforts by the psychosocial, nursing and medical staff are necessary to aid in preparing the young patients with hemoglobinopathy for independence and maturity.

Conclusion

The AYAs with hemoglobinopathies manifest age-related complications of their diseases as well as psychosocial challenges due to the process of maturation. For TM patients the cumulative effects of the disease and its treatment cause delayed puberty, reproductive dysfunction and potentially debilitating bone disease. Young SCD patients may suffer from silent brain ischemia causing mental deterioration, chronic lung disease and fertility disturbances. Improved medical therapy and accessibility of appropriate medical care insure that the vast majority of these patients will reach adulthood; they proceed through the process of maturation in terms of education, independence, interpersonal relationships and family planning, and in turn must undergo the process of transitioning from pediatric health care centers to the adult care system. The process of transitioning patients to adult health care must take into consideration the patients' preparedness, adult caretakers' expertise, transfer of medical information and the physical transfer of the patients to the adult medical service. Organized multidisciplinary transition programs will ease this process and improve the medical outcome of the patients.

References

1 Borgna-Pignatti C: The life of patients with thalassemia major. Haematologica 2010;95:345–348.
2 Ladis V, Chouliaras G, Berdoukas V, Chatziliami A, Fragodimitri C, Karabatsos F, Youssef J, Kattamis A, Karagiorga-Lagana M: Survival in a large cohort of Greek patients with transfusion-dependent beta thalassaemia and mortality ratios compared to the general population. Eur J Haematol 2011;86:332–338.
3 Platt OS, Brambilla DJ, Rosse WF, Milner PF, Castro O, Steinberg MH, Klug PP: Mortality in sickle cell disease. Life expectancy and risk factors for early death. N Engl J Med 1994;330:1639–1644.
4 Quinn CT, Rogers ZR, Buchanan GR: Survival of children with sickle cell disease. Blood 2004;103:4023–4027.
5 Modell B, Khan M, Darlison M, Westwood MA, Ingram D, Pennell DJ: Improved survival of thalassaemia major in the UK and relation to T2* cardiovascular magnetic resonance. J Cardiovasc Magn Reson 2008;10:42.
6 Rachmilewitz EA, Giardina PJ: How I treat thalassemia. Blood 2011;118:3479–3488.
7 Borgna-Pignatti C: Modern treatment of thalassaemia intermedia. Br J Haematol 2007;138:291–304.
8 Aessopos A, Farmakis D, Deftereos S, Tsironi M, Tassiopoulos S, Moyssakis I, Karagiorga M: Thalassemia heart disease: a comparative evaluation of thalassemia major and thalassemia intermedia. Chest 2005;127:1523–1530.

9 De Sanctis V, Eleftheriou A, Malaventura C: Prevalence of endocrine complications and short stature in patients with thalassaemia major: a multicenter study by the Thalassaemia International Federation (TIF). Pediatr Endocrinol Rev 2004;2(suppl 2):249–255.

10 Borgna-Pignatti C, Gamberini MR: Complications of thalassemia major and their treatment. Expert Rev Hematol 2011;4:353–366.

11 Soliman AT, Khalafallah H, Ashour R: Growth and factors affecting it in thalassemia major. Hemoglobin 2009;33(suppl 1):S116–S126.

12 Vogiatzi MG, Macklin EA, Trachtenberg FL, Fung EB, Cheung AM, Vichinsky E, Olivieri N, Kirby M, Kwiatkowski JL, Cunningham M, Holm IA, Fleisher M, Grady RW, Peterson CM, Giardina PJ: Differences in the prevalence of growth, endocrine and vitamin D abnormalities among the various thalassaemia syndromes in North America. Br J Haematol 2009;146:546–556.

13 Borgna-Pignatti C, Rugolotto S, De Stefano P, Zhao H, Cappellini MD, Del Vecchio GC, Romeo MA, Forni GL, Gamberini MR, Ghilardi R, Piga A, Cnaan A: Survival and complications in patients with thalassemia major treated with transfusion and deferoxamine. Haematologica 2004;89:1187–1193.

14 Chatterjee R, Bajoria R: Critical appraisal of growth retardation and pubertal disturbances in thalassemia. Ann NY Acad Sci 2010;1202:100–114.

15 Borgna-Pignatti C, De Stefano P, Zonta L, Vullo C, De Sanctis V, Melevendi C, Naselli A, Masera G, Terzoli S, Gabutti V, et al: Growth and sexual maturation in thalassemia major. J Pediatr 1985;106:150–155.

16 Shalitin S, Carmi D, Weintrob N, Phillip M, Miskin H, Kornreich L, Zilber R, Yaniv I, Tamary H: Serum ferritin level as a predictor of impaired growth and puberty in thalassemia major patients. Eur J Haematol 2005;74:93–100.

17 Noetzli LJ, Papudesi J, Coates TD, Wood JC: Pancreatic iron loading predicts cardiac iron loading in thalassemia major. Blood 2009;114:4021–4026.

18 Wood JC, Tyszka JM, Carson S, Nelson MD, Coates TD: Myocardial iron loading in transfusion-dependent thalassemia and sickle cell disease. Blood 2004;103:1934–1936.

19 Wood JC, Noetzl L, Hyderi A, Joukar M, Coates T, Mittelman S: Predicting pituitary iron and endocrine dysfunction. Ann NY Acad Sci 2010;1202:123–128.

20 Farmaki K, Tzoumari I, Pappa C, Chouliaras G, Berdoukas V: Normalisation of total body iron load with very intensive combined chelation reverses cardiac and endocrine complications of thalassaemia major. Br J Haematol 2010;148:466–475.

21 Singer ST, Vichinsky EP, Gildengorin G, van Disseldorp J, Rosen M, Cedars MI: Reproductive capacity in iron overloaded women with thalassemia major. Blood 2011;118:2878–2881.

22 Singer ST, Sweeters N, Vega O, Higa A, Vichinsky E, Cedars M: Fertility potential in thalassemia major women: current findings and future diagnostic tools. Ann NY Acad Sci 2010;1202:226–230.

23 Naik RP, Lanzkron S: Baby on board: what you need to know about pregnancy in the hemoglobinopathies. Hematol Am Soc Hematol Educ Program 2012, pp 208–214.

24 Safarinejad MR: Evaluation of semen quality, endocrine profile and hypothalamus-pituitary-testis axis in male patients with homozygous beta-thalassemia major. J Urol 2008;179:2327–2332.

25 Vogiatzi MG, Macklin EA, Fung EB, Vichinsky E, Olivieri N, Kwiatkowski J, Cohen A, Neufeld E, Giardina PJ: Prevalence of fractures among the thalassemia syndromes in North America. Bone 2006;38:571–575.

26 Skordis N, Toumba M: Bone disease in thalassaemia major: recent advances in pathogenesis and clinical aspects. Pediatr Endocrinol Rev 2011;8(suppl 2):300–306.

27 Lala R, Chiabotto P, Di Stefano M, Isaia GC, Garofalo F, Piga A: Bone density and metabolism in thalassaemia. J Pediatr Endocrinol Metab 1998;11(suppl 3):785–790.

28 Bielinski BK, Darbyshire PJ, Mathers L, Crabtree NJ, Kirk JM, Stirling HF, Shaw NJ: Impact of disordered puberty on bone density in beta-thalassaemia major. Br J Haematol 2003;120:353–358.

29 Vogiatzi MG, Autio KA, Mait JE, Schneider R, Lesser M, Giardina PJ: Low bone mineral density in adolescents with beta-thalassemia. Ann NY Acad Sci 2005;1054:462–466.

30 Benigno V, Bertelloni S, Baroncelli GI, Bertacca L, Di Peri S, Cuccia L, Borsellino Z, Maggio MC: Effects of thalassemia major on bone mineral density in late adolescence. J Pediatr Endocrinol Metab 2003;16(suppl 2):337–342.

31 Terpos E, Voskaridou E: Treatment options for thalassemia patients with osteoporosis. Ann NY Acad Sci 2010;1202:237–243.

32 Toumba M, Skordis N: Osteoporosis syndrome in thalassaemia major: an overview. J Osteoporos 2010;2010:537673.

33 Skordis N, Michaelidou M, Savva SC, Ioannou Y, Rousounides A, Kleanthous M, Skordos G, Christou S: The impact of genotype on endocrine complications in thalassaemia major. Eur J Haematol 2006;77:150–156.

34 Perrotta S, Cappellini MD, Bertoldo F, Servedio V, Iolascon G, D'Agruma L, Gasparini P, Siciliani MC, Iolascon A: Osteoporosis in beta-thalassaemia major patients: analysis of the genetic background. Br J Haematol 2000;111:461–466.

35 De Sanctis V: Growth and puberty and its management in thalassaemia. Horm Res 2002;58(suppl 1):72–79.

36 Scacchi M, Danesi L, Cattaneo A, Valassi E, Pecori Giraldi F, Argento C, D'Angelo E, Mirra N, Carnelli V, Zanaboni L, Cappellini MD, Cavagnini F: Growth hormone deficiency (GHD) in adult thalassaemic patients. Clin Endocrinol (Oxf) 2007;67:790–795.

37 Scacchi M, Danesi L, Cattaneo A, Valassi E, Pecori Giraldi F, Argento C, D'Angelo E, Mirra N, Carnelli V, Zanaboni L, Tampieri B, Cappellini MD, Cavagnini F: Bone demineralization in adult thalassaemic patients: contribution of GH and IGF-I at different skeletal sites. Clin Endocrinol (Oxf) 2008;69:202–207.

38 Fung EB: Nutritional deficiencies in patients with thalassemia. Ann NY Acad Sci 2010;1202:188–196.

39 Fung EB, Xu Y, Trachtenberg F, Odame I, Kwiatkowski JL, Neufeld EJ, Thompson AA, Boudreaux J, Quinn CT, Vichinsky EP: Inadequate dietary intake in patients with thalassemia. J Acad Nutr Diet 2012;112:980–990.

40 Ceci A, Baiardi P, Felisi M, Cappellini MD, Carnelli V, De Sanctis V, Galanello R, Maggio A, Masera G, Piga A, Schettini F, Stefano I, Tricta F: The safety and effectiveness of deferiprone in a large-scale, 3-year study in Italian patients. Br J Haematol 2002;118:330–336.

41 Erdogan E, Canatan D, Ormeci AR, Vural H, Aylak F: The effects of chelators on zinc levels in patients with thalassemia major. J Trace Elem Med Biol 2013;27:109–111.

42 Anapliotou ML, Kastanias IT, Psara P, Evangelou EA, Liparaki M, Dimitriou P: The contribution of hypogonadism to the development of osteoporosis in thalassaemia major: new therapeutic approaches. Clin Endocrinol (Oxf) 1995;42:279–287.

43 Lasco A, Morabito N, Gaudio A, Buemi M, Wasniewska M, Frisina N: Effects of hormonal replacement therapy on bone metabolism in young adults with beta-thalassemia major. Osteoporos Int 2001;12:570–575.

44 Skordis N, Ioannou YS, Kyriakou A, Savva SC, Efstathiou E, Savvides I, Christou S: Effect of bisphosphonate treatment on bone mineral density in patients with thalassaemia major. Pediatr Endocrinol Rev 2008;6(suppl 1):144–148.

45 Chatterjee R, Shah FT, Davis BA, Byers M, Sooranna D, Bajoria R, Pringle J, Porter JB: Prospective study of histomorphometry, biochemical bone markers and bone densitometric response to pamidronate in beta-thalassaemia presenting with osteopenia-osteoporosis syndrome. Br J Haematol 2012;159:462–471.

46 Forni GL, Perrotta S, Giusti A, Quarta G, Pitrolo L, Cappellini MD, D'Ascola DG, Borgna Pignatti C, Rigano P, Filosa A, Iolascon G, Nobili B, Baldini M, Rosa A, Pinto V, Palummeri E: Neridronate improves bone mineral density and reduces back pain in beta-thalassaemia patients with osteoporosis: results from a phase 2, randomized, parallel-arm, open-label study. Br J Haematol 2012;158:274–282.

47 Ballas SK, Kesen MR, Goldberg MF, Lutty GA, Dampier C, Osunkwo I, Wang WC, Hoppe C, Hagar W, Darbari DS, Malik P: Beyond the definitions of the phenotypic complications of sickle cell disease: an update on management. Scientific World Journal 2012;2012:949535.

48 McGann PT, Nero AC, Ware RE: Current management of sickle cell anemia. Cold Spring Harb Perspect Med 2013;3:a011817.

49 Quinn CT, Rogers ZR, McCavit TL, Buchanan GR: Improved survival of children and adolescents with sickle cell disease. Blood 2010; 115:3447–3452.

50 Hamideh D, Alvarez O: Sickle cell disease related mortality in the United States (1999–2009). Pediatr Blood Cancer 2013;60:1482–1486.

51 Vij R, Machado RF: Pulmonary complications of hemoglobinopathies. Chest 2010;138: 973–983.

52 Vichinsky EP, Styles LA, Colangelo LH, Wright EC, Castro O, Nickerson B: Acute chest syndrome in sickle cell disease: clinical presentation and course. Cooperative study of sickle cell disease. Blood 1997;89:1787–1792.

53 Vichinsky EP, Neumayr LD, Earles AN, Williams R, Lennette ET, Dean D, Nickerson B, Orringer E, McKie V, Bellevue R, Daeschner C, Manci EA: Causes and outcomes of the acute chest syndrome in sickle cell disease. National Acute Chest Syndrome Study Group. N Engl J Med 2000;342:1855–1865.

54 Styles LA, Schalkwijk CG, Aarsman AJ, Vichinsky EP, Lubin BH, Kuypers FA: Phospholipase A₂ levels in acute chest syndrome of sickle cell disease. Blood 1996;87:2573–2578.

55 Styles LA, Abboud M, Larkin S, Lo M, Kuypers FA: Transfusion prevents acute chest syndrome predicted by elevated secretory phospholipase A₂. Br J Haematol 2007;136:343–344.

56 Gladwin MT, Sachdev V, Jison ML, Shizukuda Y, Plehn JF, Minter K, Brown B, Coles WA, Nichols JS, Ernst I, Hunter LA, Blackwelder WC, Schechter AN, Rodgers GP, Castro O, Ognibene FP: Pulmonary hypertension as a risk factor for death in patients with sickle cell disease. N Engl J Med 2004;350:886–895.

57 Fonseca GH, Souza R, Salemi VM, Jardim CV, Gualandro SF: Pulmonary hypertension diagnosed by right heart catheterisation in sickle cell disease. Eur Respir J 2012;39:112–118.

58 Parent F, Bachir D, Inamo J, Lionnet F, Driss F, Loko G, Habibi A, Bennani S, Savale L, Adnot S, Maitre B, Yaici A, Hajji L, O'Callaghan DS, Clerson P, Girot R, Galacteros F, Simonneau G: A hemodynamic study of pulmonary hypertension in sickle cell disease. N Engl J Med 2011;365:44–53.

59 Colombatti R, Maschietto N, Varotto E, Grison A, Grazzina N, Meneghello L, Teso S, Carli M, Milanesi O, Sainati L: Pulmonary hypertension in sickle cell disease children under 10 years of age. Br J Haematol 2010;150:601–609.

60 Hagar RW, Michlitsch JG, Gardner J, Vichinsky EP, Morris CR: Clinical differences between children and adults with pulmonary hypertension and sickle cell disease. Br J Haematol 2008;140:104–112.

61 Minniti CP, Sable C, Campbell A, Rana S, Ensing G, Dham N, Onyekwere O, Nouraie M, Kato GJ, Gladwin MT, Castro OL, Gordeuk VR: Elevated tricuspid regurgitant jet velocity in children and adolescents with sickle cell disease: association with hemolysis and hemoglobin oxygen desaturation. Haematologica 2009;94:340–347.

62 Bernaudin F, Verlhac S, Arnaud C, Kamdem A, Chevret S, Hau I, Coic L, Leveille E, Lemarchand E, Lesprit E, Abadie I, Medejel N, Madhi F, Lemerle S, Biscardi S, Bardakdjian J, Galacteros F, Torres M, Kuentz M, Ferry C, Socie G, Reinert P, Delacourt C: Impact of early transcranial Doppler screening and intensive therapy on cerebral vasculopathy outcome in a newborn sickle cell anemia cohort. Blood 2011;117:1130–1140, quiz 1436.

63 DeBaun MR, Armstrong FD, McKinstry RC, Ware RE, Vichinsky E, Kirkham FJ: Silent cerebral infarcts: a review on a prevalent and progressive cause of neurologic injury in sickle cell anemia. Blood 2012;119:4587–4596.

64 DeBaun MR, Sarnaik SA, Rodeghier MJ, et al: Associated risk factors for silent cerebral infarcts in sickle cell anemia: low baseline hemoglobin, sex, and relative high systolic blood pressure. Blood 2012;119:3684–3690.

65 Schatz J, Brown RT, Pascual JM, Hsu L, DeBaun MR: Poor school and cognitive functioning with silent cerebral infarcts and sickle cell disease. Neurology 2001;56:1109–1111.

66 Dowling MM, Quinn CT, Rogers ZR, Buchanan GR: Acute silent cerebral infarction in children with sickle cell anemia. Pediatr Blood Cancer 2010;54:461–464.

67 Quinn CT, McKinstry RC, Dowling MM, Ball WS, Kraut MA, Casella JF, Dlamini N, Ichord RN, Jordan LC, Kirkham FJ, Noetzel MJ, Roach ES, Strouse JJ, Kwiatkowski JL, Hirtz D, DeBaun MR: Acute silent cerebral ischemic events in children with sickle cell anemia. JAMA Neurol 2013;70:58–65.

68 Vichinsky EP, Neumayr LD, Gold JI, Weiner MW, Rule RR, Truran D, Kasten J, Eggleston B, Kesler K, McMahon L, Orringer EP, Harrington T, Kalinyak K, De Castro LM, Kutlar A, Rutherford CJ, Johnson C, Bessman JD, Jordan LB, Armstrong FD: Neuropsychological dysfunction and neuroimaging abnormalities in neurologically intact adults with sickle cell anemia. JAMA 2010;303:1823–1831.

69 Hijmans CT, Fijnvandraat K, Grootenhuis MA, van Geloven N, Heijboer H, Peters M, Oosterlaan J: Neurocognitive deficits in children with sickle cell disease: a comprehensive profile. Pediatr Blood Cancer 2011;56:783–788.

70 Berthaut I, Guignedoux G, Kirsch-Noir F, de Larouziere V, Ravel C, Bachir D, Galacteros F, Ancel PY, Kunstmann JM, Levy L, Jouannet P, Girot R, Mandelbaum J: Influence of sickle cell disease and treatment with hydroxyurea on sperm parameters and fertility of human males. Haematologica 2008;93:988–993.

71 Howard J, Oteng-Ntim E: The obstetric management of sickle cell disease. Best Pract Res Clin Obstet Gynaecol 2012;26:25–36.

72 Villers MS, Jamison MG, De Castro LM, James AH: Morbidity associated with sickle cell disease in pregnancy. Am J Obstet Gynecol 2008;199:125.e121–e125.

73 American Academy of Pediatrics; American Academy of Family Physicians; American College of Physicians-American Society of Internal Medicine: A consensus statement on health care transitions for young adults with special health care needs. Pediatrics 2002;110: 1304–1306.

74 Borgna-Pignatti C, Cappellini MD, De Stefano P, Del Vecchio GC, Forni GL, Gamberini MR, Ghilardi R, Origa R, Piga A, Romeo MA, Zhao H, Cnaan A: Survival and complications in thalassemia. Ann NY Acad Sci 2005;1054:40–47.

75 Rosen DS, Blum RW, Britto M, Sawyer SM, Siegel DM: Transition to adult health care for adolescents and young adults with chronic conditions: position paper of the society for adolescent medicine. J Adolesc Health 2003; 33:309–311.

76 McPherson M, Thaniel L, Minniti CP: Transition of patients with sickle cell disease from pediatric to adult care: assessing patient readiness. Pediatr Blood Cancer 2009;52:838–841.

77 Van Staa AL, Jedeloo S, van Meeteren J, Latour JM: Crossing the transition chasm: experiences and recommendations for improving transitional care of young adults, parents and providers. Child Care Health Dev 2011;37: 821–832.

78 Smith GM, Lewis VR, Whitworth E, Gold DT, Thornburg CD: Growing up with sickle cell disease: a pilot study of a transition program for adolescents with sickle cell disease. J Pediatr Hematol Oncol 2011;33:379–382.

79 Fair CD, Sullivan K, Dizney R, Stackpole A: 'It's like losing a part of my family': transition expectations of adolescents living with perinatally acquired HIV and their guardians. AIDS Patient Care STDS 2012;26:423–429.

80 Levine L, Levine M: Health care transition in thalassemia: pediatric to adult-oriented care. Ann NY Acad Sci 2010;1202:244–247.

81 Jordan L, Swerdlow P, Coates TD: Systematic review of transition from adolescent to adult care in patients with sickle cell disease. J Pediatr Hematol Oncol 2013;35:165–169.

82 Compagno LM: Caring for adults with thalassemia in a pediatric world. Ann NY Acad Sci 2005;1054:266–272.

83 Bryant R, Young A, Cesario S, Binder B: Transition of chronically ill youth to adult health care: experience of youth with hemoglobinopathy. J Pediatr Health Care 2011;25:275–283.

84 Musallam K, Cappellini MD, Taher A: Challenges associated with prolonged survival of patients with thalassemia: transitioning from childhood to adulthood. Pediatrics 2008; 121:e1426–e1429.

85 Lebensburger JD, Bemrich-Stolz CJ, Howard TH: Barriers in transition from pediatrics to adult medicine in sickle cell anemia. J Blood Med 2012;3:105–112.

Acta Haematol 2014;132:348–362
DOI: 10.1159/000360197

Published online: September 10, 2014

Adherence-Related Issues in Adolescents and Young Adults with Hematological Disorders

Avi Leader[a, b]   Pia Raanani[a, b]

[a]Institute of Hematology, Davidoff Center, Beilinson Hospital, Rabin Medical Center, Petah Tikva, and
[b]Sackler School of Medicine, Tel Aviv University, Tel Aviv, Israel

Key Words

Adherence · Adolescents and young adults · Compliance

Abstract

Nonadherence to medical recommendations is a widespread problem well documented in a multitude of clinical settings. Nonadherence may adversely affect clinical outcomes such as survival and quality of life and increase health-care-related costs. An understanding of the factors driving nonadherence is key to developing effective adherence-enhancing interventions (AEIs). There are ongoing attempts in contemporary adherence research to better define the various components of adherence, to find optimal measures of adherence and correlations with clinical outcomes, and to create a classification system for AEIs. Nonadherence is also widely prevalent among adolescents and young adults (AYAs) with chronic hematological diseases, affecting up to 50% of patients and increasing with age. Combined use of objective (i.e. electronic monitoring, EM) and subjective (i.e. self-report) measures of adherence may be the preferred approach to assess adherence. The unique physical, social and emotional aspects of the AYA life stage are closely related to intricate causes of nonadherence in AYAs such as problems in transition to adult care. Until proven otherwise, the empirical target in AYAs with hematological disorders should be perfect adherence. Multilevel AEIs, EM feedback and behavioral interventions are among the most effective types of AEIs. Despite the magnitude of the problem, only a handful of AEIs have been evaluated among AYAs with hematological disorders. Thus, this is a field with unmet needs warranting high-quality trials using standardized and well-specified assessment methods and interventions. This review discusses the prevalence, definition, causes and clinical implications of nonadherence among AYAs with hematological disorders, along with strategies to measure and improve adherence.

© 2014 S. Karger AG, Basel

Introduction

Nonadherence to treatment recommendations is common in general medical practice [1] and is also widespread among adolescents and young adults (AYAs) with cancer, especially those taking self-administered treatment such as oral chemotherapy [2–4]. Nonadherence to medical treatment is associated with adverse clinical outcomes [5–9], increased health-care-related financial burden [10, 11] and reduced quality of life [12–14]. The im-

Avi Leader, MD
Institute of Hematology, Davidoff Center
Beilinson Hospital, Rabin Medical Center
39 Jabotinsky Street, Petah Tikva 49100 (Israel)
E-Mail avileader@yahoo.com

portance of adherence to medical treatment is highlighted by the World Health Organization which considers nonadherence to be a major public health concern [15].

The high stakes involved in the treatment of hematological disorders should intuitively be a motivator for adherence but in reality have a complex interplay with various aspects of the AYA life stage. One of the proposed explanations for inferior treatment outcomes among AYAs with cancer, including acute myeloid leukemia and acute lymphoblastic leukemia (ALL), compared to the advances made in the treatment of childhood cancers, is suboptimal adherence to treatment regimens in AYAs [16]. Consequently, promotion of adherence has been recognized as one of the markers of quality of cancer care for AYAs with cancer [17]. Inconsistencies in the definition of the age of AYAs (from 12–16 years up to 24–39 years old) affect the quality of evidence on all aspects of health care for AYAs, including the field of adherence [18].

The aim of this review is to provide an understanding of the existing literature and its limitations regarding the definition, measurement methods, prevalence, clinical importance and causes of nonadherence among AYAs with hematological disorders, as well as a review of relevant adherence-enhancing interventions (AEIs). There are some key areas of adherence which lack adequate evidence relating to the specialized patient population of AYAs with hematological disorders. In such cases, we rely upon the literature on adolescents with cancer, AYAs with nonhematological chronic disease and children or older patients with hematological disorders, and attempt to extrapolate this data to AYAs with hematological disorders. When hard evidence is lacking, we hypothesize using experience gained by us and others through working with AYAs.

Search Strategy

The NIH PubMed electronic database was searched for articles published before August 31, 2013, using filters for 'Humans' and 'English'. A search aimed at identifying articles on adherence in AYAs with hematological disorders yielded 69 articles. A search of studies related to adherence in children with hematological disorders found 773 papers. While these searches were the main source of the review, a search of adherence among AYAs in general and older adults with hematological disorders was also performed (see online suppl. table 1 for the detailed search terms; for all online suppl. material, see www.

karger.com/doi/10.1159/000360197). The focus was placed upon publications from the past 10 years. Moreover, reference lists of articles identified by this search strategy were searched, and relevant articles were selected for review. All publication types were reviewed, but more focus was placed upon studies which were larger and more methodologically sound. The tables summarizing relevant studies in the field of adherence among AYAs focused mainly upon studies published in the last 10 years, as older studies have been summarized in tabular form in other recent reviews [19, 20].

General Adherence Concepts

Terminology and Defining Adherence

The terms 'adherence', 'compliance', 'persistence', 'therapeutic alliance', 'concordance' and 'collaboration', among others, are often used interchangeably to describe the relationship between actual consumption of medications and the agreed-upon recommendations of a health care professional. A classic definition of compliance is 'the extent to which a person's behavior, in terms of taking medication, following diets or executing lifestyle changes, coincides with medical or health advice' [21] and suggests obedience to the health care professional [22]. In the contemporary patient-centered medical climate, adherence has become the preferable term, as it implies shared decision-making between the patient and health care provider regarding the therapeutic process, usually within a certain time period. Kyngas et al. [23] defined adherence as 'an active, intentional and responsible process of care, in which the individual works to maintain his or her health, in close collaboration with health care personnel'. We will utilize the term 'adherence' throughout this review. 'Adherence' is a heterogeneous process which varies along the timeline of implementing a medical recommendation. In an attempt to clarify this heterogeneity, 3 phases of adherence have recently been proposed: initiation, implementation and persistence. Importantly, the causes, clinical relevance [24] and possible solutions of nonadherence may differ between the 3 above phases. In addition, there are several adherence subtypes [25] demonstrating that the term 'adherence' relates to concordance not only with recommended medical regimens (i.e. pharmacoadherence) [25], but also with control of symptoms and adverse events, seeking medical help, attending clinic appointments [26], infectious precautions, prevention and reduction of late effects [27, 28] (e.g. lifestyle recommendations [29]) and interventions aimed at improving quality of life, each of which have a different role in the therapeutic regimen.

How to Assess Adherence
This is a critical aspect of adherence-related research since the quality of the adherence assessment is one of the best predictors of improving clinical outcomes [30]. Adherence measures can be divided into 3 categories: direct or indirect measures, which are either objective or subjective measures [1, 25]. *Direct measures* such as directly observed therapy and biochemical assays are *objective* and provide hard evidence that the medication has been consumed. Regarding the latter, the relationship between drug ingestion, measured levels and clinical outcomes depends upon multiple factors and needs to be researched for each drug and each patient population. *Indirect measures* which are *objective* include electronic monitoring (EM), pill-counting, medicine returned, pharmacy refill data and therapeutic outcomes. Electronic methods of measuring pill-taking have been validated in measuring adherence to drug medication and are widely considered as one of the most important means of monitoring adherence [1], in the absence of a uniform gold standard. Among other things, these indirect measures do not provide insight into the reasons behind nonadherence, and EM devices are also expensive and sometimes impractical. Moreover, therapeutic outcomes, for example, are affected by a multitude of factors besides adherence. *Subjective* measures of adherence are self-report measures (diaries, interviews, questionnaires) and can be divided into clinician-reported outcomes and patient-reported outcomes. They may be generic or disease specific, provide insight into the mechanisms behind nonadherence, and are easy and cheap to administer, but may be hampered by recall bias and efforts to please the health care provider. *Indirect* and *subjective* measures merely suggest that the health care recommendation has been carried out. Examples of each measure and their advantages and disadvantages are detailed in table 1.

Self-report measures overestimate adherence in AYAs and older adults with hematological disorders [6, 31–33] and other chronic disorders as much as twofold [31], when compared to *objective* measures such as EM, pill-counting and bioassays. For example, in the field of tyrosine kinase inhibitor (TKI) treatment in chronic myeloid leukemia (CML), such devices have been shown to reflect adherence more objectively than questionnaires and pill-counting, correlating with cytogenetic and molecular outcomes [6, 7]. This may explain why the association

between adherence and therapeutic outcomes seems to be stronger when evaluated by objective measures [9]. Among AYAs, different adherence measures may have distinct associations with clinical outcomes [9].

When interpreting results from a measure of adherence, one should consider the time frame which it represents [34] since certain time frames may display significantly stronger relationships between adherence and clinical outcome than others (e.g. past month or 24 h vs. past week, respectively, in AYAs with HIV [9]). On the other hand, recall periods longer than a month may interfere with the capture of accurate and valid adherence behavior. This is especially applicable to nonobjective adherence measures. An inherent limitation of research regarding adherence is that patients consenting to take part in a prospective trial may have a higher (or in certain circumstances lower) adherence than nonparticipants and that the act of participating in a clinical trial and monitoring adherence may change adherence-related behavior [35], especially during the first month of the study. EM, especially, has been shown to have an intervention effect which wanes over the course of up to 5 weeks [36, 37]. To counteract the latter, a 'washout' period of 30–45 days at the beginning of the trial, during which adherence is measured but not included in the analysis, may be considered [36].

In summary, each of the above methods for assessing adherence provides unique information on different aspects of adherence-related behavior, not provided by other methods. Thus, although there is no gold standard for measuring adherence [1], a deep understanding of adherence behavior can be achieved by the combined use of objective and self-report measures.

Defining Nonadherence
At present there is no consensus on what represents nonadherence, and the definition therefore varies between studies [9], precluding the comparison of results from adherence research. Nonadherence may be presented via cutoff values [33, 38] (e.g. <85%), anything other than perfect adherence [8, 39], or it may be portrayed as a continuous variable. Ideally, there should be a definition for nonadherence for each AYA disease subset, specifying the preferred adherence measure. Nonadherence should be defined according to its impact on therapeutic outcomes [40]. Since currently evidence-based recommendations cannot be made regarding adherence targets for AYAs in hematology, the empirical target should be perfect adherence, especially in light of convincing data from children and adolescents with ALL showing an increase in relapse risk when adherence to purinethol main-

Table 1. Methods for measuring treatment adherence

Type of measure	Advantage	Disadvantage	Example
Direct measures			
Direct observation	Objective, highly specific	Time and labor consuming; interferes with daily living and is thus less feasible on an outpatient basis; Hawthorne effect	Directly observed therapy among patients with tuberculosis [134]
Bioassay: serum/ urine/saliva [2, 31, 32, 135, 136]	Objective; proves that drug has been ingested; may be part of standard care; in selected cases random measures may represent extended time periods [34]; may correlate with other measures of adherence [34]	The nature of the association between adherence, measured drug levels and clinical outcomes is usually not known; other factors influence drug levels; usually a one-off measurement not reflecting daily behavior; costly; invasive; technology exists for selected drugs only; relevant only for pharmacoadherence; no insight into the cause of nonadherence	Serum levels of methotrexate, even when taken randomly, were associated with subjectively measured adherence to treatment in childhood ALL patients on maintenance therapy (n = 49) [34]
Indirect measures			
Prescription monitoring/refill records	Objective; easily obtained; standardized; inexpensive; provides information on a specific level of the pharmacoadherence process (pharmacy refill); may correlate with EM-measured adherence, adherence behaviors and clinical outcomes; most accurate measure in large populations	Provides information only on drug acquisition – consumption is assumed; may be misinterpreted if dose is changed or other sources of medication exist (e.g. free drug samples); no insight into the cause of nonadherence	Children with SCD had a prescription refill rate of 58.4% (folic acid, hydroxyurea, penicillin and asthma medications) [52]
Pill counts	Objective; inexpensive; unannounced counts correlate well with EM	Time consuming; complex computations; subject to patient interference [137]; assumption made that medication not counted was consumed; no insight into the cause of nonadherence; overestimates pharmaco-adherence	71% of children or adolescents (n = 21) with SCD were adherent (≥80% or prescribed dose) to deferasirox according to self-reports, while pill count-measured adherence was 43% because of poor bottle return [33]
EM [8, 32, 138]	Objective; time and date tracking; detects pill-dumping; more sensitive than pill-counting and subjective measures; correlated with clinical outcomes in adult CML and childhood/ adolescent ALL [8], among others	Costly; may malfunction; not effective with pillboxes or liquid medications; may be bulky and inconvenient; assumption made that medication removed from bottle was consumed; little insight into the cause of nonadherence	Statistically significant increase in risk of ALL relapse with every 5% decrease in adherence to maintenance purinethol therapy [8]
Therapeutic outcomes	Measured as part of standard care	Influenced by many other variables; poor substitute for more direct measures; low validity and reliability	MCV and HbF levels in SCD [139]
Subjective measures			
Patient-reported outcomes (e.g. diaries, questionnaires, VAS, interviews) [99, 140–143]	Simplistic; quick; inexpensive; affords insight into patterns and causes of various subtypes of nonadherence; may predict clinical outcomes; relatively specific for nonadherence; may correlate with bioassays [34] and EM	Social desirability bias [144]; recall bias; overestimates pharmacoadherence [6, 31, 32]; insensitive; performed during clinic visits around which adherence increases; generally unreliable	(1) Example of a self-report question: 'It is common that patients at times miss a few doses, for a whole range of reasons. Thinking of the past 7 days, have you missed any doses?' [69] (2) BAASIS (composed of 4 questions): designed for immunosuppressive medication [145] and adapted for CML [39] (3) VERITAS-Pro: 24-item scale which measures adherence levels among the hemophilia population. Subscales are time, dose, plan, skipping of doses and communication [13, 142] (4) Chronic disease compliance instrument: an 18-item scale measure of adherence to medical treatment of young people with cancer [32, 146]
Clinician-reported outcomes	Simplistic; quick; inexpensive; relatively specific for nonadherence; may predict clinical outcomes	Interactions with patients and knowledge of clinical outcomes may cause bias; insensitive	Physician VAS: rates patient adherence from 'never takes their medication' to 'always takes their medication' on a 10-cm VAS; promising sensitivity and specificity compared with EM (64 and 77%, respectively) and pill count (89 and 82%, respectively) when measuring adherence to antiretroviral drugs in HIV-positive adults [147]

Hawthorne effect = The alteration of behavior by the subjects because they are being observed; SCD = sickle cell disease; CML = chronic myeloid leukemia; MCV = mean corpuscular volume; HbF = hemoglobin F; BAASIS = Basel assessment of adherence to immunosuppressive medication scale; VERITAS = validated hemophilia regimen treatment adherence scale for prophylaxis; VAS = visual analog scale.

Acta Haematol 2014;132:348–362
DOI: 10.1159/000360197

tenance therapy drops below 95% [8]. Researchers should strive to create a definition based on clinically relevant associations [9, 41] from past and future clinical trials on adherence. Adherence as a continuous variable should always be analyzed and can deepen the understanding of the effects of nonadherence. Furthermore, nonadherence can be classified as low-risk and high-risk, depending on the variable which is assessed (e.g. not adhering to sun protection vs. not seeking medical care in the case of fever).

Adolescents and Young Adults

Overview of the Unique Aspects of Adherence in AYAs
The AYA life stage is a time of physical and emotional change, which is most prominent during adolescence [42]. AYAs transitioning into young adulthood strive to achieve financial and emotional independence, academic and occupational advances and meaningful long-term relationships. An integral part of this process involves coming to terms with their own actions. This developmental stage also influences the understanding of the disease and treatment. These unique aspects affect the way in which a patient in the AYA life stage deals with a new diagnosis and treatment of a life-threatening and/or chronic disease. In particular, these multiple factors may compromise an important facet of the treatment framework: adherence to medical recommendations.

Many of the barriers to adherence in AYAs are related to the intricate process of transition to adult care, which affects patients, parents and health care providers. Core themes of this transition are: leaving familiar surroundings, cultural gaps between pediatric and adult care, lack of communication between pediatric and adult care providers and lack of preparation [43]. For example, the refusal to comply with recommendations of the health care provider may just be another means of asserting their independence from adult control. Nonadherence may also be a sign of distress in this population, which is often subjected to societal prejudice. Accordingly, suspicion of nonadherence should trigger an honest, nonjudgmental and confidential dialogue regarding treatment plans and ways to accommodate the AYA's wishes and needs. As succinctly put by Butow et al. [19] in a review of adherence in AYAs with cancer: 'Addressing these issues as part of a holistic approach to working with AYA patients is necessary not only to avoid long-term complications but as insurance against nonadherence motivated by any of these real AYA concerns.'

Prevalence of Nonadherence
Nonadherence to treatment is widely prevalent in chronic diseases in all age groups, but especially in AYAs with chronic diseases where nonadherence can reach 50% [1]. AYAs with hematological disorders and other chronic illnesses such as cystic fibrosis, asthma or inflammatory bowel disease are less adherent than younger and older patients, even when disease and treatment parameters are comparable [4, 44, 45]. One surprising exception is that of bone marrow transplantation where younger patients seem to be less adherent than adolescents [46]. Nonadherence is also prevalent, somewhat counterintuitively, in the context of potentially lifesaving treatment for diseases such as cancer [47]. Objective data from a recently published, well-designed study show that 44% of children and adolescents with ALL were not fully adherent to purinethol maintenance treatment [8]. Estimates of nonadherence to oral anticancer therapy [8, 48] and preventative guidelines [29, 48] range between 27 and 63% in studies of cancer patients which include, at least in part, cohorts of adolescents or young adults [2, 3, 32, 46, 48, 49]. This variance in reported rates of nonadherence is a result of the multiple factors involved in the evaluation of adherence to medical recommendations, namely the type of study population (e.g. age, sex, demographic variables, type of disease), the type of treatment or behavior evaluated (the majority of data is on pharmacoadherence), the measure used to assess adherence and the definition of nonadherence. To highlight the importance of defining nonadherence, as discussed above, when adherence is defined as perfect adherence, more than 70% of certain AYA [50] or adult [39] hematology populations may be nonadherent according to self-report.

Nonadherence is also prevalent among AYAs with nonmalignant hematological disorders, receiving attention especially in hemophilia and sickle cell disease (SCD). Nonadherence to iron chelation among children and AYAs with SCD reaches up to approximately 30–60% [33, 51, 52], while nonadherence to hydroxyurea may be closer to 10–30% [50, 53, 54] and nonadherence to transcranial Doppler ultrasonography screening was 31% [28]. In one study, only 61% of SCD participants had attended the guideline-recommended number of clinic meetings in the previous year [26]. Adherence to acute medications, such as in the context of pain episodes in adolescents with SCD [55], seems to be higher than adherence to chronic medications (e.g. penicillin prophylaxis, iron chelation and hydroxyurea treatment, in the case of SCD) [50, 51]. Interestingly, estimates of nonadherence seem to be stable over time and are more affected by the assessment measure than by age of data.

Acta Haematol 2014;132:348–362
DOI: 10.1159/000360197

Effect of Adherence on Clinical Outcomes

Contemporary treatment guidelines for hematological disorders in AYAs emphasize the importance of treatment adherence. The logic behind this recommendation is obvious; however, there is a paucity of high-quality evidence clearly proving the association between adherence and clinical end points in hematology, especially in the field of AYAs.

The main evidence on the effect of adherence on clinical outcomes in AYAs with hematological disorders stems from studies on pediatric and adolescent ALL, SCD in AYAs, adolescents with hemophilia and cohorts of AYAs with cancer, including hematological malignancies. A recently published landmark study demonstrated an association between relapse risk and EM-measured adherence to purinethol maintenance treatment among 327 children and adolescents (>12 years) with ALL [8]. Fifty-nine percent of relapses in this study were associated with nonadherence. The clinical significance of adherence has also been recognized regarding contemporary cancer therapy which increasingly utilizes oral agents, characterized by the association between worse overall survival and nonadherence to adjuvant hormonal therapy for adults with breast cancer [56]. Notably, survivors of cancer during adolescence and young adulthood, including hematological malignancies, have an inferior health status compared to subjects with no history of cancer [57, 58] which may be mediated by nonadherence to follow-up guidelines [29, 59–62]. In addition, adherence to clotting factor prophylactic regimens is associated with improved joint outcomes [63] and less breakthrough bleeding [5], and is low among hemophilia A or B patients of all ages [63]. Finally, adherence to treatment may be associated with an improved health-related quality of life, as shown, for example, in hemophilia and SCD patients [12–14].

As a result of its association with clinical outcomes, poor adherence can also influence the results of clinical trials, leading to inaccurate estimates of true treatment efficacy [64]. Another aspect that warrants understanding is whether the association between adherence and clinical outcomes reaches a plateau above a certain adherence threshold, which could aid in defining adherence targets in trials assessing AEIs. A recent meta-analysis suggests that such a plateau may exist among AYAs with HIV regarding the association between adherence to antiretroviral therapy and virological response [9]. In contrast, no such plateau has been shown for adherence to TKIs in adults with CML [41, 65]. Such data may guide the design of future studies evaluating AEIs, regarding thresholds of adherence indicative of clinical relevance. One should also recognize that monitoring and improving adherence is accompanied by certain burdens. This process is not always desired by patients who may perceive this as a reminder of their illness and as an unnecessary burden [66], and it also demands health care system resources. Thus, like any intervention in medicine, one should be sure of its efficacy before implementing it.

In summary, improved adherence in itself should not be viewed as the main goal, but as a means of achieving optimal outcomes of therapy. In order to effectively design and validate AEIs, it must be clear which causes and outcomes of nonadherence are targeted and affected, respectively. This important goal can only be achieved if the effect of adherence on clinical outcomes in AYAs is clearly plotted.

Causes of Nonadherence

Adherence to medical therapy is a complex health behavior. Factors for nonadherence in non-AYA patients with hematological illness may be amplified in AYAs. The literature relies upon qualitative studies, often with small sample sizes involving questionnaires and in-depth interviews, and systematic reviews regarding the reasons of nonadherence, some of which present complex models of nonadherence [67, 68]. Those in the field of hematology [69, 70] may afford a unique insight into these diseases, and multicomponent tools can enable an integrated assessment of risk of nonadherence [71, 72]. One qualitative study of 6 AYA patients under maintenance therapy for ALL identified 4 critical elements affecting adherence: a desire for normalcy, egocentrism, concrete thinking and parental involvement [73]. AYAs have unique factors predisposing to nonadherence, which recur in different disease and treatment settings and are discussed in general below. When applicable, disease- and treatment-specific barriers to adherence will be noted.

Adherence is affected at multiple levels and different stages of the treatment process. In analyzing adherence to TKIs in CML, Gater et al. [68] proposed a sequential model of predisposing factors, patient interaction with physician and health care systems, adherence and persistence, and benefits of adherence, comprised of modifiable or fixed variables. The barriers to adherence in AYAs will be discussed below according to these categories, modified for AYAs.

Predisposing Factors
Patient Characteristics. Increasing age [8, 13, 74], low socioeconomic status [75–77] and financial problems

which can accompany this life stage [42] are all potential risk factors for nonadherence among AYAs. Adherence is also influenced by health status [76] and linguistic, cultural and social issues [78]. Ethnicity has a proven association with adherence among adolescents with ALL [8].

Disease Characteristics. Disease severity [79] and complications [80], along with adverse clinical experiences [76], have a negative impact on adherence.

Treatment Characteristics. Increased complexity of the therapeutic regimen [81], longer treatment duration [8], higher patient costs, unpleasant side effects [4] and fears about the effect on fertility [82] are all associated with decreased adherence. However, this association between treatment characteristics and nonadherence is not as clear in AYAs with cancer as it is in adult patients, and warrants future research.

Family and Caregiver Factors. Type of household structure and parent partnership status correlate with adherence in children and adolescents, namely decreased adherence among children of single mothers [8, 83]. Positive family relationships and open communication between family members promote adherence [84] among adolescents. On the other hand, certain patterns of parental behavior are associated with nonadherence [85], such as controlling parent-child relationships [86]. Moreover, dysfunctional family communication and family conflict can adversely affect adherence [87] to medication and disease-monitoring among adolescents. Caregiver knowledge of the disease and treatment [88] is also an important barrier to adherence.

Physician Characteristics. Data regarding TKI adherence among adults with CML have shown that longer duration of the first and subsequent clinic visits, more years of professional experience and number of active CML patients seen in the previous year all positively affected adherence [39]. There is reason to believe that these factors also influence adherence in AYAs with hematological disorders, especially the latter regarding experience treating AYAs.

Patient Interaction with Physician and Health Care Systems

Physician Interaction. The patient and caregiver interaction with the physician and health care system can influence adherence among children [89] and adults [66, 69]. Good patient-provider communication and relationships positively correlate with adherence to treatment and clinic appointments [76, 90], whereas controlling physician-patient relationships may negatively impact an adolescent's adherence to treatment [86]. In addition, inconsistencies in the physician's behavior, including nonadherence to practice guidelines and not meeting the needs of parents and adolescents, may cause nonadherence to medical treatment [91]. Clinic attendance does not ensure adherence to medical treatment [50] but has been associated with increased adherence to medical recommendations such as screening guidelines in SCD [28].

Patient Knowledge, Beliefs and Life Skills. Knowledge about the disease, knowledge about therapy and its relationship to health (e.g. instructions and effectiveness) [3, 48, 92, 93], perceptions of one's ability to influence health outcomes [94] and confidence in one's ability to meet the specific demands of cancer treatment and recovery [95], are all cognitive and motivational processes with the potential to influence treatment adherence. For example, patients are often not aware of the therapeutic effects of potentially lifesaving treatment which they are prescribed [79]. Decision-making competence [96] and patient involvement in decision-making [97], along with faith in the treatment option and physician [39], are additional barriers to adherence. Compensatory beliefs (i.e. the conviction that negative disease-related behavior may be offset by a different positive behavior) may also be present among AYAs [98].

Transitions in Care and Treatment. Transitions in patient care, such as treatment provider, treatment regimen [13] and transition away from parental involvement [42], may result in decreased adherence in AYAs. These transitions often coincide with leaving home, starting college, beginning a new job or other major changes in a patient's life.

Adherence and Persistence

Social Life, Friends and Lifestyle Factors. This category is of special importance among AYAs who have competing activities [99] and life obligations [42, 76] which may affect adherence. Supporting participation in usual activities is related to adherence [84]. Likewise, rite-of-passage events, which can be related to school, university or the patient's profession, among other things, can create adherence problems and should be supported. To achieve the above, the treatment team has to get to know the young patient.

Treatment Satisfaction. Medication side effects experienced by patients may cause nonadherence [69, 99], which is often intentional.

Unintentional Factors. Unintentional nonadherence is most commonly caused by forgetfulness which may, in some cases, explain more than 50% of nonadherence [74].

Acta Haematol 2014;132:348–362
DOI: 10.1159/000360197

Among AYAs, this may be related, for example, to alcohol consumption, preoccupation with illness and concerns about medication. Unintentional nonadherence may be more common than intentional nonadherence in children and adolescents under maintenance therapy for ALL [99], although both are important aspects of nonadherence. Other important contributors towards unintentional nonadherence include transportation difficulties [76], trouble obtaining pharmacy refills and the inconvenience of attending clinic visits [54]. Unintentional factors may interplay with lifestyle factors. Thus, unintentional nonadherence has a complex relationship with other barriers to adherence and may mediate their effect on intentional nonadherence [100].

Behavioral Aspects and Management. Growing independence and lack of appropriate social support [42] during treatment and follow-up are key factors affecting adherence in AYAs. In fact, nonadherence may merely be a means of expressing rebellion and independence. Although involvement of parents in the treatment regimen of adolescents and patient-parent agreement on allocation of responsibility for medication administration [92] are associated with increased adherence [33, 101], the transition into adulthood necessitates decreasing parental involvement, making parental involvement a complex process. Proven behavioral contributors towards nonadherence in AYA patients under leukemia maintenance therapy are the administration of therapy at bedtime and the lack of monitoring [99]. The adolescents' tendency to focus on short-term goals may explain poor adherence to recommendations aimed at preventing late effects of therapy [29, 59–62]. This short-term focus may result in reinforcement of negative adherence behavior if nonadherence yields no immediate negative consequences, or if initial adherence to treatment causes immediate adverse effects.

Emotion and Coping. Disordered emotional functioning and self-esteem are associated with adherence issues. Depression and anxiety [102] can adversely affect treatment adherence, especially intentional nonadherence [103], as seen for example in adolescents and adults with thalassemia.

Finally, the benefits of adherence balanced against the hazards of nonadherence, especially its impact on clinical outcome as discussed above, reinforce adherence to treatment.

Adherence-Enhancing Interventions

Despite the potentially grave consequences of nonadherence [104, 105], there is a paucity of evidence-based interventions for improving adherence in the hematology AYA population. Thus, our knowledge on AEIs in this population is derived from studies on AYAs and children with other chronic diseases [106]. The magnitude of the effect of AEIs varies, but a recent meta-analysis of randomized controlled trials (RCTs), assessing adherence by electronically compiled drug-dosing histories and including patients of all ages, evaluated the effect of AEIs and showed that adherence was 14.1% higher in the intervention group than in the control group [107]. AEIs should target specific barriers to adherence, which are discussed elsewhere in this review, and be adapted for the AYA patient who is continuously evolving. In one small study on AYAs with SCD, 47% preferred an individualized solution to adherence barriers [50]. Therefore, the first step towards improving adherence is identifying these barriers, ideally at the level of the individual patient. This may be facilitated by using a disease- and age-specific 'barriers to care' questionnaire [108] for patients and caregivers, which can be web-based [50], especially when initiating care for an AYA but also at care-related and development-related milestones. Thus, future interventions could be tailored, perhaps interactively [26] and based on patient preferences, to the unique needs of each AYA.

There are different types of AEIs, which target different barriers of adherence and suit different patients. We have adapted taxonomy used in previous studies and reviews to categorize these interventions [81, 107]. These categories are discussed below and examples of each type of intervention and their efficacy are presented in table 2.

Directly Observed Therapy

Directly observed therapy is mainly in use for ensuring adherence to antimycobacterial drugs in adults and adolescents. Although it is resource and time consuming, it has been proven to improve adherence in the above setting and also among adolescents with iron deficiency anemia in rural areas [109].

Web- and Telephone-Based Technologies

This represents a fast-developing method of assessing adherence and delivering various types of interventions, such as reminders, education and behavioral interventions. This technology base may enable effective, standardized and cost-effective assessment of adherence and intervention [110], especially in AYAs who are highly engaged in media-based social networking and seeking health information [111]. Web-based interventions can disperse educational material and facilitate tailored

Table 2. Examples of studies assessing AEIs in AYAs and hematology patients

Classification	Condition	Target population	Intervention	Design and effect size estimation (sample size)	Target variables (causing nonadherence)	Results
AYAs[a] in hematology[b]	Iron deficiency anemia [109]	Women and adolescent girls	DOT	RCT; 524 DOT, 523 self-treated	Multifactorial	DOT group had higher adherence (93 vs. 60%, p < 0.0001) and higher Hb
	Cancer survivors (leukemia >50%) [61, 62]	AYA (11–21 years) survivors of childhood cancer	Group-based intervention focusing on education regarding bone health [61] and protective UV behavior [62].	RCT; n = 75	Awareness of cancer late effects; perceived benefits of health-promoting behaviors; self-efficacy to lead a healthy lifestyle	Significant increase in calcium intake and sun safety practices compared to control group receiving standard leaflets
	Cancer (>65% with hematological malignancy such as leukemia or lymphoma) [32]	AYAs (13–29 years)	Behavioral intervention using a video game that addressed issues of cancer treatment and care for teenagers and young adults; behavioral objectives were translated into game structure	Multicenter RCT; n = 375; adherence assessed by EM of TMP/SMX consumption or serum metabolite levels (purinethol)	Cognitive and motivational processes: knowledge of therapy, perceived control and cancer-specific self-efficacy	Objectively measured adherence to 6MP and TMP/SMX, and self-efficacy and knowledge (TMP/SMX only), was greater in the intervention group; self-report measures of adherence were not affected
Childhood hematology[b]	SCD [132]	Children	Structured telephone-based outreach, including structured follow-up, support and education provided by nonmedical personnel	Single-center 'before-after' cohort; n = 147: postintervention adherence confirmed with baseline adherence; adherence assessed objectively from clinic records	Education; unintentional nonadherence	Attendance to comprehensive care clinic and transcranial Doppler ultrasonography improved after the intervention (improving from 80 to 90% and 34 to 49%, respectively)
	ALL [77]	Children	Structured parental education program	Single-center retrospective review of charts before (n = 164) and after (n = 119) the implementation of an institutional parental education program	Education	After introduction of the intervention, treatment refusal significantly decreased (from 14 to 2%) and event-free survival significantly increased (from 13 to 29%) among low-income families
Adults[c] in hematology	Newly diagnosed hematological malignancy [31]	Adults	Intensive one-on-one interventions incorporating training in pill-taking, education and home psychological support	n = 108; treatment with allopurinol and prednisone; design: 'before-after' cohort study; adherence measured by self-report measures and drug metabolite monitoring	Education; psychological barriers; unintentional nonadherence	Adherence to allopurinol, but not to prednisone, was improved compared to baseline in patients receiving any of the interventions

DOT = Directly observed therapy; Hb = hemoglobin; 6MP = 6-mercaptopurine; RCT = randomized controlled trials; TMP/SMX = trimethoprim-sulfamethoxazole; UV = ultraviolet.
[a] With or without children.
[b] Either alone or as part of a larger cohort (e.g. cancer cohorts).
[c] No separate data on young adults.

health promotion, peer support [112] and attendance of clinic appointments, as shown, for example, in AYA cancer survivors [113] and AYAs with SCD [26, 50].

Reminder Systems

These are potential solutions for unintentional nonadherence, usually caused by forgetfulness. The use of simple adherence aids or mnemonic devices may improve unintentional nonadherence [31]. This includes keeping the pill bottle in plain sight, associating pill-taking with a daily event (e.g. putting the medication next to one's toothbrush), receiving reminder calls or centralized text message reminders, using an alarm clock or cell phone alarm, taking medication from preloaded medication cases (including innovative technologies [114]) or using a medication scorecard or calendar.

Cognitive-Educational Interventions

The basis for these interventions is the notion that patients who understand their condition and its treatment will be empowered and more likely to adhere. Patient education is an important and proven [107] method of facilitating adherence and, for example, is effective in improving adherence to preventative medical advice in AYA survivors of childhood cancer [61, 62]. Parental education has also reduced treatment refusal and improved clinical outcomes among children with leukemia [77]. Education can be administered individually or in a group setting and may be delivered verbally, in written form and/or audiovisually. Promoting health-related quality of life is important because of extended duration (often at least 1 year) of many of the treatment regimens [14, 115]. Like other AEIs, educational interventions can have a short-term effect [62, 107] and could be augmented by other AEIs.

Behavioral Counseling Interventions

Behavioral counseling or cognitive-behavioral interventions encompass management and reduction of mood, anxiety and cognitive barriers to adherence by changing normal routines, equipping the patient with skills to execute behavior change and practicing their use. This is the most researched type of AEI for children with cancer and chronic illness and has large treatment effects in this population [116]. Through the cognitive-behavioral process of problem-solving, a person attempts to identify effective and adaptive solutions for specific problems encountered in everyday living [117]. Problem-solving for adherence behaviors can be effective in adolescents with chronic disease as shown in interventional studies, including RCTs [118]. Disease- and age-specific

video-game-based learning is effective for improving adherence among AYAs with cancer, as shown in a large, well-designed multicenter RCT which utilized objective measures of adherence as end points (>65% of patients had lymphoma or leukemia) [32]. This was achieved by targeting certain behavioral processes affecting adherence, such as self-efficacy and knowledge, while other processes remained relatively unaffected (e.g. perceived control over health, stress).

Motivational Interviewing

Motivational interviewing was designed to target the decreased motivation for carrying out health recommendations, which was thought to mediate failure of behavioral counseling. The counselor uses this approach to address discrepancies between values and behaviors by reflecting patient views on barriers and promoters of health behavior and highlighting the contrast with actual conduct. AYAs seem to be attractive candidates for such interventions because of motivational barriers that exist in this group of patients [119]. This approach has proven effective in facilitating behavioral changes and improving therapeutic markers (e.g. hemoglobin A_{1c}) among adolescents with chronic diseases such as HIV infection [120] and diabetes [121].

Electronically Monitored Adherence Feedback

EM devices attached to pill dispensers not only provide information on the degree of adherence, but represent an effective and proven means for providing feedback on medication-taking behavior and improving adherence in both children [35] and adults [107, 122]. The latter may be achieved by equipping patients with cognitive-behavioral skills such as problem-solving and using motivational interviewing [123] which are both facilitated by objective data on adherence. Therefore, EM feedback is actually a subtype of behavioral counseling. RCTs in this field indicate that there may be a possible effect on clinical outcomes [35, 122], and a recent meta-analysis highlighted the superior efficacy of EM feedback compared to other modalities in a general population [107]. A pilot case study has shown its potential in AYAs with hematological disorders [124]; however, this method is costly and may be suitable mainly for complex cases and not for the general population, unless overall cost-effectiveness superior to other AEIs is shown. In theory, feedback could also be given based upon data adherence measures other than EM. However, this needs to be proven, especially because of the questionable accuracy of some of these measures.

Social-Psychoaffective Interventions

These interventions focus on managing patients' emotions, social relationships and social support in order to facilitate behavioral change. Interventions that target psychosocial barriers to adherence, including those specifically designed for AYAs with hematological disorders (e.g. hematopoietic stem cell transplantation) [125], have the potential to influence adherence. Peer support and dedicated support groups may help deal with some of these psychosocial barriers in AYAs with cancer [112, 125]. A comprehensive care framework, addressing linguistic, cultural, social and other issues, results in high adherence in certain populations, such as children and adolescents with SCD [78]. The use of home-based therapy for certain components of the treatment regimen showed promise in children receiving maintenance therapy for ALL [83].

Family therapy intervention, a subgroup of social-psychoaffective interventions, targets family communications and conflicts which are important and complex barriers to adherence in AYAs [84, 87], often using cognitive-behavioral techniques. Interventions facilitating transition into adult care are another component which is especially important in AYAs because the onus of ensuring attendance of clinic visits may rest upon caregivers, such as parents, in younger AYAs [26], but responsibilities should be shifted to the patient as part of the transition to adulthood. For example, a structured transition program for AYAs [43] should be formulated to bridge the gap between pediatric and adult-oriented care and should be part of any multilevel intervention for improving adherence in AYAs.

Multicomponent Intervention

Cognitive-behavioral processes are a significant element of multicomponent interventions [126, 127] which, along with behavioral counseling, yielded the greatest effect sizes across the spectrum of chronic diseases in children and adolescents [116]. Multicomponent interventions incorporate cognitive-behavioral [128], educational and social skills, problem-solving and family therapy aspects. Purely educational, psychosocial or technology-based interventions have been less efficient [116].

All the above interventions should be implemented by a multidisciplinary team [31, 129] (i.e. physicians, nurses, clinical pharmacists, psychologists and social workers) throughout treatment and follow-up. Nurses in particular play a central role in the assessment and promotion of adherence, especially in adolescents [130]. Adherence may decrease over the course of therapy for hematological diseases in AYAs [3, 8], as does the efficacy of certain AEIs [106, 107], such as education, highlighting a need for continued monitoring and maintenance of adherence [131]. Structured telephone calls including structured follow-up, support and education provided by nonmedical personnel can improve adherence [132] and should be investigated as a maintainer of adherence as part of a multicomponent intervention. The optimal timing for administering all of these interventions, especially regarding AYA cancer survivors, has not been established.

There are several ongoing clinical trials assessing adherence-improving interventions in AYAs. Many of these studies have taken advantage of recent technological advances by evaluating text messaging and smartphone applications as potential tools for improving adherence in AYAs, including one such study on AYA cancer patients [133].

Conclusion

It is clear that methods to assess and improve adherence are an unmet need in the contemporary management of AYAs with hematological disorders. Well-designed prospective studies, either as a subgroup of large-scale multinational, industry-funded pharmacological trials or as stand-alone studies, will greatly further our ability to correctly manage this important facet of the treatment regimen. Moreover, when attempting to interpret results of trials evaluating the efficacy of treatment strategies, details on adherence are crucial [64]. These trials should be designed based upon experience from the field of adherence in AYAs with other chronic diseases or among patients from different age groups with hematological disorders. Such studies will carry the added value of promoting this important and often overlooked aspect among AYA patients, families and health care providers.

Disclosure Statement

The authors have no conflicts of interest to declare.

References

1 Osterberg L, Blaschke T: Adherence to medication. N Engl J Med 2005;353:487–497.
2 Smith SD, Rosen D, Trueworthy RC, Lowman JT: A reliable method for evaluating drug compliance in children with cancer. Cancer 1979;43:169–173.
3 Tebbi CK, Cummings KM, Zevon MA, Smith L, Richards M, Mallon J: Compliance of pediatric and adolescent cancer patients. Cancer 1986;58:1179–1184.
4 Partridge AH, Avorn J, Wang PS, Winer EP: Adherence to therapy with oral antineoplastic agents. J Natl Cancer Inst 2002;94:652–661.
5 Collins PW, Blanchette VS, Fischer K, Bjorkman S, Oh M, Fritsch S, Schroth P, Spotts G, Astermark J, Ewenstein B; rAHF-PFM Study Group: Break-through bleeding in relation to predicted factor VIII levels in patients receiving prophylactic treatment for severe hemophilia A. J Thromb Haemost 2009;7:413–420.
6 Marin D, Bazeos A, Mahon FX, Eliasson L, Milojkovic D, Bua M, Apperley JF, Szydlo R, Desai R, Kozlowski K, Paliompeis C, Latham V, Foroni L, Molimard M, Reid A, Rezvani K, de Lavallade H, Guallar C, Goldman J, Khorashad JS: Adherence is the critical factor for achieving molecular responses in patients with chronic myeloid leukemia who achieve complete cytogenetic responses on imatinib. J Clin Oncol 2010;28:2381–2388.
7 Ibrahim AR, Eliasson L, Apperley JF, Milojkovic D, Bua M, Szydlo R, Mahon FX, Kozlowski K, Paliompeis C, Foroni L, Khorashad JS, Bazeos A, Molimard M, Reid A, Rezvani K, Gerrard G, Goldman J, Marin D: Poor adherence is the main reason for loss of CCyR and imatinib failure for chronic myeloid leukemia patients on long-term therapy. Blood 2011; 117:3733–3736.
8 Bhatia S, Landier W, Shangguan M, Hageman L, Schaible AN, Carter AR, Hanby CL, Leisenring W, Yasui Y, Kornegay NM, Mascarenhas L, Ritchey AK, Casillas JN, Dickens DS, Meza J, Carroll WL, Relling MV, Wong FL: Nonadherence to oral mercaptopurine and risk of relapse in Hispanic and non-Hispanic white children with acute lymphoblastic leukemia: a report from the children's oncology group. J Clin Oncol 2012;30:2094–2101.
9 Kahana SY, Rohan J, Allison S, Frazier TW, Drotar D: A meta-analysis of adherence to antiretroviral therapy and virologic responses in HIV-infected children, adolescents, and young adults. AIDS Behav 2013;17:41–60.
10 Wu EQ, Johnson S, Beaulieu N, Arana M, Bollu V, Guo A, Coombs J, Feng W, Cortes J: Healthcare resource utilization and costs associated with non-adherence to imatinib treatment in chronic myeloid leukemia patients. Curr Med Res Opin 2010;26:61–69.
11 Candrilli SD, O'Brien SH, Ware RE, Nahata MC, Seiber EE, Balkrishnan R: Hydroxyurea adherence and associated outcomes among Medicaid enrollees with sickle cell disease. Am J Hematol 2011;86:273–277.
12 Du Treil S, Rice J, Leissinger CA: Quantifying adherence to treatment and its relationship to quality of life in a well-characterized haemophilia population. Haemophilia 2007;13:493–501.
13 Duncan N, Shapiro A, Ye X, Epstein J, Luo MP: Treatment patterns, health-related quality of life and adherence to prophylaxis among haemophilia A patients in the United States. Haemophilia 2012;18:760–765.
14 Fisak B, Belkin MH, von Lehe AC, Bansal MM: The relation between health-related quality of life, treatment adherence and disease severity in a paediatric sickle cell disease sample. Child Care Health Dev 2012;38:204–210.
15 World Health Organization: Adherence to long-term therapies: evidence for action. www.who.int/chp/knowledge/publications/adherence_full_report.pdf (accessed September 20, 2013).
16 Wood WA, Lee SJ: Malignant hematologic diseases in adolescents and young adults. Blood 2011;117:5803–5815.
17 Zebrack B, Mathews-Bradshaw B, Siegel S; Livestrong Young Adult Alliance: Quality cancer care for adolescents and young adults: a position statement. J Clin Oncol 2010;28:4862–4867.
18 Geiger AM, Castellino SM: Delineating the age ranges used to define adolescents and young adults. J Clin Oncol 2011;29:e492–e493.
19 Butow P, Palmer S, Pai A, Goodenough B, Luckett T, King M: Review of adherence-related issues in adolescents and young adults with cancer. J Clin Oncol 2010;28:4800–4809.
20 Kondryn HJ, Edmondson CL, Hill J, Eden TO: Treatment non-adherence in teenage and young adult patients with cancer. Lancet Oncol 2011;12:100–108.
21 Haynes R, Taylor D, Sackett D: Compliance in Health Care. London, Johns Hopkins University Press, 1979.
22 Lutfey KE, Wishner WJ: Beyond 'compliance' is 'adherence'. Improving the prospect of diabetes care. Diabetes Care 1999;22:635–639.
23 Kyngas H, Duffy ME, Kroll T: Conceptual analysis of compliance. J Clin Nurs 2000;9:5–12.
24 Bae JW, Guyer W, Grimm K, Altice FL: Medication persistence in the treatment of HIV infection: a review of the literature and implications for future clinical care and research. AIDS 2011;25:279–290.
25 Chisholm-Burns MA, Spivey CA: Pharmacoadherence: a new term for a significant problem. Am J Health Syst Pharm 2008;65:661–667.
26 Modi AC, Crosby LE, Hines J, Drotar D, Mitchell MJ: Feasibility of web-based technology to assess adherence to clinic appointments in youth with sickle cell disease. J Pediatr Hematol Oncol 2012;34:e93–e96.
27 Berkovitch M, Papadouris D, Shaw D, Onuaha N, Dias C, Olivieri NF: Trying to improve compliance with prophylactic penicillin therapy in children with sickle cell disease. Br J Clin Pharmacol 1998;45:605–607.
28 Eckrich MJ, Wang WC, Yang E, Arbogast PG, Morrow A, Dudley JA, Ray WA, Cooper WO: Adherence to transcranial Doppler screening guidelines among children with sickle cell disease. Pediatr Blood Cancer 2013;60:270–274.
29 Zwemer EK, Mahler HI, Werchniak AE, Recklitis CJ: Sun exposure in young adult cancer survivors on and off the beach: results from Project REACH. J Cancer Surviv 2012;6:63–71.
30 DiMatteo MR, Giordani PJ, Lepper HS, Croghan TW: Patient adherence and medical treatment outcomes: a meta-analysis. Med Care 2002;40:794–811.
31 Levine AM, Richardson JL, Marks G, Chan K, Graham J, Selser JN, Kishbaugh C, Shelton DR, Johnson CA: Compliance with oral drug therapy in patients with hematologic malignancy. J Clin Oncol 1987;5:1469–1476.
32 Kato PM, Cole SW, Bradlyn AS, Pollock BH: A video game improves behavioral outcomes in adolescents and young adults with cancer: a randomized trial. Pediatrics 2008;122:e305–e317.
33 Alvarez O, Rodriguez-Cortes H, Robinson N, Lewis N, Pow Sang CD, Lopez-Mitnik G, Paley C: Adherence to deferasirox in children and adolescents with sickle cell disease during 1 year of therapy. J Pediatr Hematol Oncol 2009;31:739–744.
34 Jaime-Perez JC, Gomez-Almaguer D, Sandoval-Gonzalez A, Chapa-Rodriguez A, Gonzalez-Llano O: Random serum methotrexate determinations for assessing compliance with maintenance therapy for childhood acute lymphoblastic leukemia. Leuk Lymphoma 2009;50:1843–1847.
35 Burgess SW, Sly PD, Devadason SG: Providing feedback on adherence increases use of preventive medication by asthmatic children. J Asthma 2010;47:198–201.
36 Deschamps AE, Van Wijngaerden E, Denhaerynck K, De Geest S, Vandamme AM: Use of electronic monitoring induces a 40-day intervention effect in HIV patients. J Acquir Immune Defic Syndr 2006;43:247–248.
37 Denhaerynck K, Schafer-Keller P, Young J, Steiger J, Bock A, De Geest S: Examining assumptions regarding valid electronic monitoring of medication therapy: development of a validation framework and its application on a European sample of kidney transplant patients. BMC Med Res Methodol 2008;8:5.
38 Ibrahim AR, Eliasson L, Apperley JF, Milojkovic D, Bua M, Szydlo R, Mahon FX, Kozlowsk K, Paliompeis C, Foroni L, Khorashad JS, Bazeos A, Molimard M, Reid A, Rezvani K, Gerrard G, Goldman J, Marin D: Poor adherence is the main reason for loss of CCyR and imatinib failure for CML patients on long term therapy. Blood 2011;117:3733–3736.

39 Noens L, van Lierde MA, De Bock R, Verhoef G, Zachee P, Berneman Z, Martiat P, Mineur P, Van Eygen K, MacDonald K, De Geest S, Albrecht T, Abraham I: Prevalence, determinants, and outcomes of nonadherence to imatinib therapy in patients with chronic myeloid leukemia: the ADAGIO study. Blood 2009; 113:5401–5411.

40 O'Hanrahan M, O'Malley K: Compliance with drug treatment. Br Med J (Clin Res Ed) 1981;283:298–300.

41 Marin D, Bazeos A, Mahon FX, Eliasson L, Milojkovic D, Bua M, Apperley JF, Szydlo R, Desai R, Kozlowski K, Paliompeis C, Latham V, Foroni L, Molimard M, Reid A, Rezvani K, de Lavallade H, Guallar C, Goldman J, Khorashad JS: Adherence is the critical factor for achieving molecular responses in patients with chronic myeloid leukemia who achieve complete cytogenetic responses on imatinib. J Clin Oncol 2010;28:2381–2388.

42 Windebank KP, Spinetta JJ: Do as I say or die: compliance in adolescents with cancer. Pediatr Blood Cancer 2008;50:1099–1100.

43 Van Staa AL, Jedeloo S, van Meeteren J, Latour JM: Crossing the transition chasm: experiences and recommendations for improving transitional care of young adults, parents and providers. Child Care Health Dev 2011;37: 821–832.

44 Lancaster D, Lennard L, Lilleyman JS: Profile of non-compliance in lymphoblastic leukaemia. Arch Dis Child 1997;76:365–366.

45 Burra P, Germani G, Gnoato F, Lazzaro S, Russo FP, Cillo U, Senzolo M: Adherence in liver transplant recipients. Liver Transpl 2011;17:760–770.

46 Phipps S, DeCuir-Whalley S: Adherence issues in pediatric bone marrow transplantation. J Pediatr Psychol 1990;15:459–475.

47 Accordino MK, Hershman DL: Disparities and challenges in adherence to oral antineoplastic agents. Am Soc Clin Oncol Educ Book 2013;2013:271–276.

48 Festa RS, Tamaroff MH, Chasalow F, Lanzkowsky P: Therapeutic adherence to oral medication regimens by adolescents with cancer. I. Laboratory assessment. J Pediatr 1992;120:807–811.

49 Lansky SB, Smith SD, Cairns NU, Cairns GF Jr: Psychological correlates of compliance. Am J Pediatr Hematol Oncol 1983;5:87–92.

50 Crosby LE, Barach I, McGrady ME, Kalinyak KA, Eastin AR, Mitchell MJ: Integrating interactive web-based technology to assess adherence and clinical outcomes in pediatric sickle cell disease. Anemia 2012;2012:492428.

51 Treadwell MJ, Law AW, Sung J, Hackney-Stephens E, Quirolo K, Murray E, Glendenning GA, Vichinsky E: Barriers to adherence of deferoxamine usage in sickle cell disease. Pediatr Blood Cancer 2005;44:500–507.

52 Patel NG, Lindsey T, Strunk RC, DeBaun MR: Prevalence of daily medication adherence among children with sickle cell disease: a 1-year retrospective cohort analysis. Pediatr Blood Cancer 2010;55:554–556.

53 Zimmerman SA, Schultz WH, Davis JS, Pickens CV, Mortier NA, Howard TA, Ware RE: Sustained long-term hematologic efficacy of hydroxyurea at maximum tolerated dose in children with sickle cell disease. Blood 2004; 103:2039–2045.

54 Thornburg CD, Calatroni A, Telen M, Kemper AR: Adherence to hydroxyurea therapy in children with sickle cell anemia. J Pediatr 2010;156:415–419.

55 Dampier C, Ely B, Brodecki D, O'Neal P: Characteristics of pain managed at home in children and adolescents with sickle cell disease by using diary self-reports. J Pain 2002;3: 461–470.

56 Hershman DL, Shao T, Kushi LH, Buono D, Tsai WY, Fehrenbacher L, Kwan M, Gomez SL, Neugut AI: Early discontinuation and non-adherence to adjuvant hormonal therapy are associated with increased mortality in women with breast cancer. Breast Cancer Res Treat 2011;126:529–537.

57 Pemmaraju N, Kantarjian H, Shan J, Jabbour E, Quintas-Cardama A, Verstovsek S, Ravandi F, Wierda W, O'Brien S, Cortes J: Analysis of outcomes in adolescents and young adults with chronic myelogenous leukemia treated with upfront tyrosine kinase inhibitor therapy. Haematologica 2012;97:1029–1035.

58 Tai E, Buchanan N, Townsend J, Fairley T, Moore A, Richardson LC: Health status of adolescent and young adult cancer survivors. Cancer 2012;118:4884–4891.

59 Robien K, Ness KK, Klesges LM, Baker KS, Gurney JG: Poor adherence to dietary guidelines among adult survivors of childhood acute lymphoblastic leukemia. J Pediatr Hematol Oncol 2008;30:815–822.

60 Freyer DR: Transition of care for young adult survivors of childhood and adolescent cancer: rationale and approaches. J Clin Oncol 2010; 28:4810–4818.

61 Mays D, Black JD, Mosher RB, Heinly A, Shad AT, Tercyak KP: Efficacy of the Survivor Health and Resilience Education (SHARE) program to improve bone health behaviors among adolescent survivors of childhood cancer. Ann Behav Med 2011;42:91–98.

62 Mays D, Black JD, Mosher RB, Shad AT, Tercyak KP: Improving short-term sun safety practices among adolescent survivors of childhood cancer: a randomized controlled efficacy trial. J Cancer Surviv 2011;5:247–254.

63 Berntorp E: Joint outcomes in patients with haemophilia: the importance of adherence to preventive regimens. Haemophilia 2009;15: 1219–1227.

64 Robiner WN: Enhancing adherence in clinical research. Contemp Clin Trials 2005;26: 59–77.

65 Ibrahim AR, Eliasson L, Apperley JF, Milojkovic D, Bua M, Szydlo R, Mahon FX, Kozlowski K, Paliompeis C, Foroni L, Khorashad JS, Bazeos A, Molimard M, Reid A, Rezvani K, Gerrard G, Goldman J, Marin D: Poor adherence is the main reason for loss of CCyR and imatinib failure for chronic myeloid leukemia patients on long-term therapy. Blood 2011; 117:3733–3736.

66 Sharf G, Hoffmann V, Bombaci F, Daban M, Efficace F, Guilhot J: Non-adherence in chronic myeloid leukemia: results of a global survey of 2,546 CML patients in 79 countries. Haematologica 2013;98:453.

67 Albritton K, Bleyer WA: The management of cancer in the older adolescent. Eur J Cancer 2003;39:2584–2599.

68 Gater A, Heron L, Abetz-Webb L, Coombs J, Simmons J, Guilhot F, Rea D: Adherence to oral tyrosine kinase inhibitor therapies in chronic myeloid leukemia. Leuk Res 2012;36: 817–825.

69 Eliasson L, Clifford S, Barber N, Marin D: Exploring chronic myeloid leukemia patients' reasons for not adhering to the oral anticancer drug imatinib as prescribed. Leuk Res 2011; 35:626–630.

70 Landier W, Hughes CB, Calvillo ER, Anderson NL, Briseno-Toomey D, Dominguez L, Martinez AM, Hanby C, Bhatia S: A grounded theory of the process of adherence to oral chemotherapy in Hispanic and Caucasian children and adolescents with acute lymphoblastic leukemia. J Pediatr Oncol Nurs 2011;28: 203–223.

71 Tielen M, van Staa AL, Jedeloo S, van Exel NJ, Weimar W: Q-methodology to identify young adult renal transplant recipients at risk for nonadherence. Transplantation 2008;85: 700–706.

72 Kondryn HJ, Edmondson CL, Hill JW, Eden TO: Treatment non-adherence in teenage and young adult cancer patients: a preliminary study of patient perceptions. Psychooncology 2009;18:1327–1332.

73 Malbasa T, Kodish E, Santacroce SJ: Adolescent adherence to oral therapy for leukemia: a focus group study. J Pediatr Oncol Nurs 2007; 24:139–151.

74 Hawwa AF, Millership JS, Collier PS, McCarthy A, Dempsey S, Cairns C, McElnay JC: The development of an objective methodology to measure medication adherence to oral thiopurines in paediatric patients with acute lymphoblastic leukaemia – an exploratory study. Eur J Clin Pharmacol 2009;65:1105–1112.

75 Blais L, Beauchesne MF, Levesque S: Socioeconomic status and medication prescription patterns in pediatric asthma in Canada. J Adolesc Health 2006;38:607.

76 Crosby LE, Modi AC, Lemanek KL, Guilfoyle SM, Kalinyak KA, Mitchell MJ: Perceived barriers to clinic appointments for adolescents with sickle cell disease. J Pediatr Hematol Oncol 2009;31:571–576.

77 Mostert S, Sitaresmi MN, Gundy CM, Janes V, Sutaryo S, Veerman AJ: Comparing childhood leukaemia treatment before and after the introduction of a parental education programme in Indonesia. Arch Dis Child 2010; 95:20–25.

78 Colombatti R, Montanaro M, Guasti F, Rampazzo P, Meneghetti G, Giordan M, Basso G, Sainati L: Comprehensive care for sickle cell disease immigrant patients: a reproducible model achieving high adherence to minimum standards of care. Pediatr Blood Cancer 2012; 59:1275–1279.

79 Lindvall K, Colstrup L, Loogna K, Wollter I, Gronhaug S: Knowledge of disease and adherence in adult patients with haemophilia. Haemophilia 2010;16:592–596.

80 Darkow T, Henk HJ, Thomas SK, Feng W, Baladi JF, Goldberg GA, Hatfield A, Cortes J: Treatment interruptions and non-adherence with imatinib and associated healthcare costs: a retrospective analysis among managed care patients with chronic myelogenous leukaemia. Pharmacoeconomics 2007;25:481–496.

81 McDonald HP, Garg AX, Haynes RB: Interventions to enhance patient adherence to medication prescriptions: scientific review. JAMA 2002;288:2868–2879.

82 Johnson RH, Kroon L: Optimizing fertility preservation practices for adolescent and young adult cancer patients. J Natl Compr Canc Netw 2013;11:71–77.

83 Phillips B, Richards M, Boys R, Hodgkin M, Kinsey S: A home-based maintenance therapy program for acute lymphoblastic leukemia – practical and safe? J Pediatr Hematol Oncol 2011;33:433–436.

84 Kyngas HA, Kroll T, Duffy ME: Compliance in adolescents with chronic diseases: a review. J Adolesc Health 2000;26:379–388.

85 Palmer DL, Osborn P, King PS, Berg CA, Butler J, Butner J, Horton D, Wiebe DJ: The structure of parental involvement and relations to disease management for youth with type 1 diabetes. J Pediatr Psychol 2011;36: 596–605.

86 Kyngas H, Hentinen M, Barlow JH: Adolescents' perceptions of physicians, nurses, parents and friends: help or hindrance in compliance with diabetes self-care? J Adv Nurs 1998; 27:760–769.

87 Hilliard ME, Guilfoyle SM, Dolan LM, Hood KK: Prediction of adolescents' glycemic control 1 year after diabetes-specific family conflict: the mediating role of blood glucose monitoring adherence. Arch Pediatr Adolesc Med 2011;165:624–629.

88 Bollinger LM, Nire KG, Rhodes MM, Chisolm DJ, O'Brien SH: Caregivers' perspectives on barriers to transcranial Doppler screening in children with sickle-cell disease. Pediatr Blood Cancer 2011;56:99–102.

89 Dimatteo MR: The role of effective communication with children and their families in fostering adherence to pediatric regimens. Patient Educ Couns 2004;55:339–344.

90 Ciechanowski PS, Katon WJ, Russo JE, Walker EA: The patient-provider relationship: attachment theory and adherence to treatment in diabetes. Am J Psychiatry 2001; 158:29–35.

91 Drotar D: Physician behavior in the care of pediatric chronic illness: association with health outcomes and treatment adherence. J Dev Behav Pediatr 2009;30:246–254.

92 Tebbi CK, Richards ME, Cummings KM, Zevon MA, Mallon JC: The role of parent-adolescent concordance in compliance with cancer chemotherapy. Adolescence 1988;23: 599–611.

93 Hess SL, Johannsdottir IM, Hamre H, Kiserud CE, Loge JH, Fossa SD: Adult survivors of childhood malignant lymphoma are not aware of their risk of late effects. Acta Oncol 2011;50:653–659.

94 Blotcky AD, Cohen DG, Conatser C, Klopovich P: Psychosocial characteristics of adolescents who refuse cancer treatment. J Consult Clin Psychol 1985;53:729–731.

95 Chesney MA, Ickovics JR, Chambers DB, Gifford AL, Neidig J, Zwickl B, Wu AW: Self-reported adherence to antiretroviral medications among participants in HIV clinical trials: the AACTG adherence instruments. Patient Care Committee and Adherence Working Group of the Outcomes Committee of the Adult AIDS Clinical Trials Group (AACTG). AIDS Care 2000;12:255–266.

96 Miller VA, Drotar D: Decision-making competence and adherence to treatment in adolescents with diabetes. J Pediatr Psychol 2007;32:178–188.

97 Sawyer SM, Aroni RA: Self-management in adolescents with chronic illness. What does it mean and how can it be achieved? Med J Aust 2005;183:405–409.

98 Rabiau MA, Knauper B, Nguyen TK, Sufrategui M, Polychronakos C: Compensatory beliefs about glucose testing are associated with low adherence to treatment and poor metabolic control in adolescents with type 1 diabetes. Health Educ Res 2009;24:890–896.

99 Mancini J, Simeoni MC, Parola N, Clement A, Vey N, Sirvent N, Michel G, Auquier P: Adherence to leukemia maintenance therapy: a comparative study among children, adolescents, and adults. Pediatr Hematol Oncol 2012;29:428–439.

100 Gadkari AS, McHorney CA: Unintentional non-adherence to chronic prescription medications: how unintentional is it really? BMC Health Serv Res 2012;12:98.

101 Berg CA, King PS, Butler JM, Pham P, Palmer D, Wiebe DJ: Parental involvement and adolescents' diabetes management: the mediating role of self-efficacy and externalizing and internalizing behaviors. J Pediatr Psychol 2011;36:329–339.

102 Mednick L, Yu S, Trachtenberg F, Xu Y, Kleinert DA, Giardina PJ, Kwiatkowski JL, Foote D, Thayalasuthan V, Porter JB, Thompson AA, Schilling L, Quinn CT, Neufeld EJ, Yamashita R, Thalassemia Clinical Research Network: Symptoms of depression and anxiety in patients with thalassemia: prevalence and correlates in the thalassemia longitudinal cohort. Am J Hematol 2010;85:802–805.

103 Wray J, Waters S, Radley-Smith R, Sensky T: Adherence in adolescents and young adults following heart or heart-lung transplantation. Pediatr Transplant 2006;10:694–700.

104 Koren G, Ferrazini G, Sulh H, Langevin AM, Kapelushnik J, Klein J, Giesbrecht E, Soldin S, Greenberg M: Systemic exposure to mercaptopurine as a prognostic factor in acute lymphocytic leukemia in children. N Engl J Med 1990;323:17–21.

105 Relling MV, Hancock ML, Boyett JM, Pui CH, Evans WE: Prognostic importance of 6-mercaptopurine dose intensity in acute lymphoblastic leukemia. Blood 1999;93: 2817–2823.

106 Kahana S, Drotar D, Frazier T: Meta-analysis of psychological interventions to promote adherence to treatment in pediatric chronic health conditions. J Pediatr Psychol 2008;33:590–611.

107 Demonceau J, Ruppar T, Kristanto P, Hughes DA, Fargher E, Kardas P, De Geest S, Dobbels F, Lewek P, Urquhart J, Vrijens B; ABC project team: Identification and assessment of adherence-enhancing interventions in studies assessing medication adherence through electronically compiled drug dosing histories: a systematic literature review and meta-analysis. Drugs 2013;73:545–562.

108 Seid M, Opipari-Arrigan L, Gelhard LR, Varni JW, Driscoll K: Barriers to care questionnaire: reliability, validity, and responsiveness to change among parents of children with asthma. Acad Pediatr 2009;9:106–113.

109 Bharti S, Bharti B, Naseem S, Attri SV: A community-based cluster randomized controlled trial of 'directly observed home-based daily iron therapy' in lowering prevalence of anemia in rural women and adolescent girls. Asia Pac J Public Health 2013, Epub ahead of print.

110 Stinson J, Wilson R, Gill N, Yamada J, Holt J: A systematic review of Internet-based self-management interventions for youth with health conditions. J Pediatr Psychol 2009;34: 495–510.

111 Skinner H, Biscope S, Poland B, Goldberg E: How adolescents use technology for health information: implications for health professionals from focus group studies. J Med Internet Res 2003;5:e32.

112 Zebrack B, Chesler MA, Kaplan S: To foster healing among adolescents and young adults with cancer: what helps? What hurts? Support Care Cancer 2010;18:131–135.

113 Murphy MH: Health promotion in adolescent and young adult cancer survivors: mobilizing compliance in a multifaceted risk profile. J Pediatr Oncol Nurs 2013;30:139–152.

114 Charles T, Quinn D, Weatherall M, Aldington S, Beasley R, Holt S: An audiovisual reminder function improves adherence with inhaled corticosteroid therapy in asthma. J Allergy Clin Immunol 2007;119:811–816.

115 Hommel KA, Davis CM, Baldassano RN: Medication adherence and quality of life in pediatric inflammatory bowel disease. J Pediatr Psychol 2008;33:867–874.

116 Graves MM, Roberts MC, Rapoff M, Boyer A: The efficacy of adherence interventions for chronically ill children: a meta-analytic review. J Pediatr Psychol 2010;35:368–382.

117 D'Zurilla T, Nezu A: Problem-Solving Therapy: A Positive Approach to Clinical Intervention, ed 3. New York, Springer, 2007.

118 Fitzpatrick SL, Schumann KP, Hill-Briggs F: Problem solving interventions for diabetes self-management and control: a systematic review of the literature. Diabetes Res Clin Pract 2013;100:145–161.

119 Suarez M, Mullins S: Motivational interviewing and pediatric health behavior interventions. J Dev Behav Pediatr 2008;29:417–428.

120 Naar-King S, Parsons JT, Murphy D, Kolmodin K, Harris DR; ATN 004 Protocol Team: A multisite randomized trial of a motivational intervention targeting multiple risks in youth living with HIV: initial effects on motivation, self-efficacy, and depression. J Adolesc Health 2010;46:422–428.

121 Channon SJ, Huws-Thomas MV, Rollnick S, Hood K, Cannings-John RL, Rogers C, Gregory JW: A multicenter randomized controlled trial of motivational interviewing in teenagers with diabetes. Diabetes Care 2007;30:1390–1395.

122 De Bruin M, Hospers HJ, van Breukelen GJ, Kok G, Koevoets WM, Prins JM: Electronic monitoring-based counseling to enhance adherence among HIV-infected patients: a randomized controlled trial. Health Psychol 2010;29:421–428.

123 Rosen MI, Rigsby MO, Salahi JT, Ryan CE, Cramer JA: Electronic monitoring and counseling to improve medication adherence. Behav Res Ther 2004;42:409–422.

124 Hilliard ME, Ramey C, Rohan JM, Drotar D, Cortina S: Electronic monitoring feedback to promote adherence in an adolescent with Fanconi anemia. Health Psychol 2011;30:503–509.

125 Cooke L, Chung C, Grant M: Psychosocial care for adolescent and young adult hematopoietic cell transplant patients. J Psychosoc Oncol 2011;29:394–414.

126 Ellis DA, Frey MA, Naar-King S, Templin T, Cunningham P, Cakan N: Use of multisystemic therapy to improve regimen adherence among adolescents with type 1 diabetes in chronic poor metabolic control: a randomized controlled trial. Diabetes Care 2005;28:1604–1610.

127 Stark LJ, Janicke DM, McGrath AM, Mackner LM, Hommel KA, Lovell D: Prevention of osteoporosis: a randomized clinical trial to increase calcium intake in children with juvenile rheumatoid arthritis. J Pediatr Psychol 2005;30:377–386.

128 Dahl J, Gustafsson D, Melin L: Effects of a behavioral treatment program on children with asthma. J Asthma 1990;27:41–46.

129 Santoleri F, Sorice P, Lasala R, Rizzo RC, Costantini A: Patient adherence and persistence with imatinib, nilotinib, dasatinib in clinical practice. PLoS One 2013;8:e56813.

130 Khair K: Minimizing joint damage: the role of nurses in promoting adherence to hemophilia treatment. Orthop Nurs 2010;29:193–200.

131 Kripalani S, Yao X, Haynes RB: Interventions to enhance medication adherence in chronic medical conditions: a systematic review. Arch Intern Med 2007;167:540–550.

132 Patik M, Phillips L, Kladny B, Captain A, Gettig E, Krishnamurti L: Structured telephone-based outreach using nonmedical personnel can improve adherence to comprehensive care in families of children with sickle cell disease. Am J Hematol 2006;81:462–464.

133 Johnson RH, Macpherson CF: Use of a smartphone medication reminder application to promote adherence to oral medications by adolescents and young adults (AYA) with cancer. www.ClinicalTrials.gov (accessed September 20, 2013, NCT01618344).

134 Mkopi A, Range N, Lwilla F, Egwaga S, Schulze A, Geubbels E, van Leth F: Adherence to tuberculosis therapy among patients receiving home-based directly observed treatment: evidence from the United Republic of Tanzania. PLoS One 2012;7:e51828.

135 Rakhmanina NY, van den Anker JN, Soldin SJ, van Schaik RH, Mordwinkin N, Neely MN: Can therapeutic drug monitoring improve pharmacotherapy of HIV infection in adolescents? Ther Drug Monit 2010;32:273–281.

136 Guilfoyle SM, Crimmins NA, Hood KK: Blood glucose monitoring and glycemic control in adolescents with type 1 diabetes: meter downloads versus self-report. Pediatr Diabetes 2011;12:560–566.

137 Cramer JA, Mattson RH, Prevey ML, Scheyer RD, Ouellette VL: How often is medication taken as prescribed? A novel assessment technique. JAMA 1989;261:3273–3277.

138 Weinstein C, Staudinger H, Scott I, Amar NJ, LaForce C: Dose counter performance of mometasone furoate/formoterol inhalers in subjects with asthma or COPD. Respir Med 2011;105:979–988.

139 Brandow AM, Panepinto JA: Monitoring toxicity, impact, and adherence of hydroxyurea in children with sickle cell disease. Am J Hematol 2011;86:804–806.

140 Arnold E, Heddle N, Lane S, Sek J, Almonte T, Walker I: Handheld computers and paper diaries for documenting the use of factor concentrates used in haemophilia home therapy: a qualitative study. Haemophilia 2005;11:216–226.

141 Lewin AB, LaGreca AM, Geffken GR, Williams LB, Duke DC, Storch EA, Silverstein JH: Validity and reliability of an adolescent and parent rating scale of type 1 diabetes adherence behaviors: the Self-Care Inventory (SCI). J Pediatr Psychol 2009;34:999–1007.

142 Duncan N, Kronenberger W, Roberson C, Shapiro A: VERITAS-Pro: a new measure of adherence to prophylactic regimens in haemophilia. Haemophilia 2010;16:247–255.

143 Von Mackensen S, Campos IG, Acquadro C, Strandberg-Larsen M: Cross-cultural adaptation and linguistic validation of age-group-specific haemophilia patient-reported outcome (PRO) instruments for patients and parents. Haemophilia 2013;19:e73–e83.

144 Marlowe D, Crowne DP: Social desirability and response to perceived situational demands. J Consult Psychol 1961;25:109–115.

145 Cleemput I, Dobbels F: Measuring patient-reported outcomes in solid organ transplant recipients: an overview of instruments developed to date. Pharmacoeconomics 2007;25:269–286.

146 Kyngas HA, Skaar-Chandler CA, Duffy ME: The development of an instrument to measure the compliance of adolescents with a chronic disease. J Adv Nurs 2000;32:1499–1506.

147 Walsh JC, Mandalia S, Gazzard BG: Responses to a 1-month self-report on adherence to antiretroviral therapy are consistent with electronic data and virological treatment outcome. AIDS 2002;16:269–277.

Acta Haematol 2014;132:363–374
DOI: 10.1159/000360213

Published online: September 10, 2014

Nursing Care for Adolescents and Young Adults with Cancer: Literature Review

Juliet Dreyer[a]   Irit Schwartz-Attias[b]

[a]Institute of Hematology, Davidoff Cancer Center, Beilinson Hospital, Rabin Medical Center, and [b]Department of Pediatric Hematology-Oncology, Schneider Children's Medical Center, Petah Tikva, Israel

Key Words

Adherence · Adolescents and young adults · Nursing · Quality of life · Symptoms

Abstract

Cancer patients belonging to the adolescent and young adult (AYA) age group have unique and very specific needs, which require special attention from the caring staff. The difficulty in maintaining the personal and professional development at this age is both natural and normal. Adding to this, coping with a life-threatening disease turns this stage in life into a period with many dilemmas and challenges of quite a complex nature. AYA patients have to deal with issues above and beyond the disease itself, which create a very complex coping picture. On top of that, prognosis for this age group has not improved in recent years, unlike the situation in other age groups like children and adults. The literature on this subject is extensive and comprehensive. However, most of the papers on this subject are very specific and narrow in their approach, each dealing with a specific topic. In this article, we bring together many different papers which make a wide and comprehensive picture of the subject of AYAs coping with cancer, coupled with recommendations for the caring staff. In this review we focus on the various aspects of the disease and treatments in AYAs, based on the conceptual model of quality of life proposed by Ferrell and colleagues [Cancer Nurs 1992;15:153–160; Cancer Nurs 1992;15:247–253], including physical, social, emotional and spiritual aspects. From the psychological standpoint, most of the papers discuss the negative aspects; however, in this article we try to include some articles from the positive psychology school of thought. From our findings it is apparent that there is an opportunity and need to further explore research in this regard. It is apparent that taking a unique approach to AYA cancer patients is needed in order to deal with the unique needs of this age group. This article aims at putting a framework around this issue, with actionable recommendations for the caring staff.   © 2014 S. Karger AG, Basel

Introduction

Adolescents and young adult (AYA) cancer patients aged 16–39 years are a unique group of patients with specific and complex needs which require our special attention. These patients are distinct from their younger and older counterparts in their cognitive, psychosocial and emotional developmental stage. This influences their perceptions of their disease and symptom experience.

Juliet Dreyer, RN
Bone Marrow Unit, Institute of Hematology, Davidoff Cancer Center
Beilinson Hospital, Rabin Medical Center
39 Jabotinsky Street, Petah Tikva 49100 (Israel)
E-Mail julietd@clalit.org.il

The World Health Organization defines adolescents as those between 10 and 19 years of age [1], but many other age ranges have been proposed. The Surveillance, Epidemiology and End Results program of the National Cancer Institute reports cancer incidence in 5-year brackets (e.g. 10–14 years and 15–19 years), and adolescents have been assigned to the quintile of 15–19 years of age [2].

AYAs with cancer are considered a 'high-risk' group. According to the National Cancer Institute, this group has not enjoyed the same survival improvements over the last several decades as older and younger cohorts [3]. This disadvantage has been attributed to a longer diagnostic period, poorer involvement in clinical trials, distinct cancer biology, inappropriate place of care and protocol differences between adult and children's regimens [4, 5].

Research of this unique group of patients has been intensified in the past decade in order to try and improve the quality of treatment and its results. This research has shed light on the physical and emotional needs of these patients, and forced the health care personnel treating this unique group of patients to further understand the challenges they face and tailor the treatment accordingly.

The aim of this review is to highlight the main aspects AYA cancer patients face when trying to cope with their disease. In this review we focused on the various aspects of the disease and treatments in AYAs, based on the conceptual model of quality of life proposed by Ferrell and colleagues [6, 7], including physical, social, emotional and spiritual aspects.

Aspects of Disease and Treatments in AYAs Based on the Quality of Life Model

Physical Aspects

The physical symptoms caused by the cancer disease and its treatment affect patients of all ages, yet the different age groups vary from one another in the type of symptoms and their intensity. Adolescents consider the physical side effects of treatment as the worst aspect of cancer, significantly affecting their quality of life [8].

The most common symptoms that were found to be frequent in adolescents during the treatment period were: fatigue, sleep disorders, nausea/eating disorders, pain and changes in physical appearance.

Fatigue

In reviewing the literature regarding physical symptoms, the symptom most frequently reported is fatigue [9]. It is experienced during the diagnostic period, hospitaliza-tion and treatment period and into the recovery period [10]. Fatigue was reported by many AYA patients as a distressing symptom which disturbed their daily routine up to 2 years after receiving treatment. The fatigue affects the AYA patients physically, psychologically and emotionally, causing stress and constraints on the patients' lifestyle, affecting the well-being and quality of life [10–13].

The main factor inducing fatigue is the treatment itself [14]. The adolescents' regular lifestyle activities, such as studying, socializing and physical activity, also have a major effect on their fatigue [10, 11, 15, 16]. Moderate or intense physical activity may contribute to fatigue, although the contrary is also true. Inactivity and boredom may also make fatigue worse [10, 11, 16]. Findings from several studies showed a predictable pattern of fatigue within a cycle of chemotherapy treatment, where fatigue peaks during the week after chemotherapy administration and slowly declines reaching its lowest level just before administration of the next chemotherapy course [11, 17–20].

As fatigue is a symptom experienced during and after treatment, much emphasis should be put onto diagnosis and intervention. Very few studies have tested interventions to manage fatigue or prevent it in this unique group of patients. There is need for further research in this field.

Sleep Disorders

Erickson et al. [21] reviewed the literature exploring the symptoms reported most frequently by AYA patients. Sleep disorders were found to be amongst the most frequently reported symptoms. When compared to healthy adolescents, AYA patients receiving chemotherapy reported a higher degree of problems with sleep quality. This was also true when compared to themselves before cancer diagnoses. Adolescents receiving chemotherapy had worse sleep hygiene (sleep-related habits) than healthy adolescents [20, 22]. Sleep disorders were apparent in all stages of sleep – i.e. difficulties in falling asleep, remaining asleep and regaining sleep [20, 22] as well as daytime sleepiness and decreased alertness [23].

Several reasons are reported for nocturnal awakenings including some of the treatment agents, hydration protocols that lead to urinary frequency, other symptoms (such as pain, nausea, vomiting), nightmares, hunger or thirst, being worried or use of medications such as dexametha-sone [24]. In a research conducted by Hinds et al. [25] on a group of patients receiving dexamethasone, age had a significant association with the change in sleep duration. Older patients spent less time in bed and had less sleep during the day than younger patients.

Acta Haematol 2014;132:363–374
DOI: 10.1159/000360213

Although nighttime sleep disturbance is commonly reported and clinically relevant for adolescents with cancer, it has received little research attention [22]. It is important to assess the adolescents' sleeping habits and sleep quality prior to the initiation of treatment. This will enable us to have a baseline for comparison during the treatment and to plan the intervention accordingly. Not much is known about interventions to improve sleep quality and sleep hygiene, and there is room for more research.

Nausea/Eating Disorders

During the past years there has been much progress in antiemetic therapy, but nausea and vomiting still remain some of the main disturbing symptoms experienced by the AYA cancer population. Furthermore, this symptom was reported as inadequately controlled by medications. Holdsworth et al. [26] found that more than half of the chemotherapy regimens received by adolescents were graded as moderately to severely emetogenic. In their review they report that more than 50% of the patients had uncontrolled nausea. Other causes for nausea and vomiting include radiotherapy, use of pain medication such as opioids, constipation, dehydration and changes in electrolyte balance and causes related to the tumor itself such as intra-abdominal tumors.

Despite advances in antiemetic therapy, adolescents still experience anticipatory, acute and delayed nausea associated with chemotherapy. Prevalence rates of acute nausea during chemotherapy in the reviewed studies ranged from 50 to 100%, and delayed nausea occurred in 29–100% [21]. Ramini et al. [27] found that some AYA patients felt that nurses did not listen or help manage the nausea and vomiting.

As a result of nausea and vomiting, many of the patients experience eating problems. The sight, sound or smell of food worsens nausea. There are several other causes for eating disorders among AYA patients such as anorexia, taste changes and dry mouth, although nausea and vomiting are the barriers that appear to affect eating the most [28]. Although these eating problems are monitored and treated during hospitalization, they are overlooked when adolescents are discharged. There is a need for a long-term intervention plan for eating disorders. In a research conducted by Rodgers et al. [29], adolescents after bone marrow transplantation provided advice to other patients and caregivers regarding strategies to try and overcome the eating problems. Different strategies were tried by the adolescents such as eating familiar food and taking control over the oral intake.

Pain

Pain has been reported by the AYA patients mainly at the time of diagnosis. At this stage the pain is mostly graded as severe. Otherwise, on average, pain is reported on a mild to moderate level [30–33]. Unrelieved pain impairs quality of life and is related to poor outcomes such as wound healing, infection and death [30]. Studies show that undertreatment of pain remains a problem despite major advances in pain management [31, 34].

The cause of pain is associated with several factors including hospitalization. Collins et al. [31] found that hospitalization was associated with higher levels of pain. Other factors associated with pain include: depression, anxiety, race and gender [21]. At the time of diagnosis, pain is associated mainly with the cancer itself. Following this period, pain is associated with the different treatments and procedures [30, 32, 35]. When examining the pattern of pain during the cycle of chemotherapy there does not seem to be a specific pattern [21].

The literature regarding pain is not satisfactory. From the studies that do exist, the strength of evidence is low to very low. There is much need for more studies in this field examining the cause of pain and the pharmacological and nonpharmacological interventions.

Changes in Physical Appearance

Changes in physical appearance occur due to scarring, bruising, changes in the skin, presence of a central venous catheter and perception of an 'ill look'. However, adolescents were particularly concerned with hair loss, weight loss or weight gain with associated stretch marks [36–39]. Changes in physical appearance made patients feel 'ugly', 'different' and less 'normal' than before treatment and made them worry about the effect of their appearance on other aspects of their lives [36–39].

Loss of hair due to chemotherapy can be very traumatic. Adolescents reported alopecia causing stress when interacting with their peers and threatening their sense of body image [40]. Taylor et al. [9] reviewed the literature in order to identify the themes affecting the AYA cancer experience. They reported hair loss to be the most common side effect impacting the patient's self-esteem. Since hair loss is extremely evident and cannot be concealed, patients are identified by all the surroundings, including strangers, as oncological patients.

Hilton et al. [41] examined the similarity of these effects between men and women having cancer in early adulthood (aged 18–38). Hair loss prevailed as a major factor in young adults' cancer experience. Young men appear to have as much difficulty as women in adjusting to

Acta Haematol 2014;132:363–374
DOI: 10.1159/000360213

chemotherapy-induced alopecia and to other people's reaction to them.

Changes in physical appearance caused the young patients to change the way they interacted with society, altering the levels of exposure to the public, due to their anticipation of negative reactions and an increased sense of self-conscience [39]. It is important that the nurses be aware and sensitive to this aspect of the physical side effects. During the patients' education regarding side effects, this point is often perceived as extremely difficult, creating an extensive emotional crisis due to self-image and stigma. At this juncture, the nursing staff plays a key role in containment, guidance and presentation of options for solutions, leading to mitigation of extreme emotions which accompany this symptom.

Late Physical Effects

AYA cancer patients may experience a variety of late physical effects such as learning disabilities, loss of memory and attention disorders from the cognitive adverse effects of the treatment. These manifestations may affect school and work performance. AYA patients can also have disturbed endocrine function, body image disruptions as well as sexual problems, obesity, osteopenia and secondary malignancies [42, 43].

Fertility is also a main concern for AYA patients. The preservation of the reproductive capabilities is paramount to most of the young patients. Many of those surviving the treatment will maintain the capabilities to reproduce. Having said that, in certain cases which include total-body irradiation, radiation to the gonads and chemotherapy regimens containing high-dose alkylators can place women at risk for acute ovarian failure or premature menopause and men at risk for temporary or permanent azoospermia [44].

Given the above, it is extremely important to provide the patients with as much information as possible about the risk of infertility. Since the information is vast and sometimes nonconsistent and contradictory, it is important to supply accurate and relevant information to the patients, also regarding ethical issues relating to the subject. It may be wise to have a dedicated team to tackle this issue, rather than to rely on the treating oncologist.

Social Support Aspects

Social support is perceived as extremely important in any age group or health condition. Cobb [45] defined this term as a state where the individual feels a sense of belonging to a social network with a joint commitment. In addition, social support leads the individual to believing that he or she is loved and accepted and that there is someone who appreciates and takes care of them. Social support during the years of adolescence is considered as one of the most important developmental tasks. The young adults have a variety of many social tasks during the years of adolescence which challenge and occupy them, helping define the final identity. These tasks are not simple for them and require special skill sets, energy and interaction with individuals of the same age group. When an adolescent is diagnosed with cancer, the social difficulties surmount, and in addition to social challenges, he or she is required to face physical and emotional hardships. The period of coping with the disease can negatively impact the social stability and impede the tasks which the adolescent has set for himself. Although according to the literature, the social harm can last for many years after surviving the disease, in this article we will focus on the social support aspects during the treatment period [10, 46–50]. Stegenga and Ward-Smith [51] conducted a research among young adults aged 10–17 years and found that adolescents who are in the stage of intensive treatments report that their parents and friends are the main resources for support.

In a study of cancer patients aged 18–35 years, who became ill after the age of 18 years, support elements of positive and negative nature were evaluated. From a compilation of the questionnaires, it was found that out of 156 subjects, 91 were positive and 65 negative. The researchers divided the subjects into 11 actions which contribute to effective coping and 9 actions which have insulting and derogative implications. The highest emphasis was given to social support and interpersonal relationships such as: positive attention from the surrounding people and promotion of 'normal' life. The participants pointed out that when they received special attention they felt a sense of belonging which led to a general positive feeling. From their point of view, the positive attention, which included tenderness, letters, gifts and visits from friends and colleagues, sent a message of caring and commitment to assist [52].

Family Support

A very important source of social support is the family of the AYA patient. Family flexibility, and its desire to preserve the normal state of the adolescent, was found to be imperative to the creation of good psychological adaptation. On the other hand, adolescents report that family relations can be a source of hardship, depending on the nature of the situation [53]. The parents' understanding of the kind of support needed can mitigate friction be-

Acta Haematol 2014;132:363–374
DOI: 10.1159/000360213

tween them and the adolescent patient. Parent adaptation combined with adolescent temperament predicts in a very efficient manner the adolescent's adaptation to the situation of cancer diagnosis [54].

Group Support

Social support is also achieved by support groups. For AYA patients this method is a good way to ease the difficulties related to dealing with the disease. In a literature review by Treadgold and Kuperberg [55], a number of articles were reviewed, all of which claiming that support groups are a very useful way of sharing experiences, thus enhancing the sense of hope [56–58]. In these groups cancer is the main link point of its individuals, and it gives them a safe place where they can have a sense of 'normalcy' which they have lost since being diagnosed with cancer [46, 59, 60]. In a world where there is high accessibility to the world of AYAs and technological advancement plays a key role, it is also apparent how influential the Internet and social networking are as a source of information and support. The media have a lot of advantages; however, there is a lot of controversy about their effect. One approach is that this kind of support enables its users for only partial emotional exposure whereas face-to-face group support obliges the individual to be more exposed, more confronted [61]. The need to express feelings in writing and read them before submitting inhibits spontaneous and associative expression [62].

Health Care Professional Care Role in Social Support

In a research conducted by Olsen and Harder [63], the researchers focused on social integration processes in which oncology nurses working in adolescent wards were involved. From the research it has come to light that nurses working with this unique population play an important role in the process of bridging the gap between the sick adolescent's world and the social world to which he/she belongs, and that nurses should do this using creative imagination (in contrast to their peers working with adult populations). The researchers claim that although physically the adult and the adolescent are of similar dimensions, the adolescent still has one foot in childhood and the other in young adulthood, a fact which obliges the nurse to have a deep understanding of the specific needs and to know how to act in a manner which will not create antagonism. This can be done by active listening, open communication and goal-focused guidance. Important support should also come from the attending physician, which has a great impact on the adolescent's perception of his/her disease. Open and direct communication will contribute to the development of a trust relationship between the adolescent and the physician. On the other hand, indirect communication, mainly through the parents, can cause noneffective coping and a negative feeling by the patient [52].

When treating AYAs it is recommended to have a team that knows and understands the connection between the adolescent's adaptation to the situation and the interfamily relationships and that could initiate a discussion about their fears and help them in choosing the appropriate course of treatment. It is important to empower the patient and to have support groups for the AYA population. The team must be aware of the risk factors: parental stress, parental posttraumatic stress, nonflexible family function and coping styles.

Research also recommends the establishment of support groups not only for the AYA, but also for their friends, in order to strengthen the friendship bond, which is considered very important. We should offer the possibility for Internet-centered support that can be a source of support for patients who refuse to take part in face-to-face support groups due to limitations of distance, mobility, physical self-image, etc.

Despite the plethora of research concerning support groups, it is important to continue this research, while putting an emphasis on support groups on the web and media. In addition, it is desirable that this research focuses on the evident differences between AYA patients relating to age, family status, career, multicultural effect, etc.

There is a need to establish integration programs for the adolescent returning to school, which should consist of information given to the school faculty and staff as well as to the other students. This can put the parents at ease and give the patient the stepping stone he/she needs to increase his/her self-esteem. It is recommended to conduct discussions with the patient regarding his/her future goals in education and career.

Psychological Aspects

The adolescence and early adulthood periods are a major phase in the formation of a person's identity, the search for the unique 'me'. Erickson divides this period into two parts: the ages of 12–18 and 18–35 years. The first period is called 'identity versus identity confusion', where the young person forms a personal and social identity. According to Erickson, this stage is very important, and the meaningful figures during this stage would be the group of equals. If during this stage the individual fails to form his identity, identity confusion (self-doubt and role confusion) will occur, creating a sense of self-destruction, social apathy, etc.

The next stage, the age of 18–35 years, is defined by Erickson as 'early maturity – intimacy versus loneliness'. In this phase, the person solidifies himself and his stature by productive occupation and by severing old dependency relationships and ties, such as academic and parental figures. At this stage the individual has to make very important decisions such as profession and spouse choices [64]. Diagnosis of cancer in this phase inhibits the normal psychological and social development.

Coping with cancer has a great influence on the subjective well-being of AYAs, during treatment and for many years after [65, 66]. Research conducted on these groups revealed that they are more vulnerable emotionally than others [67, 68]. There is not that much research which investigated the psychological effects of cancer on AYAs, and that which has been done is limited due to the small sampling which was done [69–71].

In the review of all the literature, it is evident that there is a big impact on the psychosocial well-being within the AYA group. The psychosocial aspects include: self-esteem, body image, ability to cope, adjustment and resilience. There are several factors which influence the ability of AYAs to cope with cancer.

Age

Psychological effects vary in conjunction with the adolescent's stage of maturity and development. Age can be a risk or a protecting factor. High cognitive capabilities that are tied to a later age could be a delaying factor for the cancer adolescent [72].

Stage of Disease

AYAs exhibit many different coping styles. Adolescents who have been in the treatment conclusion stage for a longer time experience different psychological problems related to low self-esteem and social stress.

Gender

There are gender-related differences in coping with cancer. Research shows that males develop greater psychological difficulties than females in adolescence. Female patients require more information and knowledge about the disease than males [73]. Male adolescents have greater concerns in relation to their athletic future than females [74], who are more concerned about their physical appearance and relationships [75]. Despite these gender-related differences, both male and female patients reported that positive thinking, hope and belief in the future

are important [8]. Hinds et al. [75] found different definitions of hope between the genders. Females' hopes are related to financial independence, family intimacy and a positive outlook on life, whereas males are more hopeful of self-acceptance as it relates to their athletic capabilities. Hendricks-Ferguson [76] found a difference in the intensity of hope between the genders. In a research conducted on a group of 45 young male adults and 33 females between the ages of 13 and 20, it was found that female hopes were of a higher magnitude than those of the males.

For many years psychologists have been investigating and researching the psychological aspects of dealing with crisis situations, mainly focusing on weaknesses and hardships. In a large research conducted in the USA among 523 cured patients of cancer of the average age of 26, the negative aspects of cancer were investigated. From the findings of the research, it is apparent that the highest negative aspects were: financial, body image, control over life, career planning, personal relationships and family planning. The research revealed that the most negative effect is related to the physical appearance and the self-image [69]. These include changes in weight, loss of hair, changes in sexual drive, scarring and changes in skin texture and pigmentation. The fear that the body will not return to its prior state and the concern of difficulty in intimacy as a result can lead to a sense of guilt, social isolation and regression [77].

Loss of control over life as a result of cancer diagnosis was also found to have a negative effect on AYAs' lives. A low level of control results in a low level of compliance with the intensive treatment required for AYAs, whereas a high sense of life control will greatly improve the quality of life among AYA cancer patients [69].

Research shows that AYAs express a concern of their future integration in normal life, the ability to obtain health insurance, the deduction of career options and genetic and hereditary risks they may be passing on to their offspring [53, 78, 79].

Together with crises and hardships, AYAs can also experience *positive feelings* as a result of coping with cancer. In the following paragraphs we will focus mainly on these positive aspects.

In a research conducted in the USA, the positive and negative influences among cancer patients between the ages of 15 and 30 years were examined. The researchers divided the study population into 3 age groups: 15–20, 21–29, 30–39 years. In all groups, one could find positive influences as a result of coping with cancer. Among these were relationships with significant others, future planning and goal setting, and the ability to have some control over the body and its health. More than 70% of all participants in all age groups reported a positive improvement in their relationship with close family, which they saw as a positive effect on their lives. More than half reported a positive influence on religious and spiritual well-being as a result of coping with the disease [69].

Hope

Hope is a psychological and spiritual resource which helps with coping. Jeven [80] classified hope as being in the same class as coping, faith, spiritual strength and empowerment. It is an imperative part of coping with chronic illnesses [81]. Among maturing young adults hope is an influencing factor identified as assisting the patient to have the ability to respond to his illness, and to be able to adjust to the situation [82]. Hinds et al. [75], who conducted several research trials on hope among young cancer patients, claim that hope can be used as an important defensive resource in coping with cancer among AYAs.

In a separate research conducted by Ritchie [83], hope was evaluated among 45 young cancer patients in comparison with healthy adolescents. The research found that there was an equal level of hope among both groups, and the researchers claim that this supports previous claims that adolescents have the capability for positive thinking and coping. In another research conducted in Taiwan on hope levels in cancer patients aged 12–18 years, it was determined that along with physical and psychological difficulties, the patients were able to focus on their belief for a better and more optimistic future. They learned to find ways to channel positive energy through structural thinking, and believing in what they had and hoped for [84]. In a research conducted in Finland on 6 adolescent cancer patients, it was discovered that hope is directed in 2 dimensions: external and internal. The internal dimension is tied to positive approach, humor, belief in God, and dreams. The external dimension relates to future plans such as getting married, higher education and career development. It was also apparent that hope is directly linked to social support and relationship with others [85].

Research points to differences in the intensity levels of hope among AYAs, which relate to the gender and developmental stage of the individual. In a research on 78 AYA cancer patients aged 13–20 years, it was found that females reported a higher level of hope compared to males and the older age group (15–19 years) a higher level of hope compared with the younger age group (13–14 years). The caring staff should be aware of the changes within the AYA group and administer the proper psychological and emotional treatment based on age and gender [76].

Posttraumatic Growth

People who experience a crisis in their lives can feel growth during the coping phase as well as afterwards. These individuals can be successful in generating positive insights from the process for a better future [86]. Posttraumatic growth can stem from an increase in self-awareness, a clearer meaning of life and positive spiritual changes [87].

The majority of the research on posttraumatic growth focuses on adults who have experienced tragedies in their personal lives, such as natural disasters, grief or illness, such as cancer. Only recently have there been publications of research of posttraumatic growth in adolescents most of which focus on the cured population.

From the article published by Turner-Sack et al. [88], it is apparent that it is imperative to conduct such research on adolescent cancer patients. The need for this stems from other research work conducted on these populations which shows maturity and emotional growth as a result of the disease. In a research trial conducted in Canada among 31 cancer patients, it was discovered that the longer the time lapse since the end of treatment, the lower and less meaningful is the posttraumatic growth. The chances for a relapse are higher among patients reporting a lower posttraumatic growth. Focusing on positive aspects also leads to positive posttraumatic growth [88].

AYA cancer patients have unique psychological needs. The caring staff needs to enable each AYA to maximize his/her potential to become a functioning and contributing individual to society. The mere diagnosis of cancer in this group has a great influence on quality of life, interpersonal relationships and cognitive performance of the patients, which are added after conclusion of treatment. Negative psychological impacts on this age group manifest as a feeling of stress, anxiety and depression, which compels the caring staff to grant psychosocial support throughout the treatment and afterwards. It is important to support the AYAs and empower them to take a positive outlook on the situation despite the illness. Positive thinking and hope are important resources which will lead to better coping, and will enable a 'soft' return and adjustment to a normal and productive life. In an article published by Fernandez et al. [89], it is stated that a routine psychological evaluation of AYAs is imperative to mitigate severe psychological influences as well as giving AYAs timely psychosocial support. The caregivers should have expertise in the field and be attuned to the patient's needs as well as those of his family.

In the area of psychological and emotional functioning, the most crucial source of information is the patient. In some cases, it might be helpful to ask the adolescent how he/she feels the diagnosis has changed and how he/she handles and copes with information. Due to the limited research on the positive aspects of AYAs coping with cancer, it is important to extend the existing research to include personal and interpersonal growth, hope and subjective well-being.

Existential/Spiritual Aspects

Diagnosis of cancer is a difficult experience for all. It is a highly stressful experience associated with physical distress and emotional difficulties [90, 91]. Yet for adolescents this is even more challenging as this is a time when they are still developing their cognitive ability to process information and are starting to plan their future [83, 92, 93].

Psychospiritual well-being is a subjective experience that incorporates both emotional health and meaning of life. It is the affirmation of life in the relationship with God, as well as the perception that one's life has a meaning [94]. There are two dimensions to spiritual well-being: religious well-being – one's relationship with God – and existential well-being – one's sense of life purpose and life satisfaction [40].

An enhanced sense of psychospiritual well-being enables to cope more effectively with various situations such as cancer and its treatments. In a research conducted by Hendricks-Ferguson [40] examining 78 adolescents with cancer, it was evident that at the time periods of the beginning of the disease and treatment there were higher levels of spiritual well-being, religious well-being and existential well-being than during the following time periods. The highest levels of spiritual well-being and its dimensions were found in the first 2 years after diagnosis. Time since diagnosis influences the spiritual well-being. Therefore, it is very important to reassess the spiritual well-being at various time points over the cancer trajectory, from diagnosis to survivorship, and plan our intervention accordingly.

In reviewing the literature examining the various components of psychospiritual well-being, we come across several themes: self-awareness, coping and adjusting effectively with stress, relationship and connectedness with others, sense of faith, sense of empowerment and confidence and living with meaning and hope [95].

Self-Awareness

There are different attitudes regarding telling the patients the whole truth or part of it regarding their disease and prognosis. In different studies it is evident that many family members avoid sharing information about their prognosis with the patients. In several research papers it was found that awareness of dying was both comforting and distressing for the patient [95]. In reviewing the literature, we did not come across any research studying the influence of sharing the truth with AYA cancer patients. From the literature regarding adult cancer patients, it is evident that self-awareness can enhance the patient's sense of psychospiritual well-being [95]; therefore, there is a need for research in this field with AYA patients.

Coping with and Adjusting Effectively to Stress

Factors that enhance coping with and adjusting to advanced cancer include a clear sense of meaning [96] and religious faith [97]. A good relationship with the family and social support have also been found important in assisting patients to cope with advanced cancer [95]. Adolescents gain comfort and confidence from the support they receive from the health care professionals and from the psychosocial support they receive primarily from chaplains, social workers and psychologists [40]. Edmonds et al. [98] found that patients benefited from a long-term psychological intervention.

Another mechanism found to be effective in coping with and adjusting to stress is optimism. This was strongly and positively associated with well-being and negatively related to psychological distress. Psychological distress was positively associated with escape-avoidance coping [99].

Relationship and Connectedness with Others

As mentioned, having positive relationships with family, friends, other patients and health care professionals has an important positive effect on the psychospiritual well-being. This is evident in many research trials [95]. Emotional support and good communications are very important to well-being. Patients report that the feeling of connectedness with others helps enhance the sense of hope [100–102] and meaning [103], awareness of life appreciation [104], desire to live [105] and sense of personal value [106]. Health care personnel using empathy, understanding and reassurance contribute to positive psychological outcomes [95].

Sense of Faith

Sense of faith is an important component of psychospiritual well-being. Yang and Yin [106] found that in patients at the end of life religious beliefs and values of patients and families were associated with positive attitudes towards the diagnosis. Swensen et al. [97] found that faith is positively related to quality of life and psychological and spiritual well-being. It is clear that having faith such as knowing God is important for having hope [95]. The use of hope, prayer and belief in God was found to be an important coping resource for AYA cancer patients [56, 82, 107–110]. Tebbi et al. [111] compared the level of religiosity among adolescents in 3 time periods after diagnosis: less than 1 year, 1–3 years and more than 3 years. A majority of the adolescents reported that belief in God was a source of support for coping with cancer and offered a sense of security when facing death. They found that there was no significant relationship between religiosity and time since diagnosis. In a review of the difference in coping resource over time since diagnosis, Ritchie [83] found that the longer the time since diagnosis, the less likely the adolescents were to seek spiritual support as a coping resource. Similar findings were reported by Nichols [109]: adolescents seek spiritual support as a coping resource during the first stages of their cancer experience, and this decreases as they come to terms with their illness. Hendricks-Ferguson [76] found that adolescents aged 15–17 years reported a higher religious well-being than adolescents aged 18–20 years.

Sense of Empowerment and Confidence

Sense of empowerment and confidence are associated with psychospiritual well-being [95]. A major concern of the patients is work and financial worries. These are negatively associated with psychospiritual well-being. Other contributing factors include dependency, being a burden on others, loss of social role functioning and feeling emotionally irrelevant. It is necessary to maintain a sense of control over loss in order to preserve hope [76].

Living with Meaning and Hope

All aspects of psychospiritual well-being are related to hope and having a meaning to life. Hendricks-Ferguson [40] reported that there was no significant difference in the levels of hope among adolescents at several time points after cancer diagnosis. Levels of hope stayed high over time. As for living with meaning, adolescents have a need to make sense out of life and find a meaning in their suffering and illness. In order to cope with this difficulty, adolescents turn to different sources of support such as spiritual support. Hendricks-Ferguson [40] found that adolescents turn to spiritual support more during the early stages after diagnosis and treatment searching for meaning and hope. As they advance along the cancer trajectory, they depend less on the spiritual support and more on their peers.

Spiritual well-being is of major importance for adolescents when coping with cancer. Strong spiritual support for an existential and identity crisis that can occur during this time may be very helpful in patients coping with isolation, identity issues, peers who do not understand and distraught families. From the literature it is evident that resources the adolescents turn to vary over time. Important resources to enhance the different dimensions of spiritual well-being and quality of life include hope, spiritual practice, specifically having a belief in God, and private prayer [76, 85]. It is important to assess the adolescent's spiritual well-being and psychosocial resources several times over the cancer trajectory while keeping in mind that the same patient will most likely change the source of support in the different time periods. More so it is important to acknowledge the need for support also in later stages of the disease, when treatment has ended and the adolescents try to return to their social role. Nurses have a major role in assisting AYA patients by assessing the need for support, planning effective interventions, being a source of support for them and directing the adolescents to different support resources.

The young adults and adolescents suffering from cancer include a wide range of ages. This population can be divided into age subgroups, each of which has its unique goals and needs. Despite the large age difference, this group is still classified in the literature as one – AYAs, due to the similarities which can be found within these groups.

Conclusion

We can assert that treatment of AYA patients is different in many aspects from other age groups, and it poses a great challenge to the treating personnel. In recent years, the prognosis of this age group has not improved compared to other age groups like children and adults. The developmental stage in which AYAs are in poses great dilemmas concerning their future (education and career). Beyond planning for the future, cancer has a great effect on this population in physiological aspects such as body perception, self-image and mood disturbance, which greatly affect the response to treatment, personal relationships with family and spouse and the entire social environment.

It is important that the health care personnel be aware of the AYA 'style': they relate to each other and the environment around them in a different way, they may choose different ways in order to get information regarding their disease and treatment.

Research shows that despite the physical and mental challenges these patients have to face, many of them are actually able to generate growth and positive insights; however, there are not many research papers in this field.

Hence, the treating staff must act in a very creative way while having empathy and understanding of the challenges the patients are facing. Including AYAs in the decision-making process, being truthful and honest, supportive while maintaining a close contact with friends and family are only some of the elements required while treating this unique group. Proper care management which takes into account the wonderful and rich world of these patients will increase their satisfaction of the service level, which will in turn increase their positive response to treatment. We see great importance in conducting workshops for treating staff which will create a better understanding and give better tools to deal with AYA patients.

Disclosure Statement

The authors have no conflicts of interest to disclose.

References

1 World Health Organization: Maternal, newborn, child and adolescent health. 2013. http://www.who.int/maternal_child_adolescent/topics/adolescence/dev/en/index.html.
2 Bleyer A, Budd T, Montello M: Adolescent and young adult with cancer. Cancer 2006; 107:1645–1655.
3 Wood WA, Lee SJ: Malignant hematologic diseases in adolescents and young adults. Blood 2011;117:5803–5815.
4 Fern L, Davies S, Eden T, Feltbower R, Grant R, Hlawkins M, Whelan J: Rates of inclusion of teenagers and young adults in England into National Cancer Research Network clinical trials: report from the National Cancer Research Institute (NCRI) Teenage and Young Adult Clinical Studies Development Group. Br J Cancer 2008;99:1967–1974.
5 Pollock BH: Where adolescents and young adults with cancer receive their care: does it matter? J Clin Oncol 2007;25:4522–4523.
6 Ferrell B, Grant M, Schmidt GM, Rhiner M, Whitehead C, Fonbuena P, Forman SJ: The meaning of quality of life for bone marrow transplant survivors. 1. The impact of bone marrow transplant on quality of life. Cancer Nurs 1992;15:153–160.
7 Ferrell B, Grant M, Schmidt GM, Rhiner M, Whitehead C, Fonbuena P, Forman SJ: The meaning of quality of life for bone marrow transplant survivors. 2. Improving quality of life for bone marrow transplant survivors. Cancer Nurs 1992;15:247–253.
8 Enskar K, Carlsson M, Golsater M, Hamrin E: Symptom distress and life situation in adolescents with cancer. Cancer Nurs 1997;20:23–33.
9 Taylor RM, Pearce S, Gibson F, Fern L, Whelan J: Developing a conceptual model of teenage and young adult experiences of cancer through meta-synthesis. Int J Nurs Stud 2013; 50:832–846.
10 Gibson F, Mulhall AB, Richardson A, Edwards JL, Ream E, Sepion BJ: A phenomenologic study of fatigue in adolescents receiving treatment for cancer. Oncol Nurs Forum 2005;32:651–660.
11 Erickson JM, Beck SL, Christian B, Dudley WN, Hollen PJ, Albritton K, Sennett MM, Dillon R, Godder K: Patterns of fatigue in adolescents receiving chemotherapy. Oncol Nurs Forum 2010;37:444–455.
12 Lai JS, Kupst MJ, Cella D, Brown SR, Peterman A, Goldman S: Using Q-methodology to understand perceived fatigue reported by adolescents with cancer. Psychooncology 2007; 16:437–447.
13 Ream E, Gibson F, Edwards J, Seption B, Mulhall A, Richardson A: Experience of fatigue in adolescents living with cancer. Cancer Nurs 2006;29:317–326.
14 Richardson A: A critical appraisal of the factors associated with fatigue; in Armes J, Krishnasamy M, Higginson I (eds): Fatigue in Cancer. Oxford, Oxford University Press, 2004, pp 29–50.
15 Hinds PS, Hockenberry M, Rai SN, Zhang L, Razzouk BI, McCarthy K, Cremer L, Rodriguez-Galindo C: Nocturnal awakening, sleep environment interruptions and fatigue in hospitalized children with cancer. Oncol Nurs Forum 2007;34:393–402.
16 Perdikaris P, Merkouris A, Patiraki E, Tsoumakas K, Vasilatou-Kosmidis E, Matziou V: Evaluating cancer related fatigue during treatment according to children's, adolescents' and parents' perspectives in a sample of Greek young patients. Eur J Oncol Nurs 2009;13: 399–408.
17 Baggott C, Dodd M, Kennedy C, Marina N, Matthay KK, Cooper BA, Miaskowski C: Changes in children's reports of symptom occurrence and severity during a course of myelosuppressive chemotherapy. J Pediatr Oncol Nurs 2010;27:307–315.
18 Hockenberry MJ, Hooke MC, Gregurich M, McCarthy K, Sambuco G, Krull K: Symptom clusters in children and adolescents receiving cisplatin, doxorubicin, or ifosfamide. Oncol Nurs Forum 2010;37:E16–E27.
19 Walker AJ, Gedaly-Duff V, Miaskowski C, Nail L: Differences in symptom occurrence, frequency, intensity, and distress in adolescents prior to and one week after the administration of chemotherapy. J Pediatr Oncol Nurs 2010;27:259–265.
20 Walker AJ, Johnson KP, Miaskowski C, Lee KA, Gedaly-Duff V: Sleep quality and sleep hygiene behaviors of adolescents during chemotherapy. Clin Sleep Med 2010;6:439–444.
21 Erickson JM, Macpherson CF, Ameringer S, Baggott C, Linder L, Stegenga K: Symptoms and symptom clusters in adolescents receiving cancer treatment: a review of the literature. Int J Nurs Stud 2013;50:847–869.
22 Walker AJ, Pongsing Y, Nail L, Pedhiwala N, Leo M, Price J, Lee K, Gedaly-Duff V: Sleep-wake patterns of school-age children and adolescents before diagnosis and during induction chemotherapy for acute lymphocytic leukemia. J Pediatr Nurs 2011;26:e37–e44.
23 Erickson JM, Beck SL, Christian BR, Dudley W, Hollen PJ, Albritton KA, Sennett M, Dillon RL, Godder K: Fatigue, sleep-wake disturbances, and quality of life in adolescents receiving chemotherapy. J Pediatr Hematol Oncol 2011;33:e17–e25.
24 Walker AJ, Johnson KP, Miaskowski C, Gedaly-Duff V: Nocturnal sleep-wake parameters of adolescents at home following cancer chemotherapy. Biol Res Nurs 2012;14:236–241.
25 Hinds PS, Hockenberry MJ, Gattuso JS, Srivastava DK, Tong X, Jones H, West N, McCarthy KS, Sadeh A, Ash M, Fernandez C, Pui CH: Dexamethasone alters sleep and fatigue in pediatric patients with acute lymphoblastic leukemia. Cancer 2007;110:2321–2330.
26 Holdsworth MT, Raisch DW, Frost J: Acute and delayed nausea and emesis control in pediatric oncology patients. Cancer 2006;106: 931–940.

27 Ramini SK, Brown R, Buckner EB: Embracing changes: adaptation by adolescents with cancer. Pediatr Nurs 2008;34:72–79.
28 Iestra JA, Fibbe WE, Zwinderman AH, van Staveren WA, Kromhout D: Body weight recovery, eating difficulties and compliance with dietary advice in the first year after stem cell transplantation: a prospective study. Bone Marrow Transplant 2002;29:417–424.
29 Rodgers C, Young A, Hockenberry M, Binder B, Symes L: The meaning of adolescents' eating experiences during bone marrow transplant recovery. J Pediatr Oncol Nurs 2010;27: 65–72.
30 Ameringer S: Barriers to pain management among adolescents with cancer. Pain Manag Nurs 2010;11:224–233.
31 Collins JJ, Byrnes ME, Dunkel IJ, Lapin J, Nadel T, Thaler HT, Polyak T, Rapkin B, Portenoy RK: The measurement of symptoms in children with cancer. J Pain Symptom Manage 2000;19:363–377.
32 Jacob E, Hesselgrave J, Sambuco G, Hockenberry M: Variations in pain, sleep, and activity during hospitalization in children with cancer. J Pediatr Oncol Nurs 2007;24:208–219.
33 Miller E, Jacob E, Hockenberry MJ: Nausea, pain, fatigue, and multiple symptoms in hospitalized children with cancer. Oncol Nurs Forum 2011;38:E382–E393.
34 Wolfe J, Grier HE, Klar N, Levin SB, Ellenbogen JM, Salem-Schatz S, Emanuel EJ, Weeks JC: Symptoms and suffering at the end of life in children with cancer. N Engl J Med 2000; 342:326–333.
35 Calissendorff-Selder M, Ljungman G: Quality of life varies with pain during treatment in adolescents with cancer. Ups J Med Sci 2006; 111:109–116.
36 Hedström M, Ljungman G, von Essen L: Perceptions of distress among adolescents recently diagnosed with cancer. J Pediatr Hematol Oncol 2005;27:15–22.
37 Larouche SS, Chin-Peuckert L: Changes in body image experienced by adolescents with cancer. J Pediatr Oncol Nurs 2006;23:200–209.
38 Wallace ML, Harcourt D, Rumsey N, Foot A: Managing appearance changes resulting from cancer treatment: resilience in adolescent females. Psychooncology 2007;16:1019–1027.
39 Williamson H, Harcourt D, Halliwell E, Frith H, Wallace M: Adolescents' and parents' experiences of managing the psychosocial impact of appearance change during cancer treatment. J Pediatr Oncol Nurs 2010;27:168–175.
40 Hendricks-Ferguson V: Hope and spiritual well-being in adolescents with cancer. West J Nurs Res 2008;30:385–401.
41 Hilton S, Hunt K, Emslie C, Salinas M, Ziebland S: Have men been overlooked? A comparison of young men and women's experiences of chemotherapy-induced alopecia. Psychooncology 2008;17:577–583.

42 Eiser C, Absolom K, Greenfield D, Snowden J, Coleman R, Hancock B, Davies H: Follow-up care for young adult survivors of cancer: lessons from pediatrics. J Cancer Surviv 2007; 1:75–86.
43 Thomas DM, Seymour JF, O'Brien T, Sawyer SM, Ashley DM: Adolescent and young adult cancer: a revolution in evolution? Intern Med J 2006;36:302–307.
44 Levine J, Canada A, Stern CJ: Fertility preservation in adolescents and young adults with cancer. J Clin Oncol 2010;28:4831–4841.
45 Cobb S: Social support as a moderator of life stress. Psychosom Med 1976;38:300–314.
46 Cassano J, Nagel K, O'Mara L: Talking with others who 'just know': perceptions of adolescents with cancer who participate in a teen group. J Pediatr Oncol Nurs 2008;25:193–199.
47 Grinyer A: The biographical impact of teenage and adolescent cancer. Chronic Illness 2007;3:265–277.
48 Kelly D, Pearce S, Mulhall A: 'Being in the same boat': ethnographic insights into an adolescent cancer unit. Int J Nurs Stud 2004;41: 847–857.
49 Lockhart IA, Berard MF: Psychological vulnerability and resilience to emotional distress: a focus group study of adolescent cancer patients. Int J Adolesc Med Health 2001;13:221–229.
50 Olsen PR, Harder I: Keeping their world together – meanings and actions created through network-focused nursing in teenager and young adult cancer care. Cancer Nursing 2009;32:493–502.
51 Stegenga K, Ward-Smith P: On receiving the diagnosis of cancer: the adolescent perspective. J Pediatr Oncol Nurs 2009;26:75–80.
52 Zebrack B, Chesler MA, Kaplan S: To foster healing among adolescents and young adults with cancer: what helps? What hurts? Support Care Cancer 2010;18:131–135.
53 Evan E, Zeltzer LK: Psychosocial dimensions of cancer in adolescents and young adults. Cancer 2006;107(suppl 7):1663–1971.
54 Barrera M, Wayland L, D'Agostino NM, Gibson J, Weksberg R, Malkin D: Developmental differences in psychological adjustment and health-related quality of life in pediatric cancer patients. Child Health Care 2003;32:215–232.
55 Treadgold CL, Kuperberg A: Been there, done that, wrote the blog: the choices and challenges of supporting adolescents and young adults with cancer. J Clin Oncol 2010;28:4842–4849.
56 Haase J: The components of courage in chronically ill adolescents. Adv Nurs Sci 1987; 9:64–80.
57 Haase J: The adolescent resilience model as a guide to interventions. J Pediatr Oncol Nurs 2004;21:289–299.
58 Meltzer LJ, Rourke MT: Oncology summer camp: benefits of social comparison. Children's Health Care 2005;34:305–314.

59 Docherty A: Experience, functions and benefits of a cancer support group. Patient Educ Couns 2004;55:87–91.
60 McGrath P: Finding from an educational support course for patients with leukemia. Cancer Pract 1999;7:198–204.
61 King R, Bambling M, Lloyd C, Gomurra R, Smith S, Reid W: Online counseling: the motives and experience of young people who choose the Internet instead of face to face or telephone counseling. Couns Psychother Res 2006;6:169–174.
62 Finfgeld DL: Therapeutic groups online: the good, the bad, and the unknown. Iss Mental Health Nurs 2000;21:241–255.
63 Olsen PR, Harder I: Caring for teenagers and young adults with cancer: a grounded theory study of network-focused nursing. Eur J Oncol Nurs 2011;15:152–159.
64 Marcia JE: Development and validation of ego identity status. J Pers Soc Psychol 1966;3:551–558.
65 Larsson G, Mattsson E, von Essen L: Aspects of quality of life, anxiety, and depression among persons diagnosed with cancer during adolescence: a long-term follow-up study. Eur J Cancer 2010;46:1062–1068.
66 Jordgarden A, Mattsson E, von Essen L: Health-related quality of life, anxiety and depression among adolescents and young adults with cancer: a prospective longitudinal study. Eur J Cancer 2007;43:1952–1958.
67 Stava CJ, Lopez A, Vassilopoulou-Sellin R: Health profiles of younger and older breast cancer survivors. Cancer 2006;107:1752–1759.
68 Mor V, Allen S, Malin M: The psychosocial impact of cancer on older versus younger patients and their families. Cancer 1994;74: 2118–2127.
69 Bellizzi KM, Smith A, Schmidt S, Keegan TH, Zebrack B, Lynch CF, Simon M: Positive and negative psychosocial impact of being diagnosed with cancer as an adolescent or young adult. Cancer 2012;15:5155–5162.
70 Decker CL: Coping in adolescents with cancer: a review of the literature. J Psychosoc Oncol 2006;24:123–140.
71 Decker CL: Social support and adolescent cancer survivors: review of literature. J Psychosoc Oncol 2007;16:1–11.
72 Sorgen KE, Manne SL: Coping in children with cancer: examining the goodness-of-fit hypothesis. Child Health Care 2002;31:191–207.
73 Decker C, Phillips CR, Haase JE: Information needs of adolescents with cancer. J Pediatr Oncol Nurs 2004;21:327–334.
74 Hinds PS: Adolescent-focused oncology nursing research. Oncol Nurs Forum 2004;31: 281–287.
75 Hinds PS, Quargnenti A, Fairclough D, Bush AJ, Betcher D, Rissmiller G, Pratt CB, Gilchrist GS: Hopefulness and its characteristics in adolescents with cancer. West J Nurs Res 1999;21:600–620.

76 Hendricks-Ferguson V: Relationships of age and gender to hope and spiritual well-being among adolescents with cancer. J Pediatr Oncol Nurs 2006;23:189–199.

77 Die-Trill M, Stuber ML: Psychological problems of curative cancer treatment; in Holland J (ed): Psycho-Oncology. New York, Oxford University Press, 1998, pp 897–906.

78 Zeltzer LK: Cancer in adolescents and young adults. Cancer 1993;71:3463–3468.

79 Keene N, Hobbie W, Ruccione K: Childhood Cancer Survivors: A Practical Guide to Your Future, ed 2. Sebastopol, O'Reilly Media, 2007.

80 Jeven RF: It All Begins with Hope. San Diego, Lura Media, 1991.

81 Parse RR: Hope: An International Human Becoming Perspective. Sudbury, Jones & Bartlett, 1999.

82 Hinds PS, Martin J: Hopefulness and the self-sustaining process in adolescents with cancer. Nurs Res 1988;37:336–340.

83 Ritchie MA: Self-esteem and hopefulness in adolescents with cancer. J Pediatr Nurs 2001;16:35–42.

84 Wu LM, Chin CC, Haase JE, Chen CH: Coping experiences of adolescents with cancer: a qualitative study. J Adv Nurs 2009;65:2358–2366.

85 Juvakka T, Kylma J: Hope in adolescents with cancer. Eur J Oncol Nurs 2009;13:193–199.

86 Tedeschi R, Park CL, Calhoun LG: Posttraumatic growth: positive changes in the aftermath of crisis. Mahwah, Erlbaum, 1998.

87 Tedeschi R, Calhoun L: Trauma and Transformation: Growing in the Aftermath of Suffering. Thousand Oaks, Sage, 1995.

88 Turner-Sack A, Menna R, Setchell SR: Posttraumatic growth, coping strategies, and psychological distress in adolescent survivors of cancer. J Pediatr Oncol Nurs 2012;29:70–79.

89 Fernandez C, Fraser GAM, Freeman C, Grunfeld E, Gupta A, Mery LS, Schacter B: Principles and recommendations for the provision of healthcare in Canada to adolescent and young adult-aged cancer patients and survivors. J Adolesc Young Adult Oncol 2011;1:54–59.

90 O'Connor AP, Wicker CA, Germino BB: Understanding the cancer patient's search for meaning. Cancer Nurs 1990;13:167–175.

91 Chiu L: A phenomenological study on searching for meaning in-life in women living with breast cancer. Hu Li Yan Jiu 1999;7:119–128.

92 Ritchie MA: Psychosocial functioning of adolescents with cancer. A developmental perspective. Oncol Nurs Forum 1992;19:1497–1501.

93 Woodgate RL: Adolescents' perspectives of chronic illness: 'it's hard'. J Pediatr Nurs 1998;13:210–223.

94 Paloutzian RF, Ellison CW: Loneliness, spiritual well-being, and the quality of life; in Peplau LA, Perlman D (eds): Loneliness: A Source Book of Current Theory, Research and Therapy. New York, Wiley, 1982.

95 Lin HR, Bauer-Wu SM: Psycho-spiritual well-being in patients with advanced cancer: an integrative review of the literature. J Adv Nurs 2003;44:69–80.

96 Taylor EJ: Factors associated with meaning in life among people with recurrent cancer. Oncol Nurs Forum 1993;20:1399–1405.

97 Swensen CH, Fuller S, Clements R: Stage of religious faith and reactions to terminal cancer. J Psychol Theol 1993;21:238–245.

98 Edmonds CV, Lockwood GA, Cunningham AJ: Psychological response to long-term group therapy: a randomized trial with metastatic breast cancer patients. Psychooncology 1999;8:74–91.

99 Miller DL, Manne SL, Taylor K, Keates J, Dougherty J: Psychological distress and well-being in advanced cancer: the effects of optimism and coping. J Clin Psychol Med Settings 1996;3:115–130.

100 Ballard A, Green T, McCaa A, Logsdon MC: A comparison of the level of hope in patients with newly diagnosed and recurrent cancer. Oncol Nurs Forum 1997;24:899–904.

101 Flemming K: The imponderable: a search for meaning. The meaning of hope to palliative care cancer patients. Int J Palliat Nurs 1997;3:14–18.

102 Benzein E, Norberg A, Saveman BI: The meaning of the lived experience of hope in patients with cancer in palliative home care. Palliat Med 2001;15:117–126.

103 Thomas J, Retsas A: Transacting self-preservation: a grounded theory of the spiritual dimensions of people with terminal cancer. Int J Nurs Stud 1999;36:191–201.

104 Mahon SM, Casperson D: Exploring the psychosocial meaning of recurrent cancer: a descriptive study. Cancer Nurs 1997;20:178–186.

105 Roud PC: Psychosocial variables associated with the exceptional survival of patients with advanced malignant disease. Int J Psychiatry Med 1986–1987;16:113–122.

106 Yang KP, Yin TJ: Defining the content domain of health related quality of life for terminally ill cancer patients. Hu Li Yan 1999;7:129–144.

107 Bull BA, Drotar D: Coping with cancer in remission: stressors and strategies reported by children and adolescents. J Pediatr Psychol 1991;16:767–782.

108 Kyngas H, Mikkonen R, Noursiainen EM, Rytilahti M, Seppanen P, Vaattovaara R, Jamsa T: Coping with the onset of cancer: coping strategies and resources of young people with cancer. Eur J Cancer Care (Engl) 2001;10:6–11.

109 Nichols ML: Social support and coping in young adolescents with cancer. Pediatr Nurs 1995;21:235–240.

110 Parry C, Chesler MA: Thematic evidence of psychosocial thriving in childhood cancer survivors. Qual Health Res 2005;15:1055–1073.

111 Tebbi CK, Mallon JC Richards ME, Bigler LR: Religiosity and locus of control of adolescent cancer patients. Psychol Rep 1987;61:683–696.

Acta Haematol 2014;132:363–374
DOI: 10.1159/000360213

Acta Haematol 2014;132:375–382
DOI: 10.1159/000360239

Published online: September 10, 2014

Peer and Romantic Relationships among Adolescent and Young Adult Survivors of Childhood Hematological Cancer: A Review of Challenges and Positive Outcomes

Rebecca H. Foster[a, b]   Marilyn Stern[c]

[a]Department of Psychology, Winona State University, Winona, Minn., [b]Behavioral Health Department, Gundersen Health System, La Crosse, Wisc., and [c]Departments of Rehabilitation and Mental Health Counseling, College of Behavioral and Community Sciences, Department of Psychology, Pediatric Epidemiology Center and Moffitt Cancer Center, University of South Florida, Tampa, Fla., USA

Key Words

Adolescents · Childhood cancer · Peers · Romantic relationships · Young adults

Abstract

This review focuses on peer and romantic relationship experiences of adolescent and young adult (AYA) survivors of childhood cancer, highlighting those surviving leukemia or lymphoma. While most AYA survivors adjust well to life following a hematological cancer diagnosis and treatment, many unique experiences, both positive and challenging, have been documented with respect to successfully navigating developmentally normative social goals. Therefore, the social implications of surviving childhood leukemia or lymphoma are explored. Specifically, the development of peer and romantic relationships, perceptions of social acceptance, parental influences and attachment, perceived vulnerabilities and body image, and risks to fertility are discussed.

© 2014 S. Karger AG, Basel

'I was diagnosed my senior year in high school. I was normal, healthy, active and happy and got pulled from a volley ball game when they found out. I was very lucky to have a mother who didn't leave my side and wonderful friends who weren't afraid to hop up in the hospital bed with me and ask if I had cute doctors. It was hard missing out on some of my senior year, but thankfully I was finished with treatment well before graduation and was sporting a spiky short haircut by the time I started my freshman year of college. I was extremely blessed to have a roommate who ([it's a] very small world) had leukemia when she was 18, and it has been amazing to have someone who truly understands and knows all the ins and outs of what I went through. Also in my freshman year, I met the guy who is soon to be my husband. I did have some fears about having to talk about the whole experience with someone who had not been there, but he cared about me so much that he cried the first time I really talked to him about it, and [he] now has two tattoo dots on his chest to match my radiation tattoos to show his support. As we are about to get married, fertility is the only issue that seems to carry over, but is one that we will deal with when the time comes. All in all, having cancer when I did was an experience that helped shape me into [who I am].'

21-year-old female survivor

'I have noticed that, compared to my peers, I deal with stressful situations much more calmly and effectively. My guess is that having essentially grown up with such a stressful experience in my past, problems that my peers saw as difficult to deal with seemed less dramatic to me in comparison to some of the treatments I experienced. Spinal taps and repeated blood tests tend to desensitize one to 'sweating the small stuff', it seems.'

18-year-old male survivor

KARGER

E-Mail karger@karger.com
www.karger.com/aha

Marilyn Stern, PhD
Departments of Rehabilitation and Mental Health Counseling
University of South Florida, 13301 Bruce B. Downs Blvd.
Tampa, FL 33612-3807 (USA)
E-Mail mstern1 @usf.edu

Introduction

The National Cancer Institute defines adolescents and young adults (AYAs) as individuals between the ages of 15 and 39, with younger AYAs, the focus of this paper, defined as those from 15 to 24 years of age [1]. Younger AYAs, simply referred to as AYAs hereafter, are more likely than older AYAs to experience hematological cancer, and while the majority of younger AYA survivors of childhood cancer adjust relatively well to life following treatment, many unique experiences are encountered with respect to developing and maintaining peer and romantic relationships [2]. Risks of difficulties in social domains exist and are due, in part, to the already complex developmental changes occurring for younger AYAs, which can be further disrupted by having experienced hematological cancer. The chronic, internal, unpredictable nature of cancer means that even when survivorship status is reached, the perceived threat does not necessarily dissipate and can impact aspects of identity and life domains far beyond those directly involving physical health status [3]. Despite challenges, positive outcomes have also been documented. Therefore, the following review examines social implications of childhood cancer, with an emphasis on younger AYAs who have survived leukemia or lymphoma. The review begins with an overview of relationship challenges related to treatment of hematological cancer, including treatment intensity and length of treatment. Following this, more specific aspects of peer and romantic relationship development are discussed, with an emphasis on perceptions of health vulnerabilities, relationships with and attachment to parents, and fertility risks. Of note, however, because most research on survivors of childhood cancer includes patients from a range of diagnostic groups, the review contains information including but not necessarily limited to survivors of hematological cancer. This highlights the need for additional research focusing exclusively on the unique needs of younger AYAs surviving childhood hematological cancer.

Cancer Treatment Intensity and Social Outcomes among AYAs

Despite the impressive advancements in cancer treatments for children surviving leukemia or lymphoma, the potentially detrimental physical and emotional late effects of lifesaving treatments on social relationships and psychosexual development cannot be dismissed [4, 5].

The severity of potential problems tends to vary based on treatment intensity, which is a collective term taking into account the diagnosis, stage or severity of the disease at diagnosis, relapse status, types of treatment modalities administered (i.e., chemotherapy, radiation, surgery, transplantation) and the number of treatment modalities utilized. Generally speaking, when treatment intensity is greater, so is the risk for significant late effects. Most childhood hematological cancer diagnoses receive an intensity rating of moderate to severe depending upon relapse status and the need for transplantation. Length of treatment varies from approximately 6 months for some types of lymphomas to 2–3 years for acute lymphoblastic leukemia (ALL), one of the most common childhood hematological cancers. Longer treatment protocols can translate into more extensive time away from typical developmental interactions with peers, potentially resulting in difficulties forming and maintaining peer and romantic relationships in the future.

While it is critically important to understand how neurocognitive deficits may relate to learning, memory, executive functioning and problem-solving capabilities, the entirety of the cancer experience, including any cognitive or physical impairment or time away from typical developmental experiences, can lead to challenges with peer and romantic relationships [6]. This was demonstrated in a recent study of AYA survivors of ALL when executive functioning, coping styles, and behavioral and social problems were explored [6]. Executive functioning included working memory, behavioral inhibition, cognitive flexibility, and self-monitoring. Results indicated that the application of cognitive restructuring, acceptance, and distraction techniques as methods of coping fully mediated the relations between working memory, cognitive flexibility, and self-monitoring and psychosocial/behavioral outcomes. In other words, being able to shift one's thinking and monitor one's mental processes was significantly related to the utilization of adaptive coping strategies. In turn, these constructs were related to better psychosocial/behavioral outcomes. Overall, the authors suggested that executive functioning difficulties could make it more difficult for survivors of ALL to cope with social stressors, such as actively addressing peer conflicts or rejection.

Studies of AYA survivors of childhood cancer have explored how treatment intensity may be related to social development and awareness. A study of adolescent survivors who underwent central nervous system treatments such as brain irradiation, intrathecal chemotherapy and/or systemic methotrexate, all commonly currently or previously utilized leukemia treatments, found that, when rated by peers, participants with higher scores on the central nervous system treatment intensity scale had fewer friendships, were less accepted by peers, were more socially sensitive, were more isolated, and were rated as being less popular than those with less intense treatments [7]. Another study of AYA survivors found that participants with a greater number of late effects were rated by their mothers as engaging in fewer social activities [5]. Greater treatment intensity was associated with greater likelihood of desiring future marriage; however, those with more severe late effects were rated as less likely to have a trusted friend. Beyond reports by parents, however, it should be noted that AYAs in the study reported functioning in social domains that was relatively similar to their same-age healthy peers. While the study demonstrated that not all research on treatment intensity finds self-perceptions of social impairment [5], collectively, results from the AYA literature suggest that childhood cancer survivors with higher-intensity treatments may be at risk of negative social outcomes.

AYA Survivors, Peer and Romantic Relationships, and Perceptions of Social Acceptance

Formation of peer and romantic relationship domains has been described as central to identity development among AYAs, as these relationships lay the groundwork for close relationships throughout adulthood [8]. Ultimately adult relationships will reflect the attachment styles developed in childhood with parents as a function of life experiences already encountered, including childhood cancer. Compromised peer and romantic relationships have been reported among AYA survivors as compared to AYAs who have not experienced cancer, with AYAs currently under treatment for and/or surviving leukemia reporting greater rates of social isolation as compared to other diagnostic groups [9], perhaps in part due to the length of treatment and time away from normative peer interactions. One study found that AYA survivors often perceive themselves as being more mature than their healthy peers, resulting in problems interacting with similarly aged peers and romantic partners [10]. AYAs have also indicated concerns that physical late effects reduce their ability to develop intimate romantic relationships [10, 11]. They worry about seeking out new friendships after losing friends to cancer deaths as well. Although these significant concerns are discussed, many participants still reported confidence in their ability to develop and maintain healthy relationships, suggesting good resiliency and perseverance in this group [10].

AYA survivors have reported delays in establishing lasting relationships, and 1 in 5 have indicated perceived restrictions in their sexual quality of life because of their cancer experience [12]. Survivors have reported feeling less experienced than their peers when it comes to romantic and/or sexual encounters. Among those going through treatment for leukemia during adolescence, delays in psychosexual development have been reported, including delays in dating, establishing committed romantic relationships, and engaging in sexual intercourse [11, 12]. Despite challenges with psychosocial development and possible risks to fertility, the majority of AYA survivors report a desire to become parents, with most reporting that they would prefer to have biological children [13]. Research has shown that survivors not only perceive themselves as physically healthy enough to be parents but often state that their cancer experience may enhance their parenting skills [12, 13].

AYA survivors of childhood cancer, including survivors of leukemia or lymphoma, commonly encounter challenges related to their physical development, including delays in physical maturation, changes in appearance due to treatment modalities (e.g., scars, dermatological problems from graft-versus-host disease, prolonged hair loss), and the risk of infertility due to certain cancer treatments [10, 12, 14]. Many of these challenges remain after cancer treatment is completed and impact perceived physical attractiveness, which, in turn, may negatively affect romantic relationships and perceptions of one's social and sexual self [11, 15, 16]. Increased physical changes have been associated with poorer body image, decreased self-worth, reduced social acceptance, and fewer intimate friendships [11, 17]. AYA survivors also participated in approximately 50% fewer social activities [17]. Diminished self-worth, higher levels of social anxiety, and more negative body image tended to increase as time since treatment ended increased, suggesting that additional difficulties with body image and social anxieties may not become evident until survivors have been off treatment for an extended time [12, 17].

Feeling one is socially accepted is of the utmost importance to AYAs. This is true regardless of whether or not an individual has survived a hematological cancer diagnosis. Not only do younger AYAs hold self-perceptions of social acceptance, they also have perceptions of their peers' levels of social acceptability and how they believe others view them. A study of adolescents with cancer attending a summer camp indicated that the adolescents with cancer perceived themselves as being more similar to the other campers with cancer than their peers without a history of cancer [18]. However, those who perceived themselves as more similar to their healthy peers felt more socially accepted. Additionally, adolescents with cancer were more likely to feel accepted by other cancer patients than by healthy peers. A more recent study of AYAs with cancer reported similar feelings and perceptions while attending supportive groups and social events [19]. During these social interactions, participants described the importance of having other patients with whom they could identify and discuss any topic. Participants added that they did not always feel understood by their healthy peers and that peers with cancer were better able to provide the support they needed.

The research in this area, however, has been inconsistent in its findings of negative perceptions of social acceptance among survivors of childhood cancer. One study of adolescent cancer survivors reported no differences in social acceptance [20]. In this study, schoolmates of childhood cancer survivors completed measures of social acceptance, loneliness, social dissatisfaction, and depression. Results suggested that while survivors were perceived as being more isolated than healthy peers, there were no differences in perceptions of social acceptance when comparing peers with/without a history of cancer. Several studies have shown similar results indicating that, in general, adolescents diagnosed with cancer are as socially accepted as their healthy peers [21].

Perceived Health Vulnerability and Social Relationships

One construct that has been implicated as important to the development of social relationships in AYA survivors of childhood cancer is perceived health vulnerability. Perceived health vulnerability refers to an individual's anxieties or concerns about personal health and how those concerns relate to adjustment [22, 23]. The impact of perceived vulnerability on developmental processes such as social skill development in AYAs with cancer has been described [22]. Using a life-span developmental approach, it has been argued that behavioral responses to significant life events like cancer depend on the interplay between past behavioral reactions and innate personality traits. Psychological plasticity enables people to mold their own development by deciding which events to in-

corporate into their life histories. When assessing perceived vulnerability in AYAs with cancer as compared to those diagnosed with diabetes and cystic fibrosis, cancer patients reported perceiving less control over future outcomes and feeling less competent to make decisions concerning their well-being. Additionally, individuals with cancer may feel less able to be autonomous and independent, which are typical markers of development among AYAs [22]. A recent study of AYA Israeli childhood cancer survivors found that those with lower perceptions of vulnerability showed a higher quality of life, including better social interactions [23].

AYA female survivors of childhood cancer tend to feel more vulnerable than males and expect poorer outcomes in the future [4, 24]. When asked to rate their feelings in relation to how likely it was that they would encounter future health problems as a result of having childhood cancer, AYA females were more likely to report a need for consistent follow-ups with a medical doctor and to perceive themselves at a greater risk for future diseases, which may make the pursuit of peer and romantic relationships feel futile if survivors believe they are vulnerable to negative outcomes. Similar gender differences have been found in other research, with AYA female cancer patients reporting greater perceived health vulnerability [4]. Higher perceived vulnerability was associated with worse scores on health-related quality of life scores in both physical and mental health domains. Overall, researchers reported that a realistic perception of vulnerabilities relating to a cancer diagnosis may be useful in motivating people to be self-efficacious about their health and in gaining the confidence to successfully adapt and lead a healthy lifestyle in the future [24]. This includes pursuing developmentally appropriate goals for peer and romantic relationships, cohabitation, marriage, and parenthood [24].

The Importance of Attachment to Parents in Establishing Future Social Relationships

Successful peer and romantic relationships in adulthood are associated with developing secure attachments in childhood (i.e., an emotional bond created between two people) [25]. A secure attachment can be influenced by any number of external and internal factors but fundamentally requires sensitivity to basic needs, receptiveness to explicit signals and an interaction that encourages continuing development. A child who is provided with these requirements is more likely to build better relation-

Acta Haematol 2014;132:375–382
DOI: 10.1159/000360239

ships with friends, seek help when necessary, and develop independence as he or she ages.

Relationships with peers, parents and romantic partners increasingly intermix as individuals enter adolescence and young adulthood [8]; however, attachment styles tend to remain relatively stable over this time period [26]. Research has shown that AYA relationships with parents are significantly related to perceived quality of both peer and romantic relationships and that attachments formulated in childhood are significantly related to the quality of current relationships with a romantic partner [27]. AYAs are just as likely to seek out their parents as compared to peers or romantic partners in asking for advice, and the quality of the parent-child relationship prior to adolescence has been found to predict the quality of romantic relationships.

Unfortunately, secure attachments are at risk of deterioration when a family's sense of normalcy is disrupted by childhood cancer [26, 28, 29]. Although opportunities for deteriorations or changes in attachment styles exist when facing cancer diagnosis, treatment and survivorship, evidence of such deteriorations has not yet been found to be unequivocal [28], and differences in AYA and parent reports exist [29]. For example, AYA survivors have reported feeling less attached to their parents than their parents perceive [29]. More specifically, AYAs endorsed poorer communication and greater feelings of alienation (both aspects of attachment) than was perceived by parents. However, although differences in ratings exist, parents' ratings of their child's sense of trust and alienation significantly contributed to AYAs' perceptions of trust and alienation within the parent-child relationship, respectively. Research has also suggested that although attachment was not significantly related to physician-rated physical sequelae, some evidence was found that quality of attachment was related to functional deficits (e.g., seizures, chronic headaches, problems with concentration, poor memory, ovarian failure and irregular menses) [28]. AYAs with functional sequelae were more likely to report feeling insecure in their relationships overall and to endorse greater ambivalence surrounding their relationships with their parents. Those whose functional sequelae developed later in life (i.e., in young adulthood or adulthood as compared to childhood or adolescence) reported greater difficulties with close relationships such as those with peers or romantic partners. Despite this, overwhelming evidence exists suggesting that if secure parental attachments can be maintained, then positive outcomes are more likely.

AYA Cancer Survivorship, Infertility Risks and Fertility Preservation

Infertility is a common sequela of childhood cancer treatment that can hinder the development of romantic relationships, alter perceptions of social acceptance, and act as a detriment to healthy identity development [12]. For survivors of leukemia or lymphoma, the level of risk tends to be associated with the type of cancer and related treatments; however, all types of therapy, including chemotherapy, surgery, irradiation therapy and/or transplantation, may carry inherent risks. Pelvic irradiation poses some of the greatest risks for infertility among both males and females, with the level of risk being related to irradiation dose, age at time of treatment, adjunctive treatment with alkylating agents, being diagnosed with Hodgkin's lymphoma and/or irradiation exposure to reproductive organs [30]. Specifically, irradiation therapy to the reproductive organs has been associated with a reduced likelihood of pregnancy, low birth weight infants, preterm births and fetal deaths [12, 30]. Acute ovarian failure, premature menopause, and uterine dysfunction are also associated risks. Moreover, the high-dose chemotherapies and full-body irradiation utilized in preparation for bone marrow or stem cell transplantation and for the treatment of hematological and other cancers place patients at a high risk of infertility [31].

The majority of AYAs diagnosed with leukemia or lymphoma will now survive into adulthood, making it pertinent that risks of infertility be discussed with patients and families at diagnosis and throughout treatment. While fertility risks and options for fertility preservation are becoming more common topics of conversation in pediatric oncology settings, research indicates that there continue to be many barriers to such discussions, which may result in medical teams failing to bring this topic to the forefront. Barriers include lack of training specific to discussing fertility risks, oncologists' unfamiliarity with community resources for fertility preservation, diffusion of responsibility to other members of the medical or psychosocial teams, and/or physician discomfort in discussing fertility risks among patients with poor prognoses [32, 33]. This lack of discussion is unfortunate for many reasons, including the fact that discussing survivorship topics, including difficult topics such as fertility risks, can provide hope for the likelihood of survivorship [34]. Additionally, most families report a desire to receive information on reproductive health regardless of patient age or prognosis [12]. Although it is typically important that treatment not be delayed to engage in fertility preservation, the increasing promotion of patient-centered care emphasizes the need for families to be fully informed of fertility risks, presented with options, and supported in decisions they may wish to pursue to promote future quality of life. While oncologists may believe they are protecting patients and families by refraining from sharing information regarding fertility risks, research indicates that AYAs may feel deceived by their medical teams and more emotionally devastated if this information is not provided until after cancer treatments are completed [12, 35].

Sperm cryopreservation has been the standard of care for male fertility preservation for several decades [12]. Sperm banking prior to cancer treatment is related to psychological relief, regardless of whether the sample is ever utilized; moreover, nearly all patients report that they would recommend cryopreservation to other cancer patients [12, 34]. The majority of patients and families also report positive impressions of sperm banking when discussed prior to cancer treatment and that they were glad that they pursued this option, even if treatment was slightly delayed to allow this process to take place [36]. Although rates of sperm banking are lower among newly diagnosed AYAs in the USA and Canada as compared to other developed countries, hospital-based interventions have successfully reduced this discrepancy. Currently, limited research exists exploring factors related to sperm banking among AYAs with cancer; however, older age, increased knowledge of fertility preservation procedures, desire to become a parent, and parental support are associated with increased sperm banking. In contrast, discomfort in discussing this topic, lack of physician recommendation, increased anxiety at diagnosis, poorer socioeconomic status/financial barriers, and being required to have a parent accompany the patient to the sperm banking facility appear to make sperm banking less likely [12, 36].

While underutilized, there are both established and experimental methods of preserving fertility among females. These include embryo cryopreservation, oocyte cryopreservation, ovarian tissue freezing and grafting, and immature oocyte preservation with in vitro maturation [12, 37]. There are also efforts made during cancer treatments to protect ovarian tissue. Embryo cryopreservation requires in vitro fertilization, which entails hormone stimulation of the ovaries. This may result in a heightened risk of future cancer and delays in treatment. Additionally, this requires the need for a sperm donor or male partner, which may not be an available option for AYA patients. Given the barriers to embryo cryopreservation, oocyte

cryopreservation is often viewed as a more favorable alternative and is no longer considered investigational.

Overall, fertility preservation has been described as highly important to AYA survivors [12]. Many AYA survivors have reported being unaware of their fertility status or risks of infertility following cancer treatment [13]. Risks of psychological distress increase with both lack of awareness and actual fertility loss, and survivors have described feeling angry about prior withholding of information, unfairness of experiencing late effects of the cancer experience, and lack of control over infertility [12, 14]. In turn, lack of knowledge of fertility status can lead to risky sexual behavior and conflicts within romantic relationships, including anxiety about being rejected or undesired by potential partners [13]. Those with problems with fertility often face challenges grieving this loss, one which may not be well understood by health care professionals, family or peers [12].

Conclusion

'I was terrified when I found out, but for some reason I couldn't imagine that I wouldn't get better. Treatment sucked, but things weren't as bad as they could have been. The worst part was having to sit at home by myself all day when all my friends were enjoying their senior year. I actually got to the point where I [was] enjoying going to the hospital because of everyone there. Since I've been in remission, life has pretty much returned to normal, although a day doesn't go by that I don't think about it and what might happen if I get sick again. Whenever I get sick or run down I freak myself out thinking that maybe it's come back, but for the most part I've [been] fine. I feel that I have a pretty good outlook on things and that I have managed to find the silver lining in what I've been through. I was able to learn a lot about myself and what I want out of life.'

20-year-old female survivor

Younger AYA survivors of childhood hematological cancers face a number of challenges related to developing and maintaining lasting peer and romantic relationships. The intensity of lifesaving treatments and length of treatment (especially among those diagnosed with ALL) often play detrimental roles in social outcomes [4, 5]. While necessary for promoting survival, lengthy and intense treatment protocols can lead to disruptions to typical developmental trajectories due to the significant time spent in medical settings, resulting in time away from peers, potential romantic partners, and more normative social environments such as school and extracurricular activities. The combined intensity and length of treatment may result in atypicalities in socialization. Although some of these outcomes may be inherently challenging, such as negative neurocognitive and physical sequelae, AYA survivors also report benefits of their cancer experiences such as increased maturity, an ability to cope with life stressors, and perceptions that they can and will have the ability to be good romantic partners and parents [12].

There are many factors associated with the development of peer and romantic relationships among AYA survivors of childhood hematological cancers that are important to consider, including perceived health vulnerabilities and body image following treatment [9, 10, 23], how attachment to parents relates to later social outcomes [28, 29], and the impact of fertility concerns on later relationships and identity development [12]. Unfortunately, much of the available literature provides findings across diagnostic groups rather than focusing on any unique challenges and positive outcomes that may exist with respect to peer and romantic relationships among AYA survivors of childhood hematological cancers. The extant literature available to date suggests that there may be a need to address peer and romantic relationship concerns within this group, possibly with a focus on early interventions provided during both active treatment and survivorship. This may be especially true with respect to providing interventions that limit disruptions to typical development, emphasize positive body image and understanding realistic perceptions of health vulnerability, and provide options for communicating fertility risks and offering preservation options regardless of prognosis. However, additional research is needed to determine specific targets of intervention among AYAs surviving childhood hematological cancers.

References

1 National Cancer Institute: A snapshot of adolescent and young adult cancers: cancers affecting adolescent and young adults (AYAs). Cancer snapshots: disease focused and other snapshots. 2013. http://www.cancer.gov/researchandfunding/snapshots/adolescent-young-adult.

2 Patenaude AF, Kupst MJ: Psychosocial functioning in pediatric cancer. J Pediatr Psychol 2005;30:9–27.

3 Gurevich M, Devins G, Rodin G: Stress response symptoms and cancer: conceptual and assessment issues. Psychosomatics 2002;43:259–281.

4 Absolom K, Eiser C, Michel G, Walters SJ, Hancock BW, Coleman RE, Snowden JA, Greenfield DM: Follow-up care for cancer survivors: views of the younger adult. Br J Cancer 2009;101:561–567.

5 Gerhardt CA, Vannatta K, Valerius KS, Correll J, Noll RB: Social and romantic outcomes in emerging adulthood among survivors of childhood cancer. J Adolesc Health 2007;40:462.e9–462.e15.

6 Campbell LK, Scaduto M, Van Slyke D, Niarhos F, Whitlock JA, Compas BE: Executive function, coping, and behavior in survivors of acute lymphocytic leukemia. J Pediatr Psychol 2009;34:317–327.

7 Vannatta K, Gerhardt CA, Well RJ, Noll RB: Intensity of CNS treatment for pediatric cancer: prediction of social outcomes in survivors. Pediatr Blood Cancer 2007;49:716–722.

8 Collins WA, van Dulmen M: Friendships and romance in emerging adulthood: assessing distinctiveness in close relationships; in Arnett JJ, Tanner JL (eds): Emerging Adults in America: Coming of Age in the 21st Century. Washington, American Psychological Association, 2006, pp 219–237.

9 Maggiolini A, Grassi R, Adamoli L, Corbetta A, Charment GP, Provantini K, Fraschini D, Jankovic M, Spinetta J, Masera G: Self-image of adolescent survivors of long-term childhood leukemia. J Pediatr Hematol Oncol 2000;22:417–421.

10 Forsbach T, Thompson A: The impact of childhood cancer on adult survivors' interpersonal relationships. Child Care Practice 2003;9:117–128.

11 Thompson A, Long K, Marsland A: Impact of childhood cancer on emerging adult survivors' romantic relationships: a qualitative account. J Sex Med 2013;10(suppl 1):65–73.

12 Klosky JL, Foster RH, Nobel A: Pediatric oncology and reproductive health; in Quinn G, Vadaparampil S (eds): Reproductive Health and Cancer in Adolescents and Young Adults. New York, Springer Publishing Company, 2012, pp 151–164.

13 Zebrack BJ, Casillas J, Nohr L, Adams H, Zeltzer LK: Fertility issues for young adult cancer survivors of childhood cancer. Psychooncology 2004;13:689–699.

14 Langeveld N, Grootenhuis M, Voute P, De Haan R, Van Den Bos C: Quality of life, self-esteem and worries in young adult survivors of childhood cancer. Psychooncology 2004;13:867–881.

15 Leena-Riitta P, Sammallahti P, Siimes M, Aalberg VA: Childhood leukemia and body image: interview reveals impairment not found with a questionnaire. J Clin Psychol 1997;53:133–137.

16 Bellizzi K, Smith A, Schmidt S, Keegan THM, Zebrack B, Lynch CF, Deapen D, Shnorhavorian M, Tompkins BJ, Simon M: Positive and negative psychosocial impact of being diagnosed with cancer as an adolescent or young adult. Cancer 2012;118:5155–5162.

17 Pendley JS, Dahlquist LM, Dreyer Z: Body image and psychosocial adjustment in adolescent cancer survivors. J Pediatr Psychol 1997;22:29–43.

18 Meltzer LJ, Rourke MT: Oncology summer camp: benefits of social comparison. Child Health Care 2005;34:305–314.

19 Cassano J, Negel K, O'Mara L: Talking with others who 'just know': perceptions of adolescents with cancer who participate in a teen group. J Pediatr Oncol Nurs 2008;25:193–199.

20 Noll RB, Bukowski WM, Davies WH: Adjustment in the peer system of adolescents with cancer: a two-year study. J Pediatr Psychol 1993;18:351–364.

21 Gray CC, Rodrigue JR: Brief report: perceptions of young adolescents about a hypothetical new peer with cancer: an analog study. J Pediatr Psychol 2001;26:247–252.

22 Weekes D: Adolescents growing up chronically ill: a life-span developmental view. Fam Community Health 1995;17:22–34.

23 Stern M, Krivoy E, Foster RH, Bitsko M, Toren A, Ben-Arush M: Psychosocial functioning and career decision-making in Israeli adolescent cancer survivors. Pediatr Blood Cancer 2010;55:703–713.

24 Eiser C, Hill J, Blacklay A: Surviving cancer: what does it mean for you? An evaluation of a clinic based intervention for survivors of childhood cancer. Psychooncology 2000;9:214–220.

25 Ainsworth MDS: The development of infant-mother attachment; in Caldwell BM, Ricciuti HN (eds): Review of Child Development Research. Chicago, University of Chicago Press, 1973, vol 3.

26 Waters E, Merrick S, Treboux D, Crowell J, Albersheim L: Attachment security in infancy and early adulthood: a twenty-year longitudinal study. Child Dev 2000;71:684–689.

27 Owens G, Crowell JA, Pan H, Treboux D, O'Connor E, Waters E: The prototype hypothesis and the origins of attachment working models: adult relationship with parents and romantic partners; in Waters E, Vaughn B, Posada G, Kondo-Ikemura K (eds): Constructs, Cultures, and Caregiving: New Growing Points of Attachment Theory. Chicago, University of Chicago Press, 1995, pp 216–233.

28 Joubert D, Sadéghi MR, Elliott M, Devins GM, Laperrière N, Rodin G: Physical sequelae and self-perceived attachment in adult survivors of childhood cancer. Psychooncology 2002;10:284–292.

29 Foster RH, Stern M, Russell C, Shivy V, Bitsko MJ, Dillon R, Klosky JL, Godder K: Examining the influence of optimism and perceived health vulnerability on parent-adolescent attachment among survivors of pediatric cancer. J Adolesc Young Adult Oncol 2012;1: 181–187.

30 Green DM, Kawashima T, Stovall M, Leisenring W, Sklar CA, Mertens AC, Donaldson SS, Byrne J, Robison LL: Fertility of female survivors of childhood cancer: a report from the Childhood Cancer Survivor Study. J Clin Oncol 2009;16:2677–2685.

31 Critchley H, Thomson AB, Wallace WH: Ovarian and uterine function and reproductive potential; in Wallace WH, Green DM (eds): Late Effects of Childhood Cancer. London, Arnold, 2004.

32 Quinn GP, Vadaparampil ST: Fertility preservation research group. Fertility preservation and adolescent/young adult cancer patients: physician communication challenges. J Adolesc Health 2009;44:394–400.

33 Vadaparampil ST, Quinn GP, King L, Wilson C, Nieder M: Barriers to fertility preservation among pediatric oncologists. Patient Educ Couns 2008;72:402–410.

34 Saito K, Suzuki K, Iwasaki A, Yumura Y, Kubota Y: Sperm cryopreservation before cancer chemotherapy helps in the emotional battle against cancer. Cancer 2005;104:521–524.

35 Nieman CL, Kinahan KE, Yount SE, Rosenbloom SK, Yost KJ, Hahn EA, Volpe T, Dilley KJ, Zoloth L, Woodruff TK: Fertility preservation and adolescent cancer patients: lessons from adult survivors of childhood cancer and their parents. Cancer Treat Res 2007;138: 201–217.

36 Ginsberg JP, Ogle SK, Tuchman LK, Carlson CA, Reilly MM, Hobbie WL, Rourke M, Zhao H, Meadows AT: Sperm banking for adolescent and young adult cancer patients: sperm quality, patient, and parent perspectives. Pediatr Blood Cancer 2008;50:594–598.

37 Levine J, Canada A, Stern CJ: Fertility preservation in adolescents and young adults with cancer. J Clin Oncol 2010;28:4831–4841.

Acta Haematol 2014;132:383–390
DOI: 10.1159/000360202

Published online: September 10, 2014

Survivorship in Adolescents and Young Adults

Ashwin Kishtagari   Montreh Tavakkoli   Jae H. Park

Leukemia Service, Department of Medicine, Memorial Sloan-Kettering Cancer Center, New York, N.Y., USA

Key Words

Adolescents and young adults · Chronic health conditions · Secondary malignancies · Survivorship

Abstract

In the USA, approximately 26,000 adolescents and young adults (AYAs) aged 15–29 years are diagnosed with cancer every year. The cure rate among this population exceeds 80%, resulting in a growing number of AYA cancer survivors. AYA cancer survivors suffer from a wide range of long-term treatment-related toxicities that adversely affect quality of life and increase the risk of premature death. Therefore, it is important to recognize the unique medical needs of the AYA cancer survivors and develop a cost-effective and systemic approach to screen and prevent cancer treatment-related sequelae and the adverse health outcomes.

© 2014 S. Karger AG, Basel

Introduction

In the USA, about 26,000 adolescents and young adults (AYAs) aged 15–29 years are diagnosed with cancer every year [1], and the cure rate of AYA cancers now exceeds 80% [2], resulting in a growing and large number of AYA cancer survivors with unique medical needs and an excess risk of chronic health conditions [3–5]. Much of our understanding of long-term health status, morbidity and

mortality after cancer in AYAs has emanated from the Childhood Cancer Survivor Study (CCSS) due to the limited number of studies and lack of a cohort in North America that is solely focused on the AYA population. Chronic disease in AYA cancer survivors can involve multiple organ systems and may not become clinically evident for many years. Late mortality in childhood cancer survivors is significantly increased (standardized mortality ratio, SMR = 19.4), mainly from subsequent cancers (SMR = 9.2), pulmonary (SMR = 8.8) and cardiac (SMR = 7.0) diseases [6]. Oeffinger et al. [3] subsequently reported the cumulative incidence of 73.4 and 42.4% for a chronic health condition and severe, disabling or life-threatening conditions, respectively, 30 years after the cancer diagnosis in childhood cancer survivors (mean age 26.6, range 18–48 years). Survivors exposed to radiation therapy (RT), chemotherapy or combination therapy (chemotherapy + RT) were all found to have elevated risks of severe or life-threatening conditions, and the incidence increased over time, suggesting that the cohort continues to face new-onset morbidity as they age and even 20–25 years after their treatment. In this section of the review series on AYAs, we describe secondary malignancies and chronic health conditions that often complicate the management of AYA survivors of hematological malignancies.

A.K. and M.T. contributed equally to this work.

© 2014 S. Karger AG, Basel
0001–5792/14/1324–0383$39.50/0

Jae H. Park
Memorial Sloan-Kettering Cancer Center
1275 York Avenue
New York, NY 10065 (USA)
E-Mail parkj6@mskcc.org

Secondary Malignancies

Treatment modalities for hematological malignancies commonly include high doses of chemotherapy, RT or a combinatorial modality of chemotherapy and RT. While these agents have improved overall survival from primary malignancies, the potential to introduce mutations at sublethal doses in healthy cells may lead to the development of secondary cancers (SCs). Furthermore, AYAs have a greater life expectancy following treatment for their primary cancer [7], and are at a higher risk of developing SCs than the general population and their adult counterparts [8, 9].

In a registry-based report of a Nordic cohort of 47,697 childhood cancer survivors, the overall risk of SCs was 2.3-fold higher compared to the general population [10]. Two other large registry-based studies of a US cohort of 14,581 and a UK cohort of 16,541 childhood cancer survivors reported a 6.4-fold and 5.8-fold greater risk of SCs than that in the general population [11, 12].

The risk and type of SC depend on the type of primary cancer, the therapeutic regimen and the cumulative doses of chemotherapy and/or RT [8]. The use of chemotherapy is frequently associated with the development of myelodysplasia and acute myeloid leukemia, and RT tends to increase the risk of solid SCs. Chemotherapy-induced myelodysplasia and acute myeloid leukemia have a shorter latency and are associated with alkylating agents or topoisomerase II inhibitors. Radiation-induced solid tumors usually have a latency period longer than 10 years and account for the largest burden of SCs [13].

Hodgkin's Lymphoma

In a British cohort of 6,798 patients diagnosed with Hodgkin's lymphoma (HL) between 15 and 34 years of age, the 20-year cumulative risk of developing SCs was 13% for patients treated with chemotherapy alone and 18% for patients treated with chemotherapy + RT [14]. In another study performed on 1,641 patients diagnosed with HL at ages ≤20, the cumulative risk of SCs was 1.9% at 10 years, 6.9% at 20 years and 18% at 30 years [15]. A Dutch cohort study of 1,253 patients diagnosed with HL at ages <40 reported that age at the time of original cancer diagnosis was an important predictor of risk for SCs, with the highest risk observed in patients diagnosed at ages <20 (relative risk, RR = 12.7), followed by patients diagnosed at the age of 21–30 (RR = 6.9) and at the age of 31–39 (RR = 4.6) [16].

Among those diagnosed between 21 and 39 years of age, the greatest increase in SCs was seen in breast, thyroid, lung and gastrointestinal carcinomas, followed by bone/soft tissue cancer, non-HL (NHL) and leukemia [9, 17]. Of these malignancies, the most common SC in AYA HL survivors is breast cancer [15]. The increased risk of breast cancer is largely attributed to irradiation to the breast field and the use of alkylating agents, and is associated with the cumulative radiation dose and number of cycles of alkylating chemotherapy. In a study of 770 patients diagnosed with HL at ages <41, an increased risk of breast cancer was reported with radiation doses ≥38.5 Gy [18]. In another study of 3,817 1-year female survivors of HL diagnosed at ≤30 years of age and treated with a chest radiation dose ≥40 Gy in the absence of an alkylating agent, the risk of secondary breast cancer at the age of 35, 45 and 55 years was 1.4, 11.1 and 29%, respectively [19].

The incidence of secondary thyroid cancer in AYA HL survivors has been reported to be 18- to 36-fold higher than that of the general population [20, 21]. A modest increase in the risk of NHL and acute leukemia has been observed among patients diagnosed with HL at ≤40 years of age, with the 25-year cumulative risk of 3.5% for NHL (95% confidence interval, CI = 2.0–6.0%) and 3.3% for acute leukemia (95% CI = 2.1–5.3%) [16]. Notably, the risk of secondary NHL and acute leukemia plateaus after 20 years following HL treatment, unlike secondary solid tumors whose risk continues to increase even after 25 years of the primary cancer treatment [20, 22].

Non-Hodgkin's Lymphoma

In the USA, NHL is the fourth most common malignancy among adolescents with a 5-year event-free survival of >90% [23]. However, studies among AYA patients with NHL and their development of SCs are limited. A study involving 1,082 5-year NHL survivors diagnosed between 0 and 21 years of age (median age 10 years) suggested that the increase in therapy-related mortality among NHL survivors continues >20 years following treatment [24]. Furthermore, a study involving 28,131 NHL survivors found that those between 20 and 39 years of age at diagnosis were at a higher risk of developing secondary solid cancers relative to those ≥40 years of age [23].

Acute Lymphoblastic Leukemia

Acute leukemia accounts for 11 and 5% of the malignancies encountered among 15- to 19- and 20- to 29-year-olds, respectively [7]. The most data on the risk of SCs in survivors of acute lymphoblastic leukemia (ALL) comes from the CCSS [25, 26]. According to these studies, patients diagnosed with ALL at 0–20 years of age have a 14- and 19-fold increased risk of developing SCs and brain

Acta Haematol 2014;132:383–390
DOI: 10.1159/000360202

tumors, respectively [25]. The utilization of cranial irradiation significantly increases the risk of developing SCs relative to nonirradiated patients (3.5 vs. 1.2%) [25]. The most common malignancies encountered in these patients include brain (24%) and thyroid cancers (22%) [26].

Pulmonary Complications

Increased occurrences of pulmonary toxicity and compromise in pulmonary function have been reported in AYA cancer survivors, particularly those who received high-dose systemic chemotherapy, hematopoietic stem cell transplantation and RT [27–30]. Survivors of ALL, acute myeloid leukemia, NHL and HL are 4.2, 24.9, 10.8 and 9.1 times more likely to die of pulmonary disease than the general population, respectively [31]. A study from the CCSS showed that 12,000 cancer survivors treated with chest radiation had a 5-fold increased risk of abnormal chest wall development (RR = 5; 95% CI = 2.7–9.4), a 4-fold excess risk of developing lung fibrosis (RR = 4.3; 95% CI = 2.9–6.6) and a 2-fold excess risk of pneumonia (RR = 2.2; 95% CI = 1.5–7.0), compared with siblings [30].

Radiation to fields involving the lungs causes direct damage to lung tissue and can lead to late pulmonary toxicities such as pulmonary fibrosis, pneumonitis, reduction of diffusing capacity of the lung for carbon monoxide, obstructive and restrictive lung diseases, bronchiolitis obliterans, bronchiectasis and chronic bronchitis [32]. More importantly, long-term and late pulmonary toxicities from radiation can result in asymptomatic pulmonary diseases detected by pulmonary function tests or radiographic images, reported in more than 30% of patients with HL [33–35]. Of the 25 HL survivors treated with standard mantle radiation before the age of 35 years, 60% had an abnormal chest radiograph, 89% had an abnormal pulmonary function test and 72% had a reduced diffusing capacity of the lung for carbon monoxide at a mean follow-up of 9 years [36]. These changes have been detected months to years after RT.

In addition to radiation to lung fields, chemotherapeutic agents such as bleomycin and alkylating agents are responsible for pulmonary disease in cancer survivors. Bleomycin, an antibiotic chemotherapy agent frequently used in HL treatment, is a prototype for chemotherapy-related lung injury, presenting as interstitial pneumonitis and pulmonary fibrosis [37]. It is characterized by impairment of gas diffusion between alveoli and pulmonary capillaries, evidenced by a reduction in the diffusing capacity of the lung for carbon monoxide in pulmonary function tests. Bleomycin toxicity is dose dependent and is exacerbated by concurrent RT [38]. Above 400 units/m^2 of bleomycin in the absence of other risk factors, 10% of patients experience fibrosis [38]. Busulfan and melphalan, often used as conditioning agents for hematopoietic stem cell transplantation, are known to cause diffuse interstitial pulmonary fibrosis in a dose-dependent manner as well. Busulfan toxicity is most predictable in doses exceeding 500 mg and may be associated with a progressive, potentially fatal restrictive lung disease [39, 40].

In determining the at-risk population of developing late and long-term pulmonary toxicities, it is important to consider age at diagnosis, cumulative radiation doses, volume of lung in the radiation field, cumulative bleomycin dose and presence of renal dysfunction [41]. Age at diagnosis (15–21 years vs. <15 years) and pulmonary toxic chemotherapy alone or combined with chest radiation are associated with a significantly increased RR of pulmonary fibrosis, pulmonary insufficiency, chronic cough, pleurisy, shortness of breath and recurrent pneumonia [30]. Furthermore, it is important to recognize that the cumulative incidence of these pulmonary toxicities increases up to 15–20 years after diagnosis.

Cardiotoxicity

Cardiac disease constitutes the second most common cause of death among AYAs following SCs [3, 6, 42]. Chest-directed RT is associated with an increased risk of myocardial infarction, congestive heart failure (CHF), valvular heart disease and arrhythmias [43–46]. Anthracycline chemotherapy increases the risk of heart failure [46, 47]. While many clinical trials are attempting to limit exposure to these cardiotoxic therapies, these agents remain an important component of curative regimens in childhood hematological malignancies. Therefore, it is critical to recognize the long-term and late therapy-related cardiotoxicities and reduce modifiable risk factors that may further increase the risk of serious cardiac events in AYA survivors.

Radiation induces microvascular changes within the myocardium and fibrosis of the myocardium, pericardium and cardiac valves [48–50]. In a cohort of 1,474 survivors of HL younger than 41 years at treatment, irradiation to the mediastinum was associated with 2- to 7-fold increased risks of cardiotoxicity (i.e. myocardial infarction, CHF and valvular disease) compared to the age-matched general population [44]. Other studies involving large cohorts of survivors of hematological malignancies similarly reported increased risks of myocardial infarction, CHF, pericardial disease and valvular disease, predominantly aortic stenosis, compared to either sibling cohorts or general populations [43, 45]. Interestingly, the radiation-induced cardiotoxicity was observed 10–20 years after radiotherapy [43], and anthracyclines significantly added to the elevated risks of CHF and valvular disorders [44].

Anthracycline-associated cardiotoxicity is caused by direct damage to the myoepithelium and is strongly related to the cumulative dose [51, 52]. A study of 607 childhood cancer survivors reported the 5% estimated risk of CHF after a median follow-up time of 6.3 years and significantly higher incidences in those who received >300 mg/m^2 anthracyclines [52]. Other studies reported symptomatic dilated cardiomyopathy and asymptomatic progressive disorder in as many as 20% of cancer survivors 15–20 years after exposure [53–55].

In addition to cumulative doses of radiation and anthracyclines, younger age at treatment appears to be the major risk factor for developing therapy-related cardiotoxicities [44, 56]. The higher risk in the younger patients may be related to cardiovascular tissue more vulnerable to radiation and chemotherapy, and low background incidence rates of cardiovascular disease.

More recently, Armstrong et al. [57] evaluated the relative contribution of modifiable cardiovascular risk factors on the development of major cardiac events in adult survivors of childhood cancer. Among 10,724 5-year survivors (median age = 33.7 years), the cumulative incidence of coronary artery disease, CHF, valvular disease and arrhythmia by 45 years of age was 5.3, 4.8, 1.5 and 1.3%, respectively. The risk of each cardiac event increased with an increasing number of cardiovascular risk factors (i.e. hypertension, dyslipidemia, diabetes, obesity). In this study, hypertension was independently associated with risk of cardiac death (RR = 5.6; 95% CI = 3.2–9.7), and chest-directed RT combined with hypertension resulted in potentiation of the risk of the major cardiac events beyond that anticipated on the basis of an additive expectation [57]. This latter finding suggests an importance and a need for careful screening of AYA survivors for an early detection of cardiovascular risk factors as recommended in the long-term follow-up guidelines from the Children's Oncology Group [58].

Neurotoxicity

Previously, cranial irradiation was the most widely utilized tool for eliminating leukemia and NHL cells in cerebrospinal fluid. Due to the significant neurotoxicity associated with cranial irradiation, this prophylactic measure has been widely replaced with the intensification of systemic chemotherapy and the use of intrathecal chemotherapy, leaving cranial irradiation as a last resort for patients with cranial relapse. Nevertheless, systemic and intrathecal treatment for cranial prophylaxis is also associated with neurotoxicity, particularly late cognitive deficits, but to a significantly lesser degree.

The treatment-related neurotoxicities associated with leukemia and NHL include neurocognitive dysfunctions, psychiatric conditions, peripheral neuropathy, seizures, transient ischemic attacks, strokes, encephalopathy, ataxia, leukoencephalopathy, cerebral atrophy and neuroendocrine-system-related changes. Due to an only limited amount of information available for neurotoxicity of AYA cancer survivors, the descriptions in this section are limited to studies performed in children and older adults.

The frequency of neurotoxicity among those who receive cranial radiation ranges from 30 to 70%, with the most common toxicities being cerebral atrophy, demyelination, leukoencephalopathy and neurocognitive defects and less commonly stroke, peripheral neuropathy, ototoxicity and neuropathic pain. A meta-analysis of 28 studies involving the long-term neurocognitive deficits of childhood ALL found that these survivors consistently experienced significant deficits in global function (intellectual functioning, academic achievement) and specific neurocognitive abilities [59], and a study of 141 childhood ALL survivors reported a learning disability in 18% of the cohort [60]. The risk of neurocognitive deficits from cranial radiation increases with female sex and younger age at diagnosis [61].

While stroke is an uncommon side effect observed in childhood cancer survivors, the risk is significantly elevated among patients treated for hematological malignancies relative to the general population. In a retrospective study on 2,201 5-year survivors of HL, irradiation of the neck and mediastinum was associated with an increased risk of stroke and transient ischemic attack (a cumulative incidence of 7% at 30 years following HL treatment) while chemotherapy alone posed no threat to the development of cerebrovascular disease (hazard ratio = 2.5, 95% CI = 1.1–5.6 years) [62]. The incidence was higher among those <21 years of age (incidence rate = 3.8) compared to those 21–30 years of age (incidence rate =

Acta Haematol 2014;132:383–390
DOI: 10.1159/000360202

3.1) [62]. The risk of stroke also appears to be dependent on a cumulative radiation dose, with the highest possible risk associated with cranial irradiation of ≥50 Gy and less so with ≥30 Gy [63].

While high-dose systemic chemotherapy is associated with only subtle long-term neurocognitive deficits (attention, executive functioning), its use increases the risk of peripheral neuropathy, psychiatric conditions and neuroendocrine changes. In a cross-sectional study performed on 80 survivors of ALL between 5 and 18 years of age with a 3-year follow-up, 34% had developed neuropathy, most commonly symmetric motor axonal polyneuropathy seen in 24% of the children [64]. In a study on 5,736 survivors of childhood leukemia, HL and NHL, patients frequently reported depression and somatic distress that was added by intensive chemotherapy [65]. Similarly, the CCSS reported an increased risk of psychiatric conditions among patients treated for ALL and NHL, with a significant increase in depression and somatic distress relative to sibling controls [66].

Lastly, cranial irradiation, hematopoietic stem cell transplantation and chemotherapy are associated with changes in the neuroendocrine system that seem to play a role in physical inactivity, obesity, visceral adiposity, insulin resistance, dyslipidemia and poor cardiopulmonary fitness seen in childhood survivors of hematological malignancies. While this finding is significantly elevated with cranial radiation, it is attenuated and associated with a later onset among those who have been treated with chemotherapy alone [67].

Endocrine Effects

The endocrine system is particularly susceptible to the long-term effects of cancer therapy. Endocrine dysfunction is one of the most common long-term effects of cancer therapy and the risk increase with time. Cranial or spinal RT, total body irradiation and target-organ irradiation involving the neck, abdomen, pelvis and testes are associated with endocrine and late effects in survivors of AYA cancers [68], and affect the normal function of the hypothalamic-pituitary-adrenal axis, thyroid gland and gonads [69, 70].

Pituitary dysfunction may develop several years after treatment and can be progressive [71]. Growth hormone (GH) secretion is the most vulnerable to irradiation, followed by gonadotropins, adrenocorticotropic hormone and thyrotropin [72]. AYA cancer survivors treated with an RT dose of ≥18 Gy to the hypothalamic-pituitary-adre-

nal axis are at greater risk for GH deficiency, whereas those treated with RT doses of ≥40 Gy to the hypothalamic-pituitary-adrenal axis are at risk for developing central hypothyroidism, gonadotropin deficiency and central adrenal insufficiency [68]. GH deficiency can be observed within 5 years after treatment with RT doses >30 Gy, whereas in patients treated with lower doses (18–24 Gy) it may not be evident for 10 years or more [68]. Childhood ALL survivors who received prophylactic cranial irradiation at doses of 18–25 Gy were found to have abnormalities of GH secretion up to 25 years after their treatment [73].

AYA cancer survivors are also at an increased risk of developing secondary thyroid cancers, hypothyroidism and, to a lesser extent, hyperthyroidism [5, 74, 75]. The prevalence of hypothyroidism following radiation to the neck/mediastinum has been estimated to be as high as 47% after 26 years of follow-up [76]. The risk of thyroid dysfunction also appears to be dose dependent. In a recent CCSS study of ALL survivors with thyroid dysfunction, an increased risk of hypothyroidism was associated with >20 Gy conformal RT in addition to any spinal RT [74].

Issues regarding gonadal dysfunction and fertility are discussed in more detail elsewhere in this issue.

AYA Screening and Surveillance Recommendations

AYA cancer survivors suffer from a wide risk of late and long-term treatment-related toxicities that adversely affect quality of life and increase the risk of premature death. Therefore, it is important to anticipate and screen for late treatment effects and apply timely interventions in order to prevent or ameliorate cancer treatment-related sequelae and the adverse health outcomes.

To this end, the Children's Oncology Group developed risk-based, exposure-related long-term follow-up guidelines for survivors of childhood, adolescent and young adult cancers. Implementation of these guidelines is intended to standardize and enhance follow-up care childhood and AYA cancer survivors. The entire guidelines can be downloaded at www.survivorshipguidelines.org.

While recommendations for the active surveillance and follow-up of AYA survivors of hematological malignancies are of importance from a clinical standpoint, it is also critical to address the issue from a more practical perspective to ensure adherence to these guidelines. For instance, cancer centers experience a significant loss to follow-up of AYA cancer survivors, and AYAs, like other healthy individuals, receive a majority of their care through primary care practitioners [77–79]. However, primary care physicians may be unfamiliar with the long-term toxicities and appropriate surveillance measures necessitated for the early detection and prevention of chronic illness among AYA cancer survivors [69]. One study conducted on 1,174 family practitioners found that 84% of primary care physicians had cared for ≤2 childhood cancer survivors within the past 5 years. Of these, 48% never, or almost never, received a treatment summary from the patients' referring cancer center. Furthermore, only 33 and 27% were comfortable caring for survivors of HL and ALL. However, their most important discovery was in the failure of 84–90% of primary care physicians to identify the appropriate follow-up care for a case presentation of childhood HL [80]. Similarly, a lower than anticipated rate of compliance with the breast cancer surveillance guideline was reported in female childhood cancer survivors at high risk of developing secondary breast cancer [63.5% of those aged 25–39 years and 23.5% of those aged 40–50 years, 81], largely attributed to the lack of training among providers in posttransitional health care and the loss of communication among providers and their patients.

One solution to this problem may lie in the development of a personalized 1-page survivorship guide that is created by the patients' oncologist at the completion of treatment, and is directly mailed to survivors in an automated fashion on an annual or biannual basis. The survivorship guide would include the recommended screens based on the treatment regimens and cumulative doses provided for the treatment of the AYA malignancy, and provide age-specific screening guidelines based on the anticipated long-term toxicities. Support for the utilization of such a program stems from the recent findings of Oeffinger et al. [82]. According to this study, 72 survivors of HL who were diagnosed between 27 and 55 years of age and at a high risk of developing secondary breast cancer and cardiomyopathy, and who had not been screened with mammography or echocardiograms for ≥2 years, were sent a 1-page survivorship care plan with recommendations for surveillance. At a 6-month follow-up, 41% of the patients were screened with mammography and 20% had been screened with an echocardiogram. The 9 physicians enrolled in the study failed to use the resources provided, but were responsive to patients' requests for the screens.

While additional studies are required to determine the effectiveness of such an approach over consecutive years, the 1-page Cancer Treatment Summary and Survivorship Care Plan may overcome multiple issues in the transition of survivorship care to their primary health care providers and provide a cost-effective means towards minimizing loss to follow-up and improving surveillance among AYA cancer survivors.

References

1 Bleyer A, Viny A, Barr R: Cancer in 15- to 29-year-olds by primary site. Oncologist 2006;11:590–601.
2 Oeffinger KC, Tonorezos ES: The cancer is over, now what? Understanding risk, changing outcomes. Cancer 2011;117:2250–2257.
3 Oeffinger KC, Mertens AC, Sklar CA, Kawashima T, Hudson MM, Meadows AT, Friedman DL, Marina N, Hobbie W, Kadan-Lottick NS, Schwartz CL, Leisenring W, Robison LL: Chronic health conditions in adult survivors of childhood cancer. N Engl J Med 2006;355:1572–1582.
4 Mody R, Li S, Dover DC, Sallan S, Leisenring W, Oeffinger KC, Yasui Y, Robison LL, Neglia JP: Twenty-five-year follow-up among survivors of childhood acute lymphoblastic leukemia: a report from the Childhood Cancer Survivor Study. Blood 2008;111:5515–5523.
5 Diller L, Chow EJ, Gurney JG, Hudson MM, Kadin-Lottick NS, Kawashima TI, Leisenring WM, Meacham LR, Mertens AC, Mulrooney DA, Oeffinger KC, Packer RJ, Robison LL, Sklar CA: Chronic disease in the Childhood Cancer Survivor Study cohort: a review of published findings. J Clin Oncol 2009;27:2339–2355.
6 Mertens AC, Liu Q, Neglia JP, Wasilewski K, Leisenring W, Armstrong GT, Robison LL, Yasui Y: Cause-specific late mortality among 5-year survivors of childhood cancer: the Childhood Cancer Survivor Study. J Natl Cancer Inst 2008;100:1368–1379.
7 Soliman H, Agresta SV: Current issues in adolescent and young adult cancer survivorship. Cancer Control 2008;15:55–62.
8 Curtis RE, Freedman DM, Ron E, Ries LAG, Hacker DG, Edwards BK, Tucker MA, Fraumeni JF Jr: New Malignancies among Cancer Survivors: SEER Cancer Registries, 1973–2000. Bethesda, National Cancer Institute, 2006.
9 Swerdlow AJ, Barber JA, Hudson GV, Cunningham D, Gupta RK, Hancock BW, Horwich A, Lister TA, Linch DC: Risk of second malignancy after Hodgkin's disease in a collaborative British cohort: the relation to age at treatment. J Clin Oncol 2000;18:498–509.
10 Olsen JH, Möller T, Anderson H, Langmark F, Sankila R, Tryggvadóttir L, Winther JF, Rechnitzer C, Jonmundsson G, Christensen J, Garwicz S: Lifelong cancer incidence in 47,697 patients treated for childhood cancer in the Nordic countries. J Natl Cancer Inst 2009;101:806–813.
11 Neglia JP, Friedman DL, Yasui Y, Mertens AC, Hammond S, Stovall M, Donaldson SS, Meadows AT, Robison LL: Second malignant neoplasms in five-year survivors of childhood cancer: childhood cancer survivor study. J Natl Cancer Inst 2001;93:618–629.
12 Jenkinson HC, Hawkins MM, Stiller CA, Winter DL, Marsden HB, Stevens MCG: Long-term population-based risks of second malignant neoplasms after childhood cancer in Britain. Br J Cancer 2004;91:1905–1910.
13 Bhatia S, Sklar C: Second cancers in survivors of childhood cancer. Nat Rev Cancer 2002;2:124–132.
14 Swerdlow AJ, Higgins CD, Smith P, Cunningham D, Hancock BW, Horwich A, Hoskin PJ, Lister TA, Radford JA, Rohatiner AZS, Linch DC: Second cancer risk after chemotherapy for Hodgkin's lymphoma: a collaborative British cohort study. J Clin Oncol 2011;29:4096–4104.

15 Sankila R, Garwicz S, Olsen JH, Döllner H, Hertz H, Kreuger A, Langmark F, Lanning M, Möller T, Tulinius H: Risk of subsequent malignant neoplasms among 1,641 Hodgkin's disease patients diagnosed in childhood and adolescence: a population-based cohort study in the five Nordic countries. Association of the Nordic Cancer Registries and the Nordic Society of Pedia. J Clin Oncol 1996;14:1442–1446.

16 Van Leeuwen FE, Klokman WJ, Veer MB, Hagenbeek A, Krol AD, Vetter UA, Schaapveld M, van Heerde P, Burgers JM, Somers R, Aleman BM: Long-term risk of second malignancy in survivors of Hodgkin's disease treated during adolescence or young adulthood. J Clin Oncol 2000;18:487–497.

17 Dores GM, Metayer C, Curtis RE, Lynch CF, Clarke EA, Glimelius B, Storm H, Pukkala E, van Leeuwen FE, Holowaty EJ, Andersson M, Wiklund T, Joensuu T, van't Veer MB, Stovall M, Gospodarowicz M, Travis LB: Second malignant neoplasms among long-term survivors of Hodgkin's disease: a population-based evaluation over 25 years. J Clin Oncol 2002; 20:3484–3494.

18 Van Leeuwen FE, Klokman WJ, Stovall M, Dahler EC, van't Veer MB, Noordijk EM, Crommelin MA, Aleman BMP, Broeks A, Gospodarowicz M, Travis LB, Russell NS: Roles of radiation dose, chemotherapy, and hormonal factors in breast cancer following Hodgkin's disease. J Natl Cancer Inst 2003;95: 971–980.

19 Travis LB, Hill D, Dores GM, Gospodarowicz M, van Leeuwen FE, Holowaty E, Glimelius B, Andersson M, Pukkala E, Lynch CF, Pee D, Smith SA, van't Veer MB, Joensuu T, Storm H, Stovall M, Boice JD, Gilbert E, Gail MH: Cumulative absolute breast cancer risk for young women treated for Hodgkin lymphoma. J Natl Cancer Inst 2005;97:1428–1437.

20 Von der Weid NX: Adult life after surviving lymphoma in childhood. Support Care Cancer 2008;16:339–345.

21 Sklar C, Whitton J, Mertens A, Stovall M, Green D, Marina N, Greffe B, Wolden S, Robison L: Abnormalities of the thyroid in survivors of Hodgkin's disease: data from the Childhood Cancer Survivor Study. J Clin Endocrinol Metab 2000;85:3227–3232.

22 Metayer C, Lynch CF, Clarke EA, Glimelius B, Storm H, Pukkala E, Joensuu T, van Leeuwen FE, van't Veer MB, Curtis RE, Holowaty EJ, Andersson M, Wiklund T, Gospodarowicz M, Travis LB: Second cancers among long-term survivors of Hodgkin's disease diagnosed in childhood and adolescence. J Clin Oncol 2000;18:2435–2443.

23 Bleyer A, O'Leary M, Barr R, Ries LAG (eds): Cancer Epidemiology in Older Adolescents and Young Adults 15 to 29 Years of Age, Including SEER Incidence and Survival: 1975–2000. Bethesda, National Cancer Institute, 2006, NIH Pub. No. 06–5767.

24 Bluhm EC, Ronckers C, Hayashi RJ, Neglia JP, Mertens AC, Stovall M, Meadows AT, Mitby PA, Whitton JA, Hammond S, Barker JD, Donaldson SS, Robison LL, Inskip PD: Cause-specific mortality and second cancer incidence after non-Hodgkin lymphoma: a report from the Childhood Cancer Survivor Study. Blood 2008;111:4014–4021.

25 Löning L, Zimmermann M, Reiter A, Kaatsch P, Henze G, Riehm H, Schrappe M: Secondary neoplasms subsequent to Berlin-Frankfurt-Münster therapy of acute lymphoblastic leukemia in childhood: significantly lower risk without cranial radiotherapy. Blood 2000;95: 2770–2775.

26 Perkins SM, Dewees T, Shinohara ET, Reddy MM, Frangoul H: Risk of subsequent malignancies in survivors of childhood leukemia. J Cancer Surviv 2013;7:544–550.

27 Cerveri I, Zoia MC, Fulgoni P, Corsico A, Casali L, Tinelli C, Zecca M, Giorgiani G, Locatelli F: Late pulmonary sequelae after childhood bone marrow transplantation. Thorax 1999;54:131–135.

28 Jenney ME, Faragher EB, Jones PH, Woodcock A: Lung function and exercise capacity in survivors of childhood leukaemia. Med Pediatr Oncol 1995;24:222–230.

29 Marina NM, Greenwald CA, Fairclough DL, Thompson EI, Wilimas JA, Mackert PW, Hudson MM, Stokes DC, Bozeman PM: Serial pulmonary function studies in children treated for newly diagnosed Hodgkin's disease with mantle radiotherapy plus cycles of cyclophosphamide, vincristine, and procarbazine alternating with cycles of doxorubicin, bleomycin, vinblastine, and dacarbazine. Cancer 1995;75:1706–1711.

30 Mertens AC, Yasui Y, Liu Y, Stovall M, Hutchinson R, Ginsberg J, Sklar C, Robison LL: Pulmonary complications in survivors of childhood and adolescent cancer. A report from the Childhood Cancer Survivor Study. Cancer 2002;95:2431–2441.

31 Armstrong GT, Liu Q, Yasui Y, Neglia JP, Leisenring W, Robison LL, Mertens AC: Late mortality among 5-year survivors of childhood cancer: a summary from the Childhood Cancer Survivor Study. J Clin Oncol 2009;27: 2328–2338.

32 Griese M, Rampf U, Hofmann D, Führer M, Reinhardt D, Bender-Götze C: Pulmonary complications after bone marrow transplantation in children: twenty-four years of experience in a single pediatric center. Pediatr Pulmonol 2000;30:393–401.

33 Horning SJ, Adhikari A, Rizk N, Hoppe RT, Olshen RA: Effect of treatment for Hodgkin's disease on pulmonary function: results of a prospective study. J Clin Oncol 1994;12:297–305.

34 Mefferd JM, Donaldson SS, Link MP: Pediatric Hodgkin's disease: pulmonary, cardiac, and thyroid function following combined modality therapy. Int J Radiat Oncol Biol Phys 1989;16:679–685.

35 Nysom K, Holm K, Hertz H, Hesse B: Risk factors for reduced pulmonary function after malignant lymphoma in childhood. Med Pediatr Oncol 1998;30:240–248.

36 Morgan GW, Freeman AP, McLean RG, Jarvie BH, Giles RW: Late cardiac, thyroid, and pulmonary sequelae of mantle radiotherapy for Hodgkin's disease. Int J Radiat Oncol Biol Phys 1985;11:1925–1931.

37 Eigen H, Wyszomierski D: Bleomycin lung injury in children. Pathophysiology and guidelines for management. Am J Pediatr Hematol Oncol 1985;7:71–78.

38 Samuels ML, Johnson DE, Holoye PY, Lanzotti VJ: Large-dose bleomycin therapy and pulmonary toxicity. A possible role of prior radiotherapy. JAMA 1976;235:1117–1120.

39 Jenney ME: Malignant disease and the lung. Paediatr Respir Rev 2000;1:279–286.

40 Meyer S, Reinhard H, Gottschling S, Nunold H, Graf N: Pulmonary dysfunction in pediatric oncology patients. Pediatr Hematol Oncol 2004;21:175–195.

41 O'Sullivan JM, Huddart RA, Norman AR, Nicholls J, Dearnaley DP, Horwich A: Predicting the risk of bleomycin lung toxicity in patients with germ-cell tumours. Ann Oncol 2003;14:91–96.

42 Reulen RC, Winter DL, Frobisher C, Lancashire ER, Stiller CA, Jenney ME, Skinner R, Stevens MC, Hawkins MM: Long-term cause-specific mortality among survivors of childhood cancer. JAMA 2010;304:172–179.

43 Hull MC, Morris CG, Pepine CJ, Mendenhall NP: Valvular dysfunction and carotid, subclavian, and coronary artery disease in survivors of Hodgkin lymphoma treated with radiation therapy. JAMA 2003;290:2831–2837.

44 Aleman BMP, van den Belt-Dusebout AW, De Bruin ML, van't Veer MB, Baaijens MHA, de Boer JP, Hart AAM, Klokman WJ, Kuenen MA, Ouwens GM, Bartelink H, van Leeuwen FE: Late cardiotoxicity after treatment for Hodgkin lymphoma. Blood 2007;109:1878–1886.

45 Mulrooney DA, Yeazel MW, Kawashima T, Mertens AC, Mitby P, Stovall M, Donaldson SS, Green DM, Sklar CA, Robison LL, Leisenring WM: Cardiac outcomes in a cohort of adult survivors of childhood and adolescent cancer: retrospective analysis of the Childhood Cancer Survivor Study cohort. BMJ 2009;339:b4606.

46 Van der Pal HJ, van Dalen EC, van Delden E, van Dijk IW, Kok WE, Geskus RB, Sieswerda E, Oldenburger F, Koning CC, van Leeuwen FE, Caron HN, Kremer LC: High risk of symptomatic cardiac events in childhood cancer survivors. J Clin Oncol 2012;30:1429–1437.

47 Lipshultz SE, Colan SD, Gelber RD, Perez-Atayde AR, Sallan SE, Sanders SP: Late cardiac effects of doxorubicin therapy for acute lymphoblastic leukemia in childhood. N Engl J Med 1991;324:808–815.

48 Adams MJ, Lipshultz SE: Pathophysiology of anthracycline- and radiation-associated cardiomyopathies: implications for screening and prevention. Pediatr Blood Cancer 2005; 44:600–606.

49 Veinot JP, Edwards WD: Pathology of radiation-induced heart disease: a surgical and autopsy study of 27 cases. Hum Pathol 1996;27: 766–773.

50 Stewart FA, Heeneman S, Te Poele J, Kruse J, Russell NS, Gijbels M, Daemen M: Ionizing radiation accelerates the development of atherosclerotic lesions in ApoE$^{-/-}$ mice and predisposes to an inflammatory plaque phenotype prone to hemorrhage. Am J Pathol 2006; 168:649–658.

51 Steinherz LJ: Anthracycline-induced cardiotoxicity. Ann Intern Med 1997;126:827, author reply 827–828.

52 Kremer LC, van Dalen EC, Offringa M, Ottenkamp J, Voûte PA: Anthracycline-induced clinical heart failure in a cohort of 607 children: long-term follow-up study. J Clin Oncol 2001;19:191–196.

53 Steinherz LJ, Steinherz PG, Tan CT, Heller G, Murphy ML: Cardiac toxicity 4–20 years after completing anthracycline therapy. JAMA 1991;266:1672–1677.

54 Lipshultz SE, Lipsitz SR, Sallan SE, Dalton VM, Mone SM, Gelber RD, Colan SD: Chronic progressive cardiac dysfunction years after doxorubicin therapy for childhood acute lymphoblastic leukemia. J Clin Oncol 2005;23: 2629–2636.

55 Kremer LCM, van der Pal HJH, Offringa M, van Dalen EC, Voûte PA: Frequency and risk factors of subclinical cardiotoxicity after anthracycline therapy in children: a systematic review. Ann Oncol 2002;13:819–829.

56 Hancock SL, Tucker MA, Hoppe RT: Factors affecting late mortality from heart disease after treatment of Hodgkin's disease. JAMA 1993;270:1949–1955.

57 Armstrong GT, Oeffinger KC, Chen Y, Kawashima T, Yasui Y, Leisenring W, Stovall M, Chow EJ, Sklar CA, Mulrooney DA, Mertens AC, Border W, Durand J-B, Robison LL, Meacham LR: Modifiable risk factors and major cardiac events among adult survivors of childhood cancer. J Clin Oncol 2013;31:3673–3680.

58 Landier W, Bhatia S, Eshelman DA, Forte KJ, Sweeney T, Hester AL, Darling J, Armstrong FD, Blatt J, Constine LS, Freeman CR, Friedman DL, Green DM, Marina N, Meadows AT, Neglia JP, Oeffinger KC, Robison LL, Ruccione KS, Sklar CA, Hudson MM: Development of risk-based guidelines for pediatric cancer survivors: the Children's Oncology Group Long-Term Follow-Up Guidelines from the Children's Oncology Group Late Effects Committee and Nursing Discipline. J Clin Oncol 2004;22:4979–4990.

59 Campbell LK, Scaduto M, Sharp W, Dufton L, Van Slyke D, Whitlock JA, Compas B: A meta-analysis of the neurocognitive sequelae of treatment for childhood acute lymphocytic leukemia. Pediatr Blood Cancer 2007;49:65–73.

60 Von der Weid N: Late effects in long-term survivors of ALL in childhood: experiences from the SPOG late effects study. Swiss Med Wkly 2001;131:180–187.

61 Buizer AI, de Sonneville LMJ, Veerman AJP: Effects of chemotherapy on neurocognitive function in children with acute lymphoblastic leukemia: a critical review of the literature. Pediatr Blood Cancer 2009;52:447–454.

62 De Bruin ML, Dorresteijn LDA, van't Veer MB, Krol ADG, van der Pal HJ, Kappelle AC, Boogerd W, Aleman BMP, van Leeuwen FE: Increased risk of stroke and transient ischemic attack in 5-year survivors of Hodgkin lymphoma. J Natl Cancer Inst 2009;101:928–937.

63 Bowers DC, Liu Y, Leisenring W, McNeil E, Stovall M, Gurney JG, Robison LL, Packer RJ, Oeffinger KC: Late-occurring stroke among long-term survivors of childhood leukemia and brain tumors: a report from the Childhood Cancer Survivor Study. J Clin Oncol 2006;24:5277–5282.

64 Jain P, Gulati S, Seth R, Bakhshi S, Toteja GS, Pandey RM: Vincristine-induced neuropathy in childhood ALL (acute lymphoblastic leukemia) survivors: prevalence and electrophysiological characteristics. J Child Neurol 2013, Epub ahead of print.

65 Zebrack BJ, Zeltzer LK, Whitton J, Mertens AC, Odom L, Berkow R, Robison LL: Psychological outcomes in long-term survivors of childhood leukemia, Hodgkin's disease, and non-Hodgkin's lymphoma: a report from the Childhood Cancer Survivor Study. Pediatrics 2002;110:42–52.

66 Green DM, Cox CL, Zhu L, Krull KR, Srivastava DK, Stovall M, Nolan VG, Ness KK, Donaldson SS, Oeffinger KC, Meacham LR, Sklar CA, Armstrong GT, Robison LL: Risk factors for obesity in adult survivors of childhood cancer: a report from the Childhood Cancer Survivor Study. J Clin Oncol 2012;30: 246–255.

67 Fulbright JM, Raman S, McClellan WS, August KJ: Late effects of childhood leukemia therapy. Curr Hematol Malig Rep 2011;6: 195–205.

68 Chemaitilly W, Sklar CA: Endocrine complications in long-term survivors of childhood cancers. Endocr Relat Cancer 2010;17:R141–R159.

69 Oeffinger KC, Mertens AC, Hudson MM, Gurney JG, Casillas J, Chen H, Whitton J, Yeazel M, Yasui Y, Robison LL: Health care of young adult survivors of childhood cancer: a report from the Childhood Cancer Survivor Study. Ann Fam Med 2004;2:61–70.

70 Darzy KH: Radiation-induced hypopituitarism after cancer therapy: who, how and when to test. Nat Clin Pract Endocrinol Metab 2009;5:88–99.

71 Littley MD, Shalet SM, Beardwell CG, Robinson EL, Sutton ML: Radiation-induced hypopituitarism is dose-dependent. Clin Endocrinol (Oxf) 1989;31:363–373.

72 Littley MD, Shalet SM, Beardwell CG, Ahmed SR, Applegate G, Sutton ML: Hypopituitarism following external radiotherapy for pituitary tumours in adults. Q J Med 1989;70:145–160.

73 Brennan BM, Rahim A, Mackie EM, Eden OB, Shalet SM: Growth hormone status in adults treated for acute lymphoblastic leukaemia in childhood. Clin Endocrinol (Oxf) 1998;48:777–783.

74 Chow EJ, Friedman DL, Stovall M, Yasui Y, Whitton JA, Robison LL, Sklar CA: Risk of thyroid dysfunction and subsequent thyroid cancer among survivors of acute lymphoblastic leukemia: a report from the Childhood Cancer Survivor Study. Pediatr Blood Cancer 2009;53:432–437.

75 Bhatti P, Veiga LHS, Ronckers CM, Sigurdson AJ, Stovall M, Smith SA, Weathers R, Leisenring W, Mertens AC, Hammond S, Friedman DL, Neglia JP, Meadows AT, Donaldson SS, Sklar CA, Robison LL, Inskip PD: Risk of second primary thyroid cancer after radiotherapy for a childhood cancer in a large cohort study: an update from the childhood cancer survivor study. Radiat Res 2010;174:741–752.

76 Hancock SL, McDougall IR, Constine LS: Thyroid abnormalities after therapeutic external radiation. Int J Radiat Oncol Biol Phys 1995;31:1165–1170.

77 Oeffinger KC, Eshelman DA, Tomlinson GE, Buchanan GR: Programs for adult survivors of childhood cancer. J Clin Oncol 1998;16: 2864–2867.

78 Tabone MD, Sommelet D: Childhood cancer surviving (in French). Arch Pediatr 2006;13: 607–609.

79 Shaw AK, Pogany L, Speechley KN, Maunsell E, Barrera M, Mery LS: Use of health care services by survivors of childhood and adolescent cancer in Canada. Cancer 2006;106: 1829–1837.

80 Nathan PC, Daugherty CK, Wroblewski KE, Kigin ML, Stewart TV, Hlubocky FJ, Grunfeld E, Del Giudice ME, Ward LA, Galliher JM, Oeffinger KC, Henderson TO: Family physician preferences and knowledge gaps regarding the care of adolescent and young adult survivors of childhood cancer. J Cancer Surviv 2013;7:275–282.

81 Oeffinger KC, Ford JS, Moskowitz CS, Diller LR, Hudson MM, Chou JF, Smith SM, Mertens AC, Henderson TO, Friedman DL, Leisenring WM, Robison LL: Breast cancer surveillance practices among women previously treated with chest radiation for a childhood cancer. JAMA 2009;301:404–414.

82 Oeffinger KC, Hudson MM, Mertens AC, Smith SM, Mitby PA, Eshelman-Kent DA, Ford JS, Jones JK, Kamani S, Robison LL: Increasing rates of breast cancer and cardiac surveillance among high-risk survivors of childhood Hodgkin lymphoma following a mailed, one-page survivorship care plan. Pediatr Blood Cancer 2011;56:818–824.

Acta Haematol 2014;132:391–399
DOI: 10.1159/000360238

Published online: September 10, 2014

Cardiotoxicity and Cardioprotection in Childhood Cancer

Steven E. Lipshultz[a–c]   Peter Sambatakos[a, b]   Michael Maguire[a, b]
Ruchika Karnik[a, b]   Samuel W. Ross[a, b]   Vivian I. Franco[a]   Tracie L. Miller[a, b]

[a]Department of Pediatrics, University of Miami Miller School of Medicine, and [b]Holtz Children's Hospital, Jackson Health System, Miami, Fla., and [c]Department of Pediatrics, Wayne State University School of Medicine and Children's Hospital of Michigan, Detroit, Mich., USA

Key Words
Cardioprotection · Cardiotoxicity · Childhood cancer survivors

Abstract
Children diagnosed with cancer are now living longer as a result of advances in treatment. However, some commonly used anticancer drugs, although effective in curing cancer, can also cause adverse late effects. The cardiotoxic effects of anthracycline chemotherapy, such as doxorubicin, and radiation can cause persistent and progressive cardiovascular damage, emphasizing a need for effective prevention and treatment to reduce or avoid cardiotoxicity. Examples of risk factors for cardiotoxicity in children include higher anthracycline cumulative dose, higher dose of radiation, younger age at diagnosis, female sex, trisomy 21 and black race. However, not all who are exposed to toxic treatments experience cardiotoxicity, suggesting the possibility of a genetic predisposition. Cardioprotective strategies under investigation include the use of dexrazoxane, which provides short- and long-term cardioprotection in children treated with doxorubicin without interfering with oncological efficacy, the use of less toxic anthracycline derivatives and nutritional supplements. Evidence-based monitoring and screening are need-ed to identify early signs of cardiotoxicity that have been validated as surrogates of subsequent clinically significant cardiovascular disease before the occurrence of cardiac damage, in patients who may be at higher risk.

© 2014 S. Karger AG, Basel

Introduction

In the 1970s, the 5-year survival rate of children diagnosed with cancer before the age of 15 years was less than 60% [1]. As of 2010, it is 83%, resulting in an estimated 379,000 survivors of childhood cancer in the USA [1, 2]. Although increased survival is promising, it is not free of consequences. These young survivors are in a developmental stage that makes them particularly vulnerable to adverse health effects from the potentially toxic anticancer treatments, which become apparent years later. More than 70% of childhood cancer survivors will experience a chronic health condition within the first 30 years after diagnosis [3]. Furthermore, cardiovasculature-related disease is the leading cause of morbidity and mortality after cancer recurrence and secondary malignancies in these survivors [3–5]. By the age of 45 years, the cumulative incidence of coronary artery disease, heart failure,

Steven E. Lipshultz, MD
Department of Pediatrics, Wayne State University School of Medicine
Children's Hospital of Michigan, 3901 Beaubien Blvd., Suite 1K40
Detroit, MI 48201 (USA)
E-Mail slipshultz@med.wayne.edu

valvular disease and arrhythmia among survivors is 5.3, 4.8, 1.5 and 1.3%, respectively, whereas the cumulative incidence for each among siblings is much lower: 0.9, 0.3, 0.1 and 0.4%, respectively [6].

Anthracyclines commonly used to treat hematological malignancies and solid tumors are effective but may cause persistent and progressive cardiovascular damage [7]. Furthermore, the risk increases when used in combination with radiation therapy [4, 8]. This review describes the mechanisms and course of anthracycline and radiation-induced cardiotoxicity and its risk factors in childhood cancer survivors, and discusses cardioprotective strategies to prevent or reduce long-term cardiac dysfunction.

Mechanisms of Anthracycline-Induced Cardiotoxicity

Anthracyclines, such as doxorubicin, epirubicin and daunorubicin, have substantially contributed to the improved cancer survival rates over the past 25 years in both adults and children [9]. These drugs have a range of anticancer properties that include preventing cell replication through DNA basepair intercalation and disrupting DNA uncoiling through inhibition of topoisomerase 2 activity. However, anthracyclines bind cellular membranes, which may negatively impact ion flow transport and form intracellular free radicals, which can further damage the cell [10].

Despite extensive research, the exact mechanism by which anthracyclines cause cardiotoxicity is still not fully known. Hypotheses include decreased ATP production as a consequence of decreased protein expression, impaired or destroyed mitochondria, and increased oxidative stress [10]. The oxidative stress hypothesis is the most commonly accepted hypothesis. Anthracyclines can form complexes with intracellular iron, which results in free radical formation, leading to the depletion of sulfhydryl-containing peptides, lipid peroxidation and DNA damage [10]. The heart is thought to be particularly sensitive to this stress as a result of an abundance of mitochondria in cardiomyocytes, which include high concentrations of cardiolipin. Cardiolipin's high affinity for anthracyclines allows the drugs to enter cardiomyocytes passively and accumulate in intracellular fluids to concentrations several hundred times higher than that in extracellular fluids [11]. Additionally, the heart has a reduced ability to scavenge free radicals created by the anthracyclines, given that there are lower concentrations than is normally present of catalase and glutathione peroxidase in the presence of

anthracyclines [10]. The increased stress and reduced free radical scavenging leads to cardiomyocyte-damaged DNA, reduced protein expression, damage to the cardiac sarcomere, destruction of myofilaments giving way to cell and organ damage, and left ventricular (LV) diastolic dysfunction with impaired contractility [9, 10].

Mechanisms of Radiotherapy-Induced Cardiotoxicity

Utilizing chemotherapy and radiation therapy together has been shown to improve oncological outcomes in many cancer patients, and about half of these patients now receive some amount of radiation [9]. However, much like the chemotherapeutic drugs, radiotherapy can also cause cardiotoxic side effects: myocardial fibrosis, cardiomyopathy, early coronary disease, and valvular and electrophysiological dysfunction [9]. The cardiotoxicity is believed to be caused by acute injury and inflammation leading to long-term myocardial fibrosis [10]. The risk of these cardiotoxic side effects increases two- to sixfold in patients receiving substantial chest radiation [12]. Cardiotoxicity from radiation is also dose dependent and correlates with the area of the heart exposed and the radiological technique used, as well as the patient's age, with a greater incidence in younger patients [9]. Patients receiving more than 1,500–3,500 cGy show an increased risk for cardiac disease, with high-level doses associated with myocardial ischemia as soon as 12 years after treatment [12].

Cardiotoxicity Risk Factors

Not every cancer survivor treated with anthracyclines and radiation experiences cardiotoxicity, but identifying risk factors may still help to determine which patients are at higher risk. These risk factors might help guide treatment and help clinicians determine appropriate follow-up intervals.

The risk of cardiotoxicity increases with a higher anthracycline cumulative dose. Cumulative doses greater than 500 mg/m^2 have been linked to early congestive heart failure [13]. In a study by Nysom et al. [14], after a median of 8.1 years since the end of anthracycline therapy, patients who received cumulative doses between 244 and 550 mg/m^2 experienced late anthracycline-related cardiotoxicity, as evidenced by depressed LV fractional shortening and increased LV dimension, whereas these conditions did not occur in 3 other cohorts who received

Acta Haematol 2014;132:391–399
DOI: 10.1159/000360238

Lipshultz/Sambatakos/Maguire/Karnik/
Ross/Franco/Miller

relatively lower doses (0–23, 45 and 73–301 mg/m^2). According to another recent study in adolescent patients, about 13 years after treatment, subclinical events occurred in about 30% of the patients, even at doses of 180–240 mg/m^2 [15]. These findings suggest that there is no safe dose of anthracyclines. Even doses as low as 100 mg/m^2 have been associated with reduced cardiac function [14, 16, 17].

Younger age at diagnosis is also associated with anthracycline-induced cardiotoxicity [18, 19]. Children less than 4 years of age at anthracycline exposure showed an increased risk of LV dysfunction [7]. Females have a higher risk of anthracycline-induced cardiotoxicity than do males [20]. Also, survivors with trisomy 21 are at an increased risk for LV dysfunction, even when patients with congenital cardiovascular abnormalities are excluded [21]. A number of other risk factors exist as well that will not be covered here such as preexisting risk factors for or the presence of cardiovascular disease, and noncardiac medical conditions that increase the risk of cardiovascular disease, including but not limited to endocrinopathies, infections, inflammatory conditions, obesity and metabolic diseases, failure to thrive, sedentary lifestyle, pulmonary disease, musculoskeletal disease, renal disease, hepatic disease, concomitant or prior medication usage (licit and illicit), a history of ethanol, energy drink (stimulant), complementary and alternative therapies, and tobacco use, prior treatment for cancer, prematurity and genetic disorders. These should all be evaluated and considered prior to initiating cardiotoxic cancer therapies to identify high-cardiovascular-risk populations for treatment to reduce this risk by modification of these risk factors, using cardioprotective strategies, and by minimizing the use of, or avoiding, cardiotoxic cancer therapies.

Independently of these risk factors, not all children and adolescents exposed to toxic treatments, even those who receive the same standardized chemotherapeutic regimens, experience cardiotoxicity, suggesting the possibility of a genetic predisposition [20, 22, 23]. For example, hereditary hemochromatosis is a genetic disorder associated with a mutation of the *Hfe* gene, which encodes the human hemochromatosis protein, a protein that interferes with iron metabolism and leads to iron overload and increases susceptibility to anthracycline-associated toxicity [24]. An animal study in doxorubicin-treated mice showed that *Hfe* knockout mice *(Hfe$^{-/-}$)* displayed a higher degree of mitochondrial damage and iron deposits in the heart than did wild-type mice [24, 25].

As described above, anthracyclines form complexes with intracellular iron, which result in free radical formation; therefore, iron accumulating in the heart increases the susceptibility to doxorubicin-induced cardiotoxicity. In a recent study of long-term survivors of childhood high-risk acute lymphoblastic leukemia, 10% of survivors were carriers of a mutation in the C282Y allele, one of the mutations most commonly associated with *Hfe* [24]. Furthermore, the risk of myocardial injury in survivors who were heterozygous for the C282Y allele was 9 times higher than that in noncarriers [24]. Blanco et al. [26] found that among patients with single nucleotide polymorphisms in CBR3 homozygous G genotypes *(CBR3:GG)*, exposure to low-to-moderate doses of anthracyclines increased the risk of cardiomyopathy by 5 and 3 times that of survivors with the *CBR3:GA/AA* genotypes unexposed and exposed to low-to-moderate-dose anthracyclines, respectively. Polymorphisms in CBR3 influence the synthesis of carbonyl reductases, which catalyze the reduction of anthracyclines to cardiotoxic alcohol metabolites [26]. These studies show the potential influence of genetics in identifying patients at an increased risk of anthracycline-induced cardiac effects; however, additional studies specifically designed to address and confirm these novel risk factors are needed.

Obesity is a well-known cardiac risk factor [27]. Compared with siblings, male survivors have a greater body fat and metabolic risk. Cranial irradiation and television hours are important risk factors for adiposity in pediatric cancer survivors [28]. In a study assessing the dietary trends of childhood cancer survivors, it was found that survivors consumed diets that only moderately adhered to current recommendations [29]. Dietary quality below current recommendations often leads to increased adiposity, increasing the risk for cardiovascular disease [29]. Targeting dietary consumption can decrease adiposity and lower cardiovascular risk. Furthermore, supervised physical activity should be encouraged to improve nutritional and cardiac conditions [30].

Klosky et al. [31] looked at childhood cancer survivors aged 14–20 years and found no significant difference between usage rates of tobacco, alcohol and illicit drugs, or risky sexual behavior when compared to sibling controls. Kahalley et al. [32] also found no significant difference in smoking rates between childhood cancer survivors and healthy sibling controls. However, Kahalley et al. did address the correlation between the increased incidence of smoking and health risk factors, such as peer smoking, household smoking and suicidal behavior. The risk factors noted by Kahalley et al., in addition to smoking, which is already an established risk factor for cardiovascular disease, put this patient population into a high-risk group, and they should be counseled accordingly [33].

The sex of the patient also appears to be a risk factor for cardiotoxicity. Females have higher rates of LV dysfunction than do males exposed to similar doses of doxorubicin [34]. The cause of this increased risk associated with females is not clear. It is hypothesized that because doxorubicin does not reach a high concentration in adipose tissue, females generally have a higher percent body fat and anthracycline dosages are calculated based on body surface area, female cardiomyocytes may be exposed to a higher concentration when compared to cardiomyocyte intracellular concentrations in males [35].

Monitoring and Screening

Evidence-based monitoring and screening of childhood cancer survivors is imperative in identifying early signs of cardiotoxicity in patients who may be at higher risk. Aside from obtaining a thorough medical history, baseline cardiac studies are recommended before beginning chemotherapy [36–38]. Although endomyocardial biopsy may provide useful histological information, serial biopsies are not only expensive, but also highly invasive.

Newer studies of serum cardiac biomarkers are showing promise. These biomarkers may identify several different populations, including those experiencing cardiotoxicity, as well as those who may develop future cardiotoxicity. Lipshultz et al. [39] evaluated children with acute lymphoblastic leukemia treated with doxorubicin. They monitored concentrations of cardiac troponin T, N-terminal probrain natriuretic peptide (NT-proBNP) and high-sensitivity C-reactive protein. Serum cardiac troponin T concentrations elevated in the first 90 days of treatment with anthracyclines were significantly associated with reduced LV end-diastolic posterior wall thickness, reduced LV mass and increased LV remodeling 4 years after therapy [39]. Serum NT-proBNP concentrations may indicate increasing LV wall stress, as this level rises with wall stretch. NT-proBNP concentrations were elevated in 89% of patients before treatment and in 48% of patients after treatment [39]. Overall, NT-proBNP was elevated in more patients than was cardiac troponin T, which may identify patients at risk for future cardiotoxicity, and significantly predicted late LV remodeling [39]. The authors did not find elevated high-sensitivity C-reactive protein concentrations measured during anthracycline therapy to be a reliable marker for patients who

may develop late cardiotoxicity as long-term survivors [39].

Additionally, as assessment of LV diastolic function and cardiac magnetic resonance imaging are increasingly used in pediatric cardiology, adolescent patients may benefit from its ability to identify cardiotoxicity. However, limited availability of diastolic function measurements and the availability, accessibility, high cost and lengthy studies may potentially limit widespread cardiac magnetic resonance usage.

Preventing Cardiotoxicity

Given the risk of cardiotoxicity with anthracyclines, various strategies to limit cardiac injury without reducing oncological efficacy have been explored. These are summarized below.

Continuous versus Bolus Anthracycline Infusion

In adults, cardiotoxicity assessed early after anthracycline infusion is reduced by continuous infusion, which lowers peak plasma levels in comparison with bolus infusions [40]. However, these same results were not replicated in a large prospective randomized controlled trial of children with a diagnosis of high-risk acute lymphoblastic leukemia [41]. Neither outcome with LV function nor 10-year event-free survival differed significantly between groups receiving either continuous or bolus infusion [41, 42]. This study suggests that continuous infusion of anthracyclines does not provide cardioprotection over bolus infusion in children [41].

Structural Modifications of Anthracyclines

Modifying the structural form of anthracyclines to reduce their cardiotoxicity is another experimental approach. Epirubicin, a structural analog of doxorubicin, has less overall toxicity but the same efficacy as doxorubicin. A cumulative dose of epirubicin up to 900 mg/m^2 is equivalent to only 450 mg/m^2 of doxorubicin in terms of cardiotoxicity [43].

Two separate studies of patients with breast cancer showed that epirubicin had a less toxic profile than doxorubicin [44, 45]. A meta-analysis of 5 randomized control trials comparing epirubicin to doxorubicin found no significant difference in the incidence of early clinical heart failure between control and experimental groups [46]. However, on the basis of a wide confidence interval and a low relative risk, this meta-analysis suggested a lower rate of clinical heart failure in the epirubicin treatment

Acta Haematol 2014;132:391–399
DOI: 10.1159/000360238

group [46]. All these studies were limited to adults with solid tumors. Response rates did not differ between groups [46]. In a separate study, also in adults, lower doses of epirubicin up to 360 mg/m^2 have also caused subclinical cardiotoxicity [47].

Other doxorubicin analogs, idarubicin and mitoxantrone, although they may reduce cardiac injury, do not completely eliminate the risk of cardiotoxicity [43, 48]. Studies with use of these different analogs have so far been done only in adults with breast cancer [47, 48]. To our knowledge, no studies have been conducted in adolescents that might justify the use of analogs in this group.

Liposomal Anthracyclines
Liposomal anthracyclines have a better and safer oncological profile than do conventional anthracyclines [49]. Two forms of liposomal anthracyclines are currently available: pegylated PL-ODX/Doxil/Caelyx and non-pegylated Tl-D99/Myocet.

Pegylated anthracyclines, compared to regular anthracyclines, have longer circulation times, longer half-lives, slower clearance from plasma, a smaller volume of distribution and they cannot penetrate cardiac cell tight junctions [50, 51]. These characteristics result in higher drug concentrations in tumors and lower concentrations in the heart [51]. Therefore, pegylated anthracyclines decrease cardiotoxicity while maintaining oncological efficacy. This conclusion was supported by endomyocardial biopsies of patients receiving liposomal versus conventional anthracyclines [49].

Another retrospective study showed that cumulative doses of the pegylated form, up to 500 mg/m^2, did not result in heart failure [52]. A meta-analysis of 2 other randomized controlled trials in women with metastatic breast cancer found fewer clinical and subclinical cardiac events in the group receiving liposomal anthracyclines [46]. However, no randomized controlled trials in children have been conducted to reproduce these results [51].

Only 1 randomized trial studied the use of liposomal daunorubicin as a second-line therapy in children with relapsed acute myeloid leukemia [53]. However, interpreting cardiac damage in this population is difficult because the patients had already undergone aggressive first-line therapy.

Use of Cardioprotective Agents
Dexrazoxane
Dexrazoxane is an iron-chelating agent that reduces the formation of iron-anthracycline complexes [54, 55]. Without these iron-anthracycline complexes, the genera-

tion of reactive oxygen species is limited, thus limiting the toxicity of anthracyclines [54, 55]. Dexrazoxane also interferes with topoisomerase 2β, thereby antagonizing doxorubicin-induced DNA damage [56].

A randomized controlled trial by Lipshultz et al. [54] compared children less than 18 years of age with a diagnosis of high-risk acute lymphoblastic leukemia receiving doxorubicin alone with those receiving treatment with dexrazoxane and doxorubicin. The cardiac damage, as measured by serum cardiac troponin concentrations, was significantly less in the group receiving dexrazoxane [54]. Girls treated with doxorubicin and dexrazoxane had better long-term outcomes in terms of LV fractional shortening, LV end-diastolic dimension, LV posterior wall thickness and LV pathological remodeling measurements [55]. At the same time, the rate of secondary neoplasms and 8-year event-free survival was similar, whether or not children received dexrazoxane with doxorubicin [55].

A meta-analysis by Van Dalen et al. [57] revealed statistically lower rates of heart failure in children and adult patients who had been treated with dexrazoxane when compared to those who had not. The two groups did not differ significantly in antioncological effects or in survival rates [57]. The American Society of Clinical Oncology recommends dexrazoxane in adult patients with metastatic breast cancer being treated with anthracyclines in cumulative doses greater than 300 mg/m^2 [58].

Carvedilol
Carvedilol provides cardioprotection by inhibiting reactive oxygen species, scavenging free radicals, preventing lipid peroxidation and increasing vitamin E concentrations [59]. Some of these mechanisms have been documented in in vitro studies [60]. Carvedilol reduced anthracycline-induced cardiomyopathy in rats [61]. This evidence further needs to be supported in human studies [61].

Supplements
Coenzyme Q
Coenzyme Q, an antioxidant, is an important part of the mitochondrial respiratory chain [62]. Supplementation of coenzyme Q prevented anthracycline-induced cardiotoxicity in both preclinical and clinical studies [62]. Currently, only 1 study has shown that coenzyme Q treatment has reduced the incidence of cardiotoxicity in children treated with doxorubicin [63].

L-Carnitine
The naturally occurring amino acid L-carnitine protects the heart from damage by its antioxidant action against an-

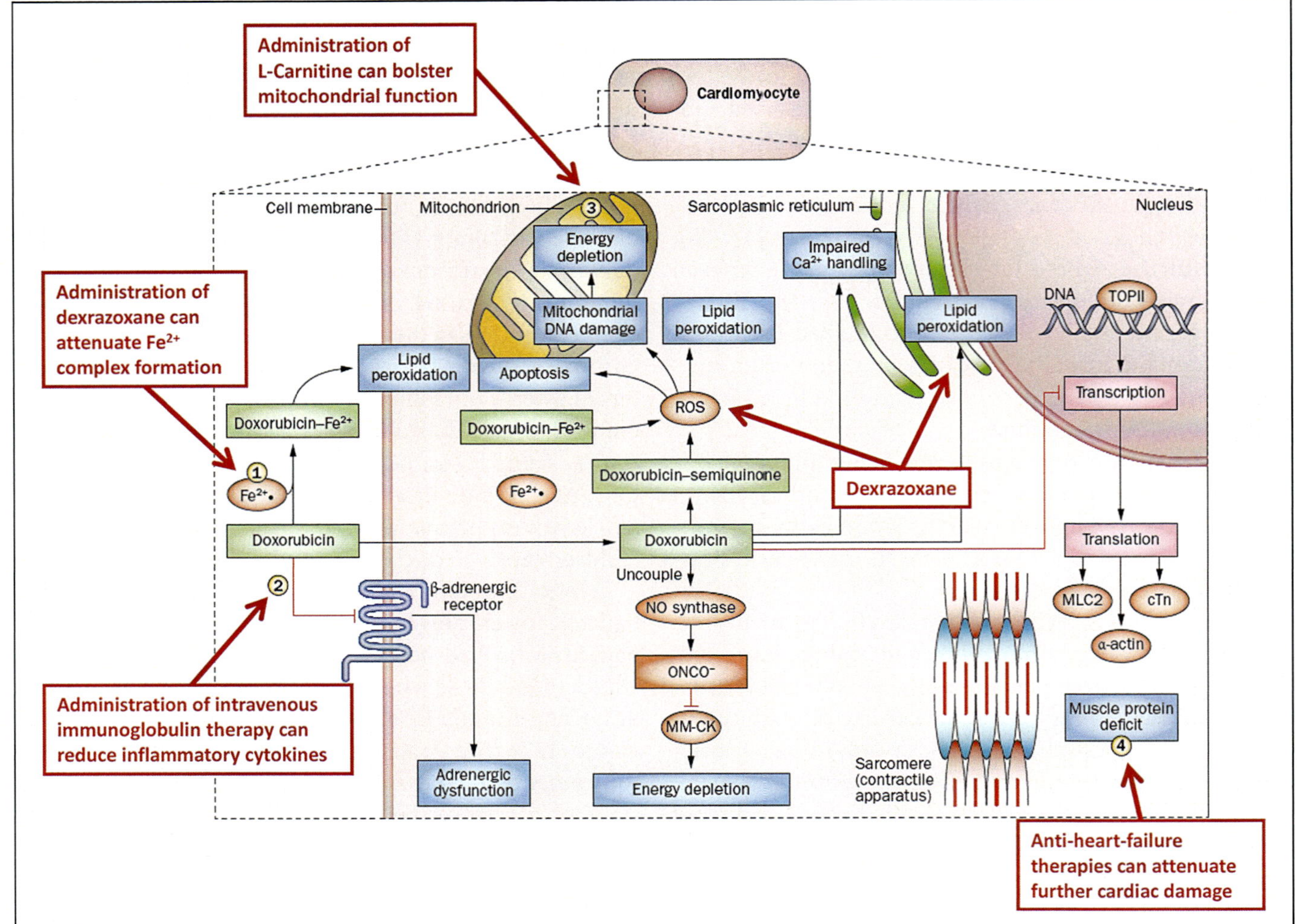

Fig. 1. Potential opportunities for targeted multiagent cardioprotection. Doxorubicin chemotherapy has a range of effects on cardiomyocytes. It induces lipid peroxidation at the cell and mitochondrial membranes by way of complexing with Fe²⁺ and induces apoptosis, mitochondrial DNA damage and energy depletion through its production of reactive oxygen species. Furthermore, it impairs Ca²⁺ processing in the sarcoplasmic reticulum and inhibits the transcription of important muscle elements, weakening the heart muscle. It also downregulates adrenergic receptors and interrupts cell signaling. We have explored 4 areas for multiagent anthracycline cardioprotection, but other mechanisms and potential targets exist as well. This figure illustrates the 4 areas we have focused on and their potential cardioprotective mechanisms and includes: (1) administration of dexrazoxane, which can prevent Fe²⁺ complex formation; (2) intravenous immunoglobulin therapy, which can reduce inflammatory cytokines; (3) L-carnitine, which can bolster mitochondrial function, and (4) anti-heart-failure therapies, such as angiotensin-converting enzyme inhibitors and β-blockers, which can prevent further damage and pathological ventricular remodeling. cTn = Cardiac troponin; MLC2 = myosin light chain 2; MM-CK = myofibrillar isoform of the creatine kinase enzyme; NO = nitric oxide; ROS = reactive oxygen species; TOPII = topoisomerase 2. Modified with permission from Lipshultz et al. [70] in Nature Publishing Group.

thracycline-induced lipid peroxidation of cardiac membranes and by reducing the ability of anthracyclines to inhibit long-chain fatty acid production [58]. Therefore, L-carnitine supplementation should protect against the acute and chronic effects of anthracycline-induced cardiotoxicity. However, there is insufficient evidence to justify the conclusion that L-carnitine is cardioprotective [46, 64].

Glutathione

Glutathione, a tripeptide thiol, is another antioxidant that scavenges free radicals. It acts as a substrate for glutathione peroxidase whose activity is interfered with by anthracyclines [65]. Thus, glutathione supplementation may protect the heart from anthracycline effects [58]. Both in vitro and animal studies have shown that gluta-

Acta Haematol 2014;132:391–399
DOI: 10.1159/000360238

thione supplementation decreases cardiac damage [66–69]. Glutathione does have potential in preventing anthracycline-induced cardiac damage.

Conclusion

Advancements in cancer therapies have undoubtedly contributed to the improved life expectancy of childhood cancer survivors. However, despite this increased survival, many survivors have a lower quality of life as a result of the adverse late effects of the same treatments that cured their cancer. Exposure to these treatments of children at a young age makes them particularly vulnerable to impaired growth and development and to an increased risk of premature cardiovascular disease. Screening for risk factors, including genetic risk factors such as *Hfe*, together with serum biomarkers, might prove useful at early stages to inform treatment decisions. However, the mechanisms of anthracycline- and radiation-induced cardiotoxicity need to be better understood to develop effective and safe cardioprotective strategies. Nevertheless, an effective cardioprotective agent, dexrazoxane, has been validated in children receiving anthracycline chemotherapy and should be incorporated into clinical trials where children with cancer receive anthracycline chemotherapy. Additional cardioprotective strategies may allow for multiagent cardioprotection to maximize oncological efficacy while minimizing toxicity and late adverse effects (fig. 1). This is particularly important since the successful treatment of childhood cancer brings about the overall quality of life during a lifespan as determined by the balance between efficacy and late effects.

References

1 American Cancer Society: Cancer Facts and Figures 2012. Atlanta, American Cancer Society, 2012.
2 Howlader N, Noone AM, Krapcho M, Garshell J, Neyman N, Altekruse SF, Kosary CL, Yu M, Ruhl J, Tatalovich Z, Cho H, Mariotto A, Lewis DR, Chen HS, Feuer EJ, Cronin KA (eds): SEER Cancer Statistics Review, 1975–2010. Bethesda, National Cancer Institute. http://seer.cancer.gov/csr/1975_2010/ (based on November 2012 SEER data submission, posted to the SEER web site, April 2013).
3 Oeffinger KC, Mertens AC, Sklar CA, Kawashima T, Hudson MM, Meadows AT, Friedman DL, Marina N, Hobbie W, Kadan-Lottick NS, Schwartz CL, Leisenring W, Robison LL; Childhood Cancer Survivor Study: Chronic health conditions in adult survivors of childhood cancer. N Engl J Med 2006;355: 1572–1582.
4 Mulrooney DA, Yeazel MW, Kawashima T, Mertens AC, Mitby P, Stovall M, Donaldson SS, Green DM, Sklar CA, Robison LL, Leisenring WM: Cardiac outcomes in a cohort of adult survivors of childhood and adolescent cancer: retrospective analysis of the Childhood Cancer Survivor Study cohort. BMJ 2009;339:b4606.
5 Tukenova M, Guibout C, Oberlin O, Doyon F, Mousannif A, Haddy N, Guérin S, Pacquement H, Aouba A, Hawkins M, Winter D, Bourhis J, Lefkopoulos D, Diallo I, de Vathaire F: Role of cancer treatment in long-term overall and cardiovascular mortality after childhood cancer. J Clin Oncol 2010;28:1308–1315.

6 Armstrong GT, Oeffinger KC, Chen Y, Kawashima T, Yasui Y, Leisenring W, Stovall M, Chow EJ, Sklar CA, Mulrooney DA, Mertens AC, Border W, Durand JB, Robison LL, Meacham LR: Modifiable risk factors and major cardiac events among adult survivors of childhood cancer. J Clin Oncol 2013;31:3673–3680.
7 Lipshultz SE, Colan SD, Gelber RD, Perez-Atayde AR, Sallan SE, Sanders SP: Late cardiac effects of doxorubicin therapy for acute lymphoblastic leukemia in childhood. N Engl J Med 1991;324:808–815.
8 Landy DC, Miller TL, Lipsitz SR, Lopez-Mitnik G, Hinkle AS, Constine LS, Adams MJ, Lipshultz SE: Cranial irradiation as an additional risk factor for anthracycline cardiotoxicity in childhood cancer survivors: an analysis from the cardiac risk factors in childhood cancer survivors study. Pediatr Cardiol 2013; 34:826–834.
9 Adão R, de Keulenaer G, Leite-Moreira A, Brás-Silva C: Cardiotoxicity associated with cancer therapy: pathophysiology and prevention. Rev Portug Cardiol (English ed) 2013;32: 395–409.
10 Diamond M, Franco V: Preventing and treating anthracycline-related cardiotoxicity in survivors of childhood cancer. Curr Cancer Ther Rev 2012;8:141–151.
11 Franco VI, Henkel JM, Miller TL, Lipshultz SE: Cardiovascular effects in childhood cancer survivors treated with anthracyclines. Cardiol Res Pract 2011;2011:134679.
12 Dillenburg RF, Nathan P, Mertens L: Educational paper: decreasing the burden of cardiovascular disease in childhood cancer survivors: an update for the pediatrician. Eur J Pediatr 2013;172:1149–1160.

13 Von Hoff DD, Layard MW, Basa P, Davis HL Jr, Von Hoff AL, Rozencweig M, Muggia FM: Risk factors for doxorubicin-induced congestive heart failure. Ann Intern Med 1979;91: 710–717.
14 Nysom K, Holm K, Lipsitz SR, Mone SM, Colan SD, Orav EJ, Sallan SE, Olsen JH, Hertz H, Jacobsen JR, Lipshultz SE: Relationship between cumulative anthracycline dose and late cardiotoxicity in childhood acute lymphoblastic leukemia. J Clin Oncol 1998;16:545–550.
15 Vandecruys E, Mondelaers V, De Wolf D, Benoit Y, Suys B: Late cardiotoxicity after low dose of anthracycline therapy for acute lymphoblastic leukemia in childhood. J Cancer Surviv 2012;6:95–101.
16 Lipshultz SE, Adams MJ: Cardiotoxicity after childhood cancer: beginning with the end in mind. J Clin Oncol 2010;28:1276–1281.
17 Van der Pal HJ, van Dalen EC, Hauptmann M, Kok WE, Caron HN, van den Bos C, Oldenburger F, Koning CC, van Leeuwen FE, Kremer LC: Cardiac function in 5-year survivors of childhood cancer: a long-term follow-up study. Arch Intern Med 2010;170:1247–1255.
18 Swain SM, Whaley FS, Ewer MS: Congestive heart failure in patients treated with doxorubicin: a retrospective analysis of three trials. Cancer 2003;97:2869–2879.
19 Lipshultz SE, Lipsitz SR, Sallan SE, Dalton VM, Mone SM, Gelber RD, Colan SD: Chronic progressive cardiac dysfunction years after doxorubicin therapy for childhood acute lymphoblastic leukemia. J Clin Oncol 2005;23: 2629–2636.

20 Krischer JP, Epstein S, Cuthbertson DD, Goorin AM, Epstein ML, Lipshultz SE: Clinical cardiotoxicity following anthracycline treatment for childhood cancer: the Pediatric Oncology Group experience. J Clin Oncol 1997;15:1544–1552.

21 Wang L, Weinshilboum R: Thiopurine S-methyltransferase pharmacogenetics: insights, challenges and future directions. Oncogene 2006;25:1629–1638.

22 Deng S, Wojnowski L: Genotyping the risk of anthracycline-induced cardiotoxicity. Cardiovasc Toxicol 2007;7:129–134.

23 Blanco JG, Leisenring WM, Gonzalez-Covarrubias VM, Kawashima TI, Davies SM, Relling MV, Robison LL, Sklar CA, Stovall M, Bhatia S: Genetic polymorphisms in the carbonyl reductase 3 gene CBR3 and the NAD(P)H: quinone oxidoreductase 1 gene NQO1 in patients who developed anthracycline-related congestive heart failure after childhood cancer. Cancer 2008;112:2789–2795.

24 Lipshultz SE, Lipsitz SR, Kutok JL, Miller TL, Colan SD, Neuberg DS, Stevenson KE, Fleming MD, Sallan SE, Franco VI, Henkel JM, Asselin BL, Athale UH, Clavell LA, Michon B, Laverdiere C, Larsen E, Kelly KM, Silverman LB: Impact of hemochromatosis gene mutations on cardiac status in doxorubicin-treated survivors of childhood high-risk leukemia. Cancer 2013;119:3555–3562.

25 Miranda CJ, Makui H, Soares RJ, Bilodeau M, Mui J, Vali H, Bertrand R, Andrews NC, Santos MM: *Hfe* deficiency increases susceptibility to cardiotoxicity and exacerbates changes in iron metabolism induced by doxorubicin. Blood 2003;102:2574–2580.

26 Blanco JG, Sun CL, Landier W, Chen L, Esparza-Duran D, Leisenring W, Mays A, Friedman DL, Ginsberg JP, Hudson MM, Neglia JP, Oeffinger KC, Ritchey AK, Villaluna D, Relling MV, Bhatia S: Anthracycline-related cardiomyopathy after childhood cancer: role of polymorphisms in carbonyl reductase genes – a report from the Children's Oncology Group. J Clin Oncol 2012;30:1415–1421.

27 Qureshi MY, Wilkinson JD, Lipshultz SE: The relationship of childhood obesity with cardiomyopathy and heart failure; in Lipshultz SE, Messiah SE, Miller TL (eds): Pediatric Metabolic Syndrome. London, Springer, 2012, pp 199–215.

28 Miller TL, Lipsitz SR, Lopez-Mitnik G, Hinkle AS, Constine LS, Adams MJ, French C, Proukou C, Rovitelli A, Lipshultz SE: Characteristics and determinants of adiposity in pediatric cancer survivors. Cancer Epidemiol Biomarkers Prev 2010;19:2013–2022.

29 Landy DC, Lipsitz SR, Kurtz JM, Hinkle AS, Constine LS, Adams MJ, Lipshultz SE, Miller TL: Dietary quality, caloric intake, and adiposity of childhood cancer survivors and their siblings: an analysis from the Cardiac Risk Factors in Childhood Cancer Survivors Study. Nutr Cancer 2013;65:547–555.

30 Miller AM, Lopez-Mitnik G, Somarriba G, Lipsitz SR, Hinkle AS, Constine LS, Lipshultz SE, Miller TL: Exercise capacity in long-term survivors of pediatric cancer: an analysis from the Cardiac Risk Factors in Childhood Cancer Survivors Study. Pediatr Blood Cancer 2013; 60:663–668.

31 Klosky JL, Howell CR, Li Z, Foster RH, Mertens AC, Robison LL, Ness KK: Risky health behavior among adolescents in the Childhood Cancer Survivor Study cohort. J Pediatr Psychol 2012;37:634–646.

32 Kahalley LS, Robinson LA, Tyc VL, Hudson MM, Leisenring W, Stratton K, Mertens AC, Zeltzer L, Robison LL, Hinds PS: Risk factors for smoking among adolescent survivors of childhood cancer: a report from the Childhood Cancer Survivor Study. Pediatr Blood Cancer 2012;58:428–434.

33 Lakier JB: Smoking and cardiovascular disease. Am J Med 1992;93(1A):8S–12S.

34 Silber JH, Jakacki RI, Larsen RL, Goldwein JW, Barber G: Increased risk of cardiac dysfunction after anthracyclines in girls. Med Pediatr Oncol 1993;21:477–479.

35 Lipshultz SE, Lipsitz SR, Mone SM, Goorin AM, Sallan SE, Sanders SP, Orav EJ, Gelber RD, Colan SD: Female sex and drug dose as risk factors for late cardiotoxic effects of doxorubicin therapy for childhood cancer. N Engl J Med 1995;332:1738–1743.

36 Bovelli D, Plataniotis G, Roila F: Cardiotoxicity of chemotherapeutic agents and radiotherapy-related heart disease: ESMO Clinical Practice Guidelines. Ann Oncol 2010;21 (suppl 5):v277–v282.

37 Trachtenberg BH, Landy DC, Franco VI, Henkel JM, Pearson EJ, Miller TL, Lipshultz SE: Anthracycline-associated cardiotoxicity in survivors of childhood cancer. Pediatr Cardiol 2011;32:342–353.

38 Gottsauner-Wolf M, Schedlmayer-Duit J, Porenta G, Gwechenberger M, Huber K, Glogar D, Probst P, Sochor H: Assessment of left ventricular function: comparison between radionuclide angiography and semiquantitative two-dimensional echocardiographic analysis. Eur J Nucl Med 1996;23:1613–1618.

39 Lipshultz SE, Miller TL, Scully RE, Lipsitz SR, Rifai N, Silverman LB, Colan SD, Neuberg DS, Dahlberg SE, Henkel JM, Asselin BL, Athale UH, Clavell LA, Laverdière C, Michon B, Schorin MA, Sallan SE: Changes in cardiac biomarkers during doxorubicin treatment of pediatric patients with high-risk acute lymphoblastic leukemia: associations with long-term echocardiographic outcomes. J Clin Oncol 2012;30:1042–1049.

40 Legha SS, Benjamin RS, Mackay B, Ewer M, Wallace S, Valdivieso M, Rasmussen SL, Blumenschein GR, Freireich EJ: Reduction of doxorubicin cardiotoxicity by prolonged continuous intravenous infusion. Ann Intern Med 1982;96:133–139.

41 Lipshultz SE, Miller TL, Lipsitz SR, Neuberg DS, Dahlberg SE, Colan SD, Silverman LB, Henkel JM, Franco VI, Cushman LL, Asselin BL, Clavell LA, Athale U, Michon B, Laverdière C, Schorin MA, Larsen E, Usmani N, Sallan SE; Dana-Farber Cancer Institute Acute Lymphoblastic Leukemia Consortium: Continuous versus bolus infusion of doxorubicin in children with ALL: long-term cardiac outcomes. Pediatrics 2012;130:1003–1011.

42 Lipshultz SE, Giantris AL, Lipsitz SR, Kimball Dalton V, Asselin BL, Barr RD, Clavell LA, Hurwitz CA, Moghrabi A, Samson Y, Schorin MA, Gelber RD, Sallan SE, Colan SD: Doxorubicin administration by continuous infusion is not cardioprotective: the Dana-Farber 91-01 Acute Lymphoblastic Leukemia protocol. J Clin Oncol 2002;20:1677–1682.

43 Barry E, Alvarez JA, Scully RE, Miller TL, Lipshultz SE: Anthracycline-induced cardiotoxicity: course, pathophysiology, prevention and management. Expert Opin Pharmacother 2007;8:1039–1058.

44 French Epirubicin Study Group: A prospective randomized phase III trial comparing combination chemotherapy with cyclophosphamide, fluorouracil, and either doxorubicin or epirubicin. J Clin Oncol 1988;6:679–688.

45 Phase III randomized study of fluorouracil, epirubicin, and cyclophosphamide versus fluorouracil, doxorubicin, and cyclophosphamide in advanced breast cancer: an Italian multicentre trial. Italian Multicentre Breast Study with Epirubicin. J Clin Oncol 1988;6:976–982.

46 Van Dalen EC, Michiels EM, Caron HN, Kremer LC: Different anthracycline derivates for reducing cardiotoxicity in cancer patients. Cochrane Database Syst Rev 2010;5:CD005006.

47 Meinardi MT, van Veldhuisen DJ, Gietema JA, Dolsma WV, Boomsma F, van den Berg MP, Volkers C, Haaksma J, de Vries EG, Sleijfer DT, van der Graaf WT: Prospective evaluation of early cardiac damage induced by epirubicin-containing adjuvant chemotherapy and locoregional radiotherapy in breast cancer patients. J Clin Oncol 2001;19:2746–2753.

48 Cowan JD, Neidhart J, McClure S, Coltman CA Jr, Gumbart C, Martino S, Hutchins LF, Stephens RL, Vaughan CB, Osborne CK: Randomized trial of doxorubicin, bisantrene, and mitoxantrone in advanced breast cancer: a Southwest Oncology Group study. J Natl Cancer Inst 1991;83:1077–1084.

49 Gabizon AA, Lyass O, Berry GJ, Wildgust M: Cardiac safety of pegylated liposomal doxorubicin (Doxil/Caelyx) demonstrated by endomyocardial biopsy in patients with advanced malignancies. Cancer Invest 2004;22:663–669.

50 Leonard RC, Williams S, Tulpule A, Levine AM, Oliveros S: Improving the therapeutic index of anthracycline chemotherapy: focus on liposomal doxorubicin (Myocet). Breast 2009;18:218–224.

51 Sieswerda E, Kremer LC, Caron HN, van Dalen EC: The use of liposomal anthracycline analogues for childhood malignancies: a systematic review. Eur J Cancer 2011;47:2000–2008.

52 Safra T, Muggia F, Jeffers S, Tsao-Wei DD, Lyass O, Henderson R, Berry G, Gabizon A: Pegylated liposomal doxorubicin (Doxil): reduced clinical cardiotoxicity in patients reaching or exceeding cumulative doses of 500 mg/m^2. Ann Oncol 2000;11:1029–1033.

53 Kaspers GJ, Zimmermann M, Reinhardt D, Gibson BE, Tamminga RY, Aleinikova O, Armendariz H, Dworzak M, Ha SY, Hasle H, Hovi L, Maschan A, Bertrand Y, Leverger GG, Razzouk BI, Rizzari C, Smisek P, Smith O, Stark B, Creutzig U: Improved outcome in pediatric relapsed acute myeloid leukemia: results of a randomized trial on liposomal daunorubicin by the International BFM Study Group. J Clin Oncol 2013;31:599–607.

54 Lipshultz SE, Rifai N, Dalton VM, Levy DE, Silverman LB, Lipsitz SR, Colan SD, Asselin BL, Barr RD, Clavell LA, Hurwitz CA, Moghrabi A, Samson Y, Schorin MA, Gelber RD, Sallan SE: The effect of dexrazoxane on myocardial injury in doxorubicin-treated children with acute lymphoblastic leukemia. N Engl J Med 2004;351:145–153.

55 Lipshultz SE, Scully RE, Lipsitz SR, Sallan SE, Silverman LB, Millter TL, Barry EV, Asselin BL, Athale U, Clavell LA, Larsen E, Moghrabi A, Samson Y, Michon B, Schorin MA, Cohen HJ, Neuberg DS, Orav EJ, Colan SD: Assessment of dexrazoxane as a cardioprotectant in doxorubicin-treated children with high-risk acute lymphoblastic leukaemia: long-term follow-up of a prospective, randomised, multicentre trial. Lancet Oncol 2010;11:950–961.

56 Lyu YL, Kerrigan JE, Lin CP, Azarova AM, Tsai YC, Ban Y, Liu LF: Topoisomerase II-beta mediated DNA double-strand breaks: implications in doxorubicin cardiotoxicity and prevention by dexrazoxane. Cancer Res 2007;67:8839–8846.

57 Van Dalen EC, Caron HN, Dickinson HO, Kremer LC: Cardioprotective interventions for cancer patients receiving anthracyclines. Cochrane Database Syst Rev 2011;6:CD003917.

58 Wouters KA, Kremer LC, Miller TL, Herman EH, Lipshultz SE: Protecting against anthracycline-induced myocardial damage: a review of the most promising strategies. Br J Haematol 2005;131:561–578.

59 Feuerstein GZ, Ruffolo RR Jr: Carvedilol, a novel multiple action antihypertensive agent with antioxidant activity and the potential for myocardial and vascular protection. Eur Heart J 1995;16(suppl F):38–42.

60 Spallarossa P, Garibaldi S, Altieri P, Fabbi P, Manca V, Nasti S, Rossettin P, Ghigliotti G, Ballestrero A, Patrone F, Barsotti A, Brunelli C: Carvedilol prevents doxorubicin-induced free radical release and apoptosis in cardiomyocytes in vitro. J Mol Cell Cardiol 2004;37:837–846.

61 Matsui H, Morishima I, Numaguchi Y, Toki Y, Okumura K, Hayakawa T: Protective effects of carvedilol against doxorubicin-induced cardiomyopathy in rats. Life Sci 1999;65:1265–1274.

62 Granados-Principal S, Quiles JL, Ramirez-Tortosa CL, Sanchez-Rovira P, Ramirez-Tortosa MC: New advances in molecular mechanisms and the prevention of Adriamycin toxicity by antioxidant nutrients. Food Chem Toxicol 2010;48:1425–1438.

63 Iarussi D, Auricchio U, Agretto A, Murano A, Giuliano M, Casale F, Indolfi P, Iacono A: Protective effect of coenzyme Q_{10} on anthracyclines cardiotoxicity: control study in children with acute lymphoblastic leukemia and non-Hodgkin lymphoma. Mol Aspects Med 1994;15(suppl):s207–s212.

64 De Leonardis V, Neri B, Bacalli S, Cinelli P: Reduction of cardiac toxicity of anthracyclines by L-carnitine: preliminary overview of clinical data. Int J Clin Pharmacol Res 1985;5:137–142.

65 Doroshow JH, Locker GY, Myers CE: Enzymatic defenses of the mouse heart against reactive oxygen metabolites: alterations produced by doxorubicin. J Clin Invest 1980;65:128–135.

66 Arrick BA, Nathan CF, Griffith OW, Cohn ZA: Glutathione depletion sensitizes tumor cells to oxidative cytolysis. J Biol Chem 1982;257:1231–1237.

67 Suttorp N, Toepfer W, Roka L: Antioxidant defense mechanisms of endothelial cells: glutathione redox cycle versus catalase. Am J Physiol 1986;251:C671–C680.

68 Mohamed HE, El-Swefy SE, Hagar HH: The protective effect of glutathione administration on Adriamycin-induced acute cardiac toxicity in rats. Pharmacol Res 2000;42:115–121.

69 Ferrari R, Ceconi C, Curello S, Cargnoni A, Alfieri O, Pardini A, Marzollo P, Visioli O: Oxygen free radicals and myocardial damage: protective role of thiol-containing agents. Am J Med 1991;91(3C):95S–105S.

70 Lipshultz SE, Cochran TR, Franco VI, Miller TL: Treatment-related cardiotoxicity in survivors of childhood cancer. Nat Rev Clin Oncol 2013;10:697–710.

Acta Haematol 2014;132:400–413
DOI: 10.1159/000360199

Published online: September 10, 2014

Fertility Preservation in Young Females with Hematological Malignancies

Moran Shapira[a, b]   Hila Raanani[a, b]   Yoram Cohen[a, b]   Dror Meirow[a, b]

[a]Fertility Preservation Center, Chaim Sheba Medical Center, Tel Hashomer, and [b]Sackler School of Medicine, Tel Aviv University, Tel Aviv, Israel

Key Words

Embryo freezing · Fertility preservation · Gonadotoxicity · Hematological malignancies · Oocyte freezing · Ovarian failure · Ovarian transplantation

Abstract

Impaired reproductive function and possible infertility are major concerns in long-term survivors of hematological malignancies. The ongoing increase in the survival rates of these patients is therefore accompanied with a growing demand for effective, safe and specifically tailored fertility preservation options. When approaching patients facing hematological malignancy, an individual evaluation of potential infertility risks and possible preventive or preserving measures should be performed. This review aims to provide up-to-date knowledge on female reproductive risks, and ovarian, uterine and genital injuries associated with therapy regimens currently used in hemato-oncological disorders. Recent progress in fertility preservation methods including ovarian tissue cryopreservation and transplantation, egg and embryo freezing, ovarian transposition and their specific role in hematological disorders are presented. The efficacy of these methods, possible risks and future challenges are critically discussed.

© 2014 S. Karger AG, Basel

Introduction

Recent years have seen major advances in the field of fertility preservation, which has gradually become an imperative aspect of a multidisciplinary approach to cancer patients. In light of the increased life expectancy of patients with hemato-oncological diseases and a growing attention to the adverse effects of long-term treatment, it is of no surprise that referrals to reproductive endocrinologists are increasingly employed [1–3]. Such a trend stresses the necessity to better estimate the potential reproductive insults of an upcoming anticancer therapy. It also represents the growing demand for effective, safe and individualized fertility preservation options, enabling a possible restoration of endocrine function and an opportunity for a future biological offspring. In this review we aim to present updated data regarding fertility risks associated with cancer therapy and available fertility preservation technologies. A particular attention will be given to the applicability of fertility preservation methods in young women and girls facing hematological malignancies, accompanied with recommended guidelines based on literature review and our own experience.

Moran Shapira and Hila Raanani contributed equally to this work.

KARGER

© 2014 S. Karger AG, Basel
0001–5792/14/1324–0400$39.50/0

E-Mail karger@karger.com
www.karger.com/aha

Dror Meirow, MD
Fertility Preservation Center, IVF Unit, Division of Obstetrics and Gynecology
Chaim Sheba Medical Center
Tel Hashomer (Israel)
E-Mail meircw@post.tau.ac.il

Cancer Treatment and Reproductive Damage

At birth, the ovary contains a fixed number of primordial follicles, commonly believed to represent the female oocyte pool for life. As women age, a gradual depletion of the primordial follicular reserve occurs due to an ongoing atresia. According to a suggested model of the human ovarian reserve, it is estimated that 81% of the variance in follicular count levels is exclusively related to age [4]. After the age of 37, ovarian reserve depletion significantly accelerates and eventually results in menopause at an average age of 50–51 years.

Both ovarian reserve and female reproductive system as a whole are subjected to numerous damaging effects of chemotherapy and radiation. Various studies have reported impaired ovarian reserve in cancer survivors treated with gonadotoxic agents, with both laboratory and sonographic measures being affected. Higher follicle-stimulating hormone levels, lower antimüllerian hormone levels and lower antral follicular count have all been described [5–8]. Both a complete and a partial depletion of follicular store may present clinically in cancer survivors. Patients suffering from a partial depletion of the follicular store experience menstrual irregularities and hormonal disturbances, whereas patients suffering from a complete follicular depletion exhibit permanent amenorrhea and climacteric symptoms [9]. Indeed, the multicenter Childhood Cancer Survivor Study has found cancer survivors to have an increased risk for premature ovarian failure, defined as irreversible cessation of menses before the age of 40 years [10]. Cancer survivors may also experience milder clinical manifestations, such as menstrual irregularities and hormonal disturbances. Altogether, this can result in diminished fertility potential and lower post-treatment birth rates [11, 12].

Age plays a crucial role in determining how resilient the ovary will be to anticancer treatment. Older patients have a diminished follicular reserve and are therefore more vulnerable to chemotherapy and radiation. Several studies demonstrate that patients who maintain ovarian function after chemotherapy are significantly younger compared to those who lost ovarian function [13]. It is also described that the effective sterilizing dose decreases with an increasing age at radiotherapy [14].

Radiotherapy-Induced Reproductive Damage

Radiation therapy with a field that includes the pelvis may entail significant consequences, with both ovaries and uterus being affected.

Ovarian Damage

The extent of ovarian damage is largely based on the patient's age, treatment dose and the irradiation field. Increasing doses of abdominal pelvic radiation are associated with an increased risk for developing premature ovarian failure. It has been estimated that half of the total number of dormant follicles are lost at doses of 2 Gy (LD_{50}) [5], and that a total radiation exposure of 20 Gy fractionated over 6 weeks produces sterility with 95% confidence in young women and children [15]. As for the radiation field impacts, in the long-term follow-up, ovarian failure has been observed to result in 90% of patients following total body irradiation (TBI) [16]. After abdominal radiation during childhood, ovarian failure rates may be as high as 97% [17].

Uterine Damage

Radiation-induced uterine damage is also dose and age dependent [18, 19]. Premenarchal patients are more likely to be affected since the growing uterus is probably more vulnerable to irradiation than the adult uterus. Radiation to the uterus carries an increased risk for spontaneous abortions, premature deliveries and low birth weight [16]. Such poor outcomes may be the consequence of various insults that have been described. A decrease in endometrial thickness and uterine length (3.2 cm on average), accompanied with diminished uterine blood flow, has been demonstrated in women who have been treated with whole abdominal therapy during their childhood [19]. Although uterine damage is usually considered irreversible, a possible improvement in uterine volume and endometrial thickness in response to hormone replacement therapy has been reported in patients previously treated with TBI [18], with older patients showing a better response to hormone replacement therapy than younger ones.

Chemotherapy-Induced Reproductive Damage

Maturing ovarian follicles comprise a prime target for chemotherapeutic agents, which specifically induce atresia and apoptosis in actively dividing granulosa cells. Clinically, this results in a temporal cessation of menses which generally resume after a period of recovery. The future fertility potential, however, is determined by the primordial follicle reserve, and the means by which chemotherapy induces damage on dormant follicles is under intense investigation. Possible mechanisms include primordial follicle apoptosis [20, 21] and blood vessel damage, resulting in local ischemia and cortical fibrosis [22]. Another suggested mechanism is follicular 'burnout'

Table 1. Ovarian function in patients treated for Hodgkin's disease

First author [ref.]	Patients, n	Follow-up, years	Parameter	Treatment	Results
Behringer [29]	405	3.2	Amenorrhea	ABVD	3.9%
				Advanced chemotherapy	23–51%
Brusamolino [27]	67	10	Fertility	ABVD	Preserved
Kiserud [104]	91	10	Parenthood	Low dose	55%
				Advanced chemotherapy	22–27%
Decanter [6]	30	1	AMH	ABVD	Normal

AMH = Antimüllerian hormone. Taken from Harel et al. [26].

[23]: loss of growing follicles due to chemotherapy results in a decrease in growth inhibitory factors which are granulosa cell derived, thus promoting primordial follicle recruitment, which themselves may be subjected to damage during further cycles of treatment. Furthermore, alkylating agents have recently been found to trigger the activation of the phosphoinositide 3-kinase pathway, which induces enhanced follicular recruitment and a resultant burnout of the ovarian follicle reserve [24]. The magnitude of ovarian failure and diminished infertility following chemotherapy depends on the patient's age and the chemotherapeutic regimen. Alkylating agents are responsible for the highest age-adjusted odds ratio of ovarian failure rates [9]. Platinum agents and taxanes are also associated with a significant risk for a diminished ovarian reserve [23], whereas methotrexate, fluorouracil, vincristine, bleomycin and dactinomycin are relatively safe [25].

Contemporary treatment protocols for acute myeloid leukemia (AML) are usually devoid of alkylating agents. Therefore, the risk of ovarian damage in AML patients, unless treated with hematopoietic stem cell transplantation, is low. According to the American Society of Clinical Oncology, the risk of permanent amenorrhea following AML therapy (anthracycline/cytarabine) or multiagent acute lymphoblastic leukemia (ALL) therapy is less than 20% [25]. The two commonly used regimens for the treatment of Hodgkin's lymphoma – ABVD (doxorubicin, bleomycin, vinblastine, dacarbazine) and escalated BEACOPP (bleomycin, etoposide, Adriamycin, cyclophosphamide, oncovin, procarbazine, prednisone) – exert a substantially different effect on fertility potential.

Table 1 [26] presents an overview of treatment-related risks of ovarian damage in Hodgkin's lymphoma. Generally, the ABVD regimen is considered to be safe in young patients, with a birth rate comparable to that of the general population [27, 28]. In contrast, the escalated BEACOPP regimen may significantly impair ovarian function, mainly due to the presence of alkylating agents. In a study of 405 Hodgkin's lymphoma patients, 19.3% had amenorrhea after a median of 3.2 years following chemotherapy. Multivariate analysis recognized escalated BEACOPP regimen, older age at treatment, higher stage of disease and absence of oral contraception as main risk factors for amenorrhea [29].

Although commonly treated with alkylating agents, non-Hodgkin's lymphoma survivors appear to be at a relatively low risk for ovarian dysfunction. According to the American Society of Clinical Oncology, the CHOP regimen (cyclophosphamide, doxorubicin, vincristine, prednisone) is associated with a relatively low risk for permanent amenorrhea (<20%) [25]. It has also been reported to result in an ovarian insufficiency rate of 5% and a pregnancy rate of 50% [30]. An additional small study found the hyper-CVAD regimen (cyclophosphamide, vincristine, doxorubicin, dexamethasone, cytarabine, methotrexate) to be associated with an ovarian insufficiency rate of 14% and a pregnancy rate of 43% [31].

Bone Marrow Transplantation-Induced Reproductive Damage

Most women undergoing bone marrow transplantation (BMT) are young patients in their reproductive years, who are therefore exposed to various reproductive adverse effects.

Ovarian Damage

Conditioning treatments prior to BMT are associated with extremely high rates of ovarian failure, ranging from 72 to 100% [16, 32–35]. Age at the time of BMT and conditioning protocol are likely to determine the extent of ovarian damage. TBI is considered to be more toxic than chemotherapy conditioning alone, with only 10–14% of women demonstrating ovarian function recovery and a reported pregnancy rate lower than 3% following treatment [36]. A fractionated protocol, however, is associated with a lower risk for ovarian failure [35]. When conditioning with chemotherapy alone, busulfan is known to be more deleterious than cyclophosphamide [37] and melphalan [34]. Indeed, according to various studies, the busulfan-induced ovarian failure rate may be as high as 100% [16, 32, 38].

Acta Haematol 2014;132:400–413
DOI: 10.1159/000360199

Uterine Damage

Treatment with TBI has been reported to result in impaired uterine blood flow and diminished uterine volume [39]. As previously discussed, such insults may result in serious adverse effects.

Vaginal Damage

Graft-versus-host disease affects about 50% of patients undergoing BMT. It may involve the lower genital tract, causing a chronic damage to the vaginal mucous membrane with resultant loss of elasticity and resilience. Patients may therefore present with dyspareunia, dysuria and burning sensation [40]. In severe cases, adhesions and scar tissue result in vaginal narrowing and outflow obstruction, and patients may demonstrate gradual cessation of menses (whether spontaneous or induced by hormone replacement therapy), accompanied by abdominal cramps due to blood collection [41, 42]. Importantly, genital involvement is not rare. In fact, a study of 213 female patients undergoing BMT reported genital graft-versus-host disease in 25% of patients [40]. Awareness of the aforementioned symptoms is of great importance, as it allows early detection and prevention of serious lesions. Possible preventive measures include local exogenous estrogen replacement, topical steroids and vaginal dilators [43, 44].

Biological Treatment Reproductive Damage

Improved understanding of the molecular mechanisms behind cancer cell proliferation has opened the door for the development of new 'targeted' therapies aimed at prolonging patients' lives without debilitating side effects. Specific targeted treatments, such as imatinib and other tyrosine kinase inhibitors, are currently considered the mainstay of treatment for patients diagnosed with chronic myeloid leukemia (CML). To date, imatinib is not considered to impair the ovarian reserve in humans, and animal studies have failed to associate imatinib with infertility [45, 46]. Moreover, several studies suggest imatinib to counteract the effects of an ongoing chemotherapy on ovarian reserve, potentially serving as an ovarian protective agent [47].

It is important to stress that according to animal studies [48] and prescribing information [49], pregnancy should be avoided during imatinib treatment, although normal live births following imatinib administration during pregnancy have been described.

Evaluation of Patients Considering Fertility Preservation

When consulting a patient facing cancer therapy, a careful evaluation of possible gonadotoxic consequences and sterilization risk should be done. Planned cancer therapy regimen, patient's age and current ovarian reserve should all be taken into account. Thereafter, according to the patient's health status and available time before cancer treatment, the most appropriate fertility preservation method should be determined and discussed with a fertility specialist.

Although a vast literature describing anticancer effects on fertility potential exists, an accurate prediction of treatment effects remains a serious challenge, since therapy regimens are constantly changing and treatment is often tailor made. Evaluation of pretreatment ovarian reserve can be done using antral follicular count combined with laboratory markers, namely follicle-stimulating hormone and antimüllerian hormone levels. These measures have been reported to predict long-term ovarian function after chemotherapy in women [50] and prepubertal girls [51].

Different types of hematological malignancies are associated with distinct challenges and concerns, which in turn influence the optimal approach to fertility preservation. Patients with leukemia often present with anemia and thrombocytopenia. Ovarian tissue harvesting may therefore be complicated by bleeding in the ovarian bed, and transvaginal egg retrieval may necessitate administration of clotting factors and platelets prior to the scheduled procedure. Lymphoma patients may present with large thoracic masses, potentially resulting in airway obstruction, interference with ventilatory pressures, inferior or superior vena cava compression and pericardial tamponade, all of which may expose the patient to serious anesthetic complications.

Options for Fertility Preservation

Gonadotropin-Releasing Hormone Agonist as an Ovarian Protectant

Since chemotherapy mostly affects rapidly proliferating cells, it might be expected that a continuous administration of a gonadotropin-releasing hormone agonist (GnRHa), resulting in a hypogonadotropic state and a decrease in follicular recruitment, will exert a protective effect on the ovarian follicular pool. Other suggested protection mechanisms are a resultant reduced ovarian perfusion [52] and upregulation of antiapoptotic molecules [53]. Practically, the efficacy of a GnRHa as an ovarian protectant is constantly under investigation, and its potential potency has yet to become a consensus. Several meta-analyses [54–56] and randomized controlled trials [57] found GnRHas to have a protective effect, based on various fertility measures. A trial conducted on 84 lymphoma patients found significantly higher antimüllerian hormone levels in women who received cotreatment with a GnRHa; however, there was no difference in the incidence of premature ovarian failure 1 year after chemotherapy (approx. 20%). Furthermore, the German Hodgkin Study Group failed to observe any ovarian protection with GnRHa cotreatment during an escalated BEACOPP regimen [58], and two additional studies failed to prove a significant effect in breast cancer patients [59, 60]. More such trials with longer follow-up periods are necessary to clarify the possible influence of GnRH analogs during chemotherapy.

Transposition of the Ovaries

When radiotherapy to the pelvis is indicated, the gonads should be transposed from the radiation field by a laparoscopic procedure. Apparently, this is not possible when the radiation field overlaps with the ovaries or when TBI is required as a conditioning treatment for BMT. Several complications may accompany the procedure, including vascular injury, fallopian tube infarction and ovarian cyst formation. Moreover, diminished blood supply to the ovary and scattered irradiation may result in a failure rate of up to 50% [26]. It is therefore our recommendation to perform a combined procedure with ovarian tissue preservation, thereby giving the patient a better chance for future fertility. When posttreatment pregnancy is desired and ovarian function exists, abdominal oocyte retrieval or repositioning of the ovaries may be performed. Alternately, if ovarian failure occurs, ovarian tissue reimplantation may be indicated. Since radiation to the pelvis may result in a significant uterine damage, surrogacy is usually indicated.

Ovarian Tissue Cryopreservation

Ovarian tissue cryopreservation (OTCP) is an extremely promising fertility preservation modality, with more than 30 live births reported so far [61, 62]. It allows the future restoration of ovarian endocrine function and fertility, and has also been shown to successfully induce puberty in prepubertal girls exposed to gonadotoxic agents [63, 64]. OTCP has the significant advantage of preserving a large number of primordial follicles, and it does not require prior hormonal stimulation. It is therefore the only option available for the prepubertal girl and may be the best option for patients who cannot postpone the initiation of potentially gonadotoxic therapy [65, 66].

Ovarian tissue storage should be offered to patients who are designated for curative therapy with a subsequent high risk for sterilization or significant ovarian damage. Young cancer patients who have recently been exposed to chemotherapy may also significantly benefit from this technology, because it mainly preserves primordial follicles which are less subjected to the deleterious effects of chemotherapy, as opposed to maturing follicles. On the other hand, patients who were not exposed to chemotherapy during the previous 6 months may undergo immature egg retrieval for in vitro maturation (IVM) prior to ovarian tissue harvesting, at the same setting. Such a combined procedure enables the preservation of two different follicle populations, that is primordial follicles and maturing antral follicles.

Importantly, ovarian follicular reserve declines with age and may be partially exhausted in the mid-30s, thus making the age of the patient an important factor which should be taken into account. At Chaim Sheba Medical Center, we offer ovarian cryopreservation before the age of 39 years and limit the procedure for infants beyond the age of 1 year, due to higher rates of anesthetic complications.

Harvesting and Transplantation

The amount of ovarian tissue to be removed for cryopreservation is somewhat under debate. Whereas several departments perform a complete oophorectomy, many others harvest half of one ovarian cortex, where most of the primordial follicles within the ovary are found. Generally, the decision of how much ovarian cortex to remove is influenced by the existing ovarian volume and the probability of future ovarian failure, according to planned anticancer treatment [66].

Although many authors recommend that transport times of the harvested tissue to the laboratory should be as reduced as possible, the Danish group reported successful results after transplantation of ovarian tissue that had been transported for 4–5 h [67]. A recent case report has even suggested that ovarian tissue can sustain a prolonged transport of 20 h [68]. In Denmark, tissue is harvested in a local hospital and transported to the center that performs cryopreservation [67, 69, 70]. When retransplantation is indicated, the frozen tissue is transported back to the local hospital, and the patient does not need to travel. Such a model promotes laboratory and clinical standardization, thus facilitating better quality control.

Transplantation of the ovarian tissue should be performed in sterilized patients with no ovarian function, once they have completed cancer treatment, are disease free and desire pregnancy. Usually, transplantation is considered only after at least 2 years of follow-up since the completion of cancer treatment. It involves autografting the thawed cortical tissue subcutaneously (heterotopic site) or more commonly into the pelvic cavity (orthotopic site), preferably on the remaining ovarian bed [62]. Orthotopic transplantation can be performed by laparoscopy or minilaparotomy, and though more invasive than heterotopic transplantation, its proven efficacy makes it the favored approach [65]. In fact, all OTCP-derived live births reported so far are the result of orthotopic transplantation. The current literature mostly describes unsuccessful heterotopic transplantation attempts, with only 1 resultant clinical pregnancy described to date [71].

A major concern with reimplantation is the possible presence of malignant cells in the transplanted ovarian tissue, which could lead to recurrence of the primary disease [72–79]. Although no ovarian autotransplantation procedures have been linked directly to oncological relapse, the magnitude of the risk of reintroduction of malignant cells is unknown. In a recent study [80] reviewing 15 years of activities in ovarian tissue cryobanking, the incidence of malignant cells found at light microscopy evaluation was very low (5/391). Interestingly, all positive samples were derived from patients with hematological malignancies, while no malignant cells were found in ovarian tissue obtained from breast cancer patients. A comprehensive review of the literature on OTCP in cancer survivors and the risk of reintroducing malignancy came to a similar conclusion [81]. While metastases were repeatedly detected in ovarian tissue obtained from patients with leukemia, no metastases were detected in ovarian tissue from Hodgkin's lymphoma and breast cancer patients.

In order to increase the safety of OTCP and reimplantation procedure, uncovering of tumor involvement in the ovaries and detection of malignant cells in ovarian tissue prior to reimplantation are vital. One of the most sensitive techniques for minimal residual disease (MRD) detection is qualitative and quantitative PCR [82]. However, specific tests can detect MRD only when there is a tumor-specific marker such as tumor-specific DNA or RNA sequences that can be PCR amplified. Unfortunately, the applicability of this sensitive method is limited since these MRD-PCR targets vary with disease category. While in CML and ALL, a specific MRD-PCR target can be found in a significant proportion of patients, in ALL such a target can be found in only 30–50% of patients [83].

Graft Function and Outcomes

Ovarian function of the graft is estimated to occur 4–6 months after transplantation. A decrease in follicle-stimulating hormone levels and elevation of estradiol can be detected within 3.5–6.5 months [61], and first menses are reported to occur in 4.7 months on average [84]. The duration of graft functioning varies from 9 to more than 86 months [84], depending on the age and ovarian reserve of the patient at the time of cryopreservation, the amount of tissue reimplanted and previous gonadotoxic treatment [85]. Both natural conception [86] and in vitro fertilization (IVF) pregnancy [62] resulting in live birth have been reported. Up until now, neither reports of adverse pregnancy outcomes nor congenital abnormalities have been reported. It is important to stress that despite its increasing use, the effectiveness of OTCP as an emerging technology remains difficult to estimate, with the current literature mainly representing successes. At Sheba Medical Center, 400 patients have undergone ovarian tissue harvesting and cryopreservation between the years 1996 and 2013. Hematological malignancies comprised the most common indication for the procedure (fig. 1). Stored ovarian tissue was transplanted in 14 patients suffering from ovarian failure, out of them 13 demonstrated an appropriate graft function after transplantation, as indicated by spontaneous menses and hormonal profiles; 4 patients have conceived, resulting in 8 pregnancies: 3 live births following IVF cycles, 2 currently ongoing 2nd- to 3rd-trimester spontaneous pregnancies and 3 additional missed abortions. Such encouraging outcomes, accompanied with worldwide reported successful experience (fig. 2), establish OTCP as an effective fertility preservation technique which should be offered routinely to any appropriate patient.

Ovarian Stimulation and IVF for Embryo and Mature Oocyte Cryopreservation

Ovarian stimulation, followed by IVF and embryo storage, represents the most established strategy for fertility preservation. Best candidates are postpubertal females who have a permanent spouse or who are willing to use donor sperm. Alternately, patients without a male partner can be offered oocyte cryopreservation, which is no longer considered to be experimental [87].

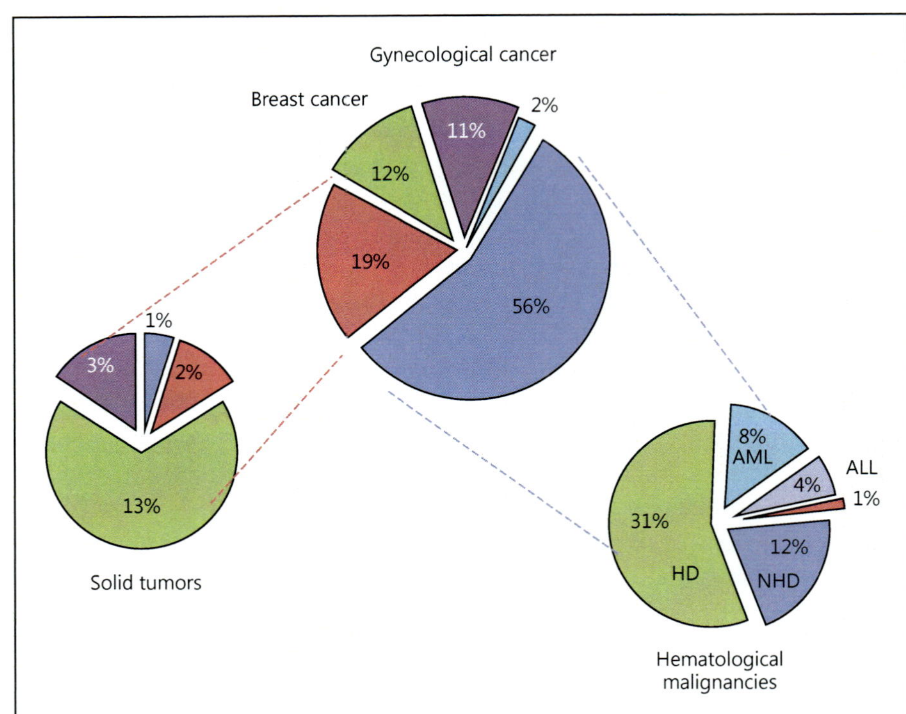

Fig. 1. Indications and diagnosis of patients who underwent OTCP at Sheba Medical Center. The different hematological indications are specified. HD = Hodgkin's disease; NHD = non-Hodgkin's disease; solid tumors = soft tissue sarcoma, bone sarcoma, colorectal cancer, lung cancer.

Timing and Protocol Selection

One of the major limitations of the utilization of IVF in cancer patients is the time frame available for ovarian stimulation. Ovarian stimulation and IVF may require several days to be completed and are therefore not applicable when urgent cancer treatment is indicated, as in the case of acute leukemia. The most established stimulation protocol in general infertility practice is the long agonist protocol. However, it requires approximately 4 weeks to be completed, and therefore, when managing cancer patients, the GnRH antagonist protocol is usually preferred. Compared with the long agonist protocol, it allows shorter duration of stimulation and, importantly, lowers the risk of ovarian hyperstimulation syndrome [88], which itself can further delay the initiation of anticancer treatment. As recently published, the antagonist protocol may be initiated in both the follicular and luteal phases of the menstrual cycle with no significantly different outcomes [89, 90], thus providing more flexibility in the patient's management.

Importantly, embryo- or oocyte-banking procedures must be completed prior to the initiation of cancer therapies. Recent chemotherapy is likely to result in a reduced response to ovarian stimulation [91]. Moreover, it carries the risk for morphologically and genetically abnormal re-trieved oocytes [91–93]. The exposure of maturing follicles to chemotherapy has been shown to have deleterious effects on reproductive outcome, including high abortion and malformation rates as indicated in animal studies [93]. Such adverse effects are not observed in primordial follicles that survive in the long term after chemotherapy exposure, as there is no increased risk of birth defects in women who conceive years after chemotherapy [94]. Thus, if fertility preservation is required and chemotherapy treatment has already begun, IVF is precluded and OTCP should be seriously considered. In any case, patients should delay attempts to conceive until at least 6 months (time needed for human oocyte maturation) after completion of treatment [91].

Outcomes – Embryo Cryopreservation

Embryo cryopreservation can virtually be performed in all IVF centers. Pregnancy rates per thawed transferred embryo are generally known within each program and are ranging from 15.3 to 38.7% in infertile couples, depending on the patient's age [95]. Since data regarding IVF pregnancy rates in cancer patients is currently limited, it is a common practice to use the aforementioned pregnancy rates when counseling cancer patients seeking fertility preservation. It is well known that malignancy

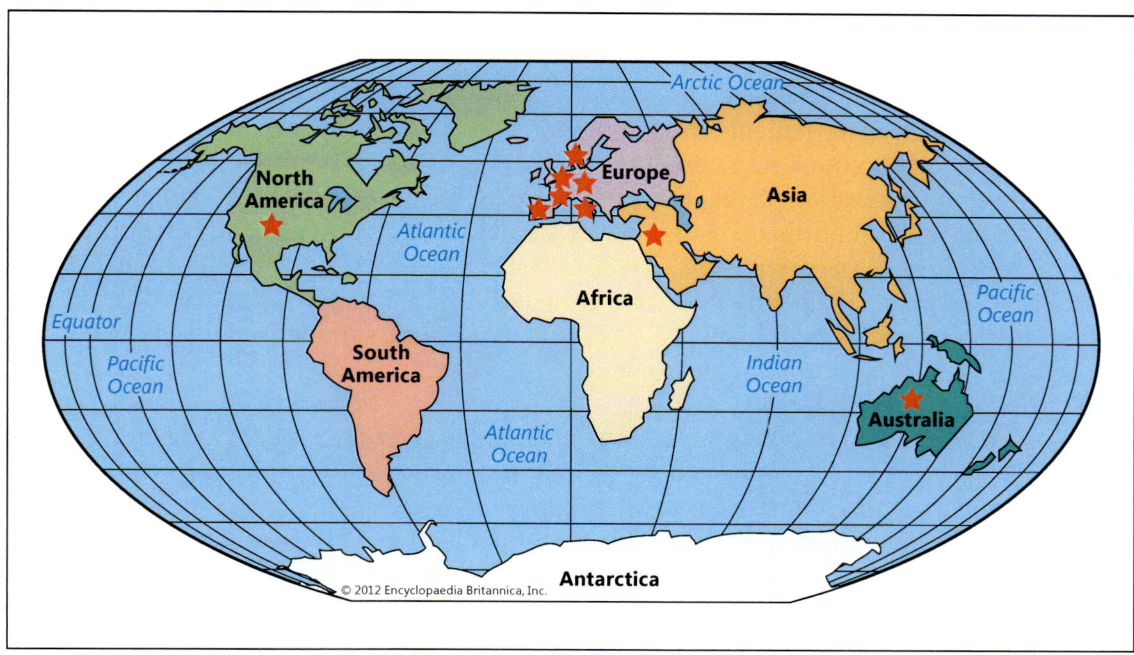

Fig. 2. Countries that reported live births after transplantation (asterisks). The number of cases or centers are not indicated.

can adversely affect fertility in males, even prior to exposure to gonadotoxic treatment. Correspondingly, there is a speculation that female cancer patients may also demonstrate impaired fertility and reduced response to IVF prior to cancer treatment. Nonetheless, as demonstrated in table 2 [65], several studies describing IVF results have not found lower responses in cancer patients, and the pregnancy rates of these patients are actually expected to be higher than those reported in infertility patients. The European registry study reported the results of 205 stimulation treatments in cancer patients [96]. 33% of the patients had lymphoma, which was the second most common diagnosis amongst the study's participants. The average of retrieved eggs was 11, and the fertilization rate was 63%. Using a German IVF registry, pregnancy rate and live birth rate per embryo were estimated to be 20 and 15%, respectively. In a smaller series, half of the patients who returned for embryo transfer ultimately had live births [97].

Outcomes – Oocyte Cryopreservation

Up until recently, the success of oocyte cryopreservation has been considered to be low. However, ongoing modifications in available techniques have resulted in continuously improving pregnancy rates. A current literature about oocyte freezing for fertility preservation is lacking, and most studies include donor populations. According to several randomized controlled trials, clinical pregnancy rates per thawed oocyte range from 4.5 to 12%, and clinical pregnancy rates per embryo transfer range from 36 to 61% [87]. Such outcomes provide good evidence that success rates with thawed oocytes are sim-

Table 2. IVF results in cancer patients

First author [ref.]	Eggs		Embryos – 2PN stage		p
	cancer	controls	cancer	controls	
Oktay [105]	12.3		5.3		
Knopman [106]	14±9	12±7			NS
Quintero [107]	13	11.5	7.4	6.8	NS
Robertson [97]	12±8	14±9	6±5	7±6	NS
Lawrenz [96]	11.6±7.7				
Domingo [108]	10.5	12.4			
	9.5–11.6	11.2–13.6			0.02
Meirow [109]					
<35 years	11		7.1		
>35 years	9.2		6		

2PN stage = 2-pronucleus stage; controls = noncancer patients; NS = nonsignificant. Taken from Chung et al. [65].

ilar to fresh oocytes. This encouraging data, however, should be viewed judiciously, as it mostly represents fertility centers with a vast experience in oocyte freezing. Indeed, when counseling patients, local success rates should be taken into account. As for perinatal outcomes after oocyte cryopreservation, data is reassuring, and an estimated congenital abnormality rate of 1.3% can be quoted according to one large study [98]. Long-term data regarding developmental outcomes is currently unavailable.

In vitro Maturation of Oocytes

In vitro maturation of oocytes represents an alternate approach to the retrieval of mature oocytes following ovarian stimulation. Immature oocytes in prophase I stage (germinal vesicle stage) are aspirated and are then cultured for up to 36 h, thereby allowing time for progression to metaphase II (MII stage) through meiosis. Mature MII oocytes can then be used for oocyte cryopreservation or alternately for IVF and embryo freezing. IVM offers several advantages, some of which are especially relevant for cancer patients seeking fertility preservation. It requires only a few preparatory steps, with minimal or no prior hormonal stimulation, and can be completed within 2–6 days without any risk for ovarian hyperstimulation syndrome. Moreover, immature oocytes can be retrieved in both the follicular and luteal phases, with no significant difference in the number of retrieved eggs, fertilization rates and resultant embryos [99–101]. As mentioned previously, IVM can also be combined with ovarian tissue cryopreservation, further increasing future fertility in selected patients. Although such favorable qualities advocate the application of IVM in fertility preservation practice, pregnancy rates in cancer patients are currently lacking, and general success rates have been discouraging, with lower success rates in IVM cycles compared to traditional IVF [102]. Incidence of obstetric complications, congenital anomalies and developmental outcomes are comparable with conceptions of infertile women undergoing IVF cycles with intracytoplasmic sperm injection, albeit these findings are based on limited data [103]. Altogether, IVM should only be performed as an experimental procedure in specialized centers for carefully selected patients [102]. Clearly, further efforts are required to improve the clinical efficacy of IVM before it can be reliably used in fertility preservation practice.

Recommended Guidelines

Each hematological malignancy presents its own particular challenges and unique set of fertility considerations. Although fertility preservation methods should be tailored to each patient specifically, fertility considerations are frequently disease dependent, and general recommendations can be made. In order to maximize the efficacy and safety of fertility preservation treatments, we have summarized the following recommendations.

Hodgkin's Lymphoma

In early-stage Hodgkin's lymphoma, the ABVD regimen, often combined with radiation to the involved field, is considered as standard treatment. As demonstrated previously, the ABVD protocol is associated with a very limited risk for ovarian failure in young patients. Therefore, for patients younger than 25 years, fertility preservation is usually unnecessary. For patients older than 25 years, we recommend to consider fertility preservation.

In advanced stage Hodgkin's lymphoma/refractory disease, recommended protocols involve alkylating agents (i.e. BEACOPP) and are therefore associated with a major risk for infertility. Ovarian tissue collection should be considered prior to treatment with the BEACOPP protocol or after up to 2 cycles of such a regimen, if reduction of tumor mass is required to allow the procedure. Importantly, MRD in Hodgkin's disease is extremely rare, and future retransplantation of the harvested tissue is safe. In some cases, immature oocyte retrieval prior to chemotherapy, followed by IVM and cryopreservation of oocytes or embryos, is optional. A GnRHa can be administered as a supplementary treatment or may be offered to patients for whom no other option is applicable.

Non-Hodgkin's Lymphoma

Although chemotherapy regimens for non-Hodgkin's lymphoma are associated with relatively low rates of ovarian damage, treatment usually includes alkylating agents and the potential risk for infertility should still be addressed. As time is often limited, we recommend ovarian tissue cryopreservation in patients with an appropriate health status.

Acute Leukemia

Both AML and ALL patients require urgent treatment, allowing no time for hormonal stimulation. These girls or young women should therefore be seriously considered for OTCP. Recommended guidelines are summarized in fig-

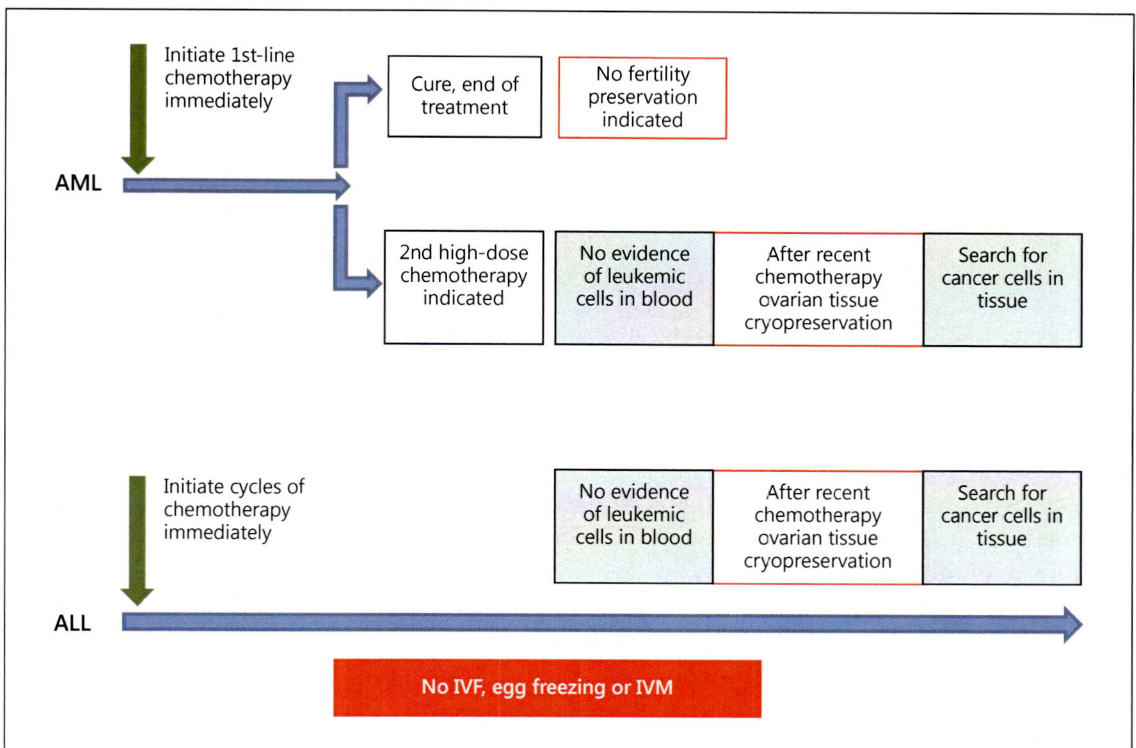

Fig. 3. Different approaches for fertility preservation in young female patients diagnosed with acute leukemia – AML, ALL. IVF and IVM are not recommended after recent exposure to chemotherapy – see text. Taken from Chung et al. [65].

ure 3 [65]. Since chemotherapy for AML is not associated with a significant ovarian damage, we recommend starting chemotherapy immediately without storing ovarian tissue. Only AML patients that subsequently will require additional high-dose chemotherapy and/or BMT are referred for ovarian tissue harvesting due to high sterilization risks. At this stage, if the blood and bone marrow are devoid of leukemic cells, the chance of finding leukemic cells in the ovary is vastly reduced. In any case, prior to reimplantation, the thawed ovarian tissue is tested for MRD using the most sensitive methods available. In ALL, the first chemotherapy courses are also typically not sterilizing. Collecting ovarian tissue may be performed after a few cycles of chemotherapy when there is no evidence of leukemic cells in the blood. In contrast, mature or immature egg collection is not recommended at this stage due to a decrease or no response to ovarian stimulation, genetically abnormal oocytes and adverse reproductive outcome such as high abortion and malformation rates as animal studies indicate.

Chronic Myeloid Leukemia

First-line medications for CML patients (hydroxyurea, 6-mercaptopurine) do not cause ovarian damage, and fer-tility preservation is generally not required. Imatinib is also considered safe in terms of fertility, though during its administration, pregnancy should be avoided due to an increased risk for congenital abnormalities. Patients who desire pregnancy and have achieved a 2-year complete/major molecular remission, may temporarily discontinue imatinib treatment in order to prevent such adverse pregnancy outcomes. BMT represents another treatment modality for CML patients, usually reserved for blast crisis or tyrosine kinase inhibitor failure. In such circumstances, fertility preservation should be seriously considered. OTCP is rather safe in these patients due to CML's distinct molecular marker which enables MRD detection.

Conclusions

Remarkable improvements in survival rates of cancer patients have created a special interest in the field of fertility preservation, offering patients advanced technologies designated to improve reproductive outcomes and overall quality of life. Significant efforts to improve our current limited understanding in toxic mechanisms of

Table 3. IVF: pros and cons

Pros	Cons
Well established	Time demanding
Relatively safe procedure	High estrogen → procoagulation state
No additional operation needed	Unsuitable for young girls
	Limited number of embryos generated per cycle
	Needs to be completed before initiation of chemotherapy

Table 4. OTCP: pros and cons

Pros	Cons
Low complication rate	Invasive procedure
Suitable from 1 to 37 years of age	Possible MRD
A delay of only 4 days in cancer therapy	
No need for hormonal stimulation	
Can be done after exposure to chemotherapy	
High posttransplantation success rate	
Restores ovarian endocrine function	
Enables induction of puberty	

antineoplastic agents are constantly being made, and are extremely essential to the further development of both emerging and well-established fertility preservation techniques. The future certainly holds several hopes and developments in the constantly changing field of fertility preservation. With the increasing reports of successful outcomes, it is likely that OTCP will become a more common practice in the near future. However, addressing the safety aspects (i.e. MRD) of this promising technique is vital and may enable an additional population of patients, especially leukemic patients, to benefit from its favorable qualities. Distinct fertility preservation measures have considerable different advantages (tables 3, 4), and every patient should accordingly be informed with her available options as indicated by age, current ovarian reserve, upcoming cancer therapy and available time before its initiation. It is essential to discuss all options before cancer therapy has begun, and early reference is of the utmost importance.

References

1 Forman EJ, Anders CK, Behera MA: A nationwide survey of oncologists regarding treatment-related infertility and fertility preservation in female cancer patients. Fertil Steril 2010;94:1652–1656.

2 Lee S, Heytens E, Moy F, Ozkavukcu S, Oktay K: Determinants of access to fertility preservation in women with breast cancer. Fertil Steril 2011;95:1932–1936.

3 Quinn GP, Vadaparampil ST, Lee JH, Jacobsen PB, Bepler G, Lancaster J, Keefe DL, Albrecht TL: Physician referral for fertility preservation in oncology patients: a national study of practice behaviors. J Clin Oncol 2009; 27:5952–5957.

4 Wallace WH, Kelsey TW: Human ovarian reserve from conception to the menopause. PLoS One 2010;5:e8772.

5 Bath LE, Wallace WH, Shaw MP, Fitzpatrick C, Anderson RA: Depletion of ovarian reserve in young women after treatment for cancer in childhood: detection by anti-mullerian hormone, inhibin B and ovarian ultrasound. Hum Reprod 2003;18:2368–2374.

6 Decanter C, Morschhauser F, Pigny P, Lefebvre C, Gallo C, Dewailly D: Anti-Müllerian hormone follow-up in young women treated by chemotherapy for lymphoma: preliminary results. Reprod Biomed Online 2010;20:280–285.

7 Partridge AH, Ruddy KJ, Gelber S, Schapira L, Abusief M, Meyer M, Ginsburg E: Ovarian reserve in women who remain premenopausal after chemotherapy for early stage breast cancer. Fertil Steril 2010;94:638–644.

8 Senapati S, Morse CB, Sammel MD, Kim J, Mersereau JE, Efymow B, Gracia CR: Fertility preservation in patients with haematological disorders: a retrospective cohort study. Reprod Biomed Online 2014;28:92–98.

9 Meirow D: Reproduction post-chemotherapy in young cancer patients. Mol Cell Endocrinol 2000;169:123–131.

10 Sklar CA, Mertens AC, Mitby P, Whitton J, Stovall M, Kasper C, Mulder J, Green D, Nicholson HS, Yasui Y, Robison LL: Premature menopause in survivors of childhood cancer: a report from the childhood cancer survivor study. J Natl Cancer Inst 2006;98:890–896.

11 Critchley HO, Wallace WH: Do survivors of childhood cancer have increased incidence of premature menopause? Nat Clin Pract Oncol 2007;4:84–85.

12 Wallace WH, Anderson RA, Irvine DS: Fertility preservation for young patients with cancer: who is at risk and what can be offered? Lancet Oncol 2005;6:209–218.

13 Brusamolino E, Lunghi F, Orlandi E, Astori C, Passamonti F, Barate C, Pagnucco G, Baio A, Franchini P, Lazzarino M, Bernasconi C: Treatment of early-stage Hodgkin's disease with four cycles of ABVD followed by adjuvant radio-therapy: analysis of efficacy and long-term toxicity. Haematologica 2000;85: 1032–1039.

14 Wallace WH, Thomson AB, Saran F, Kelsey TW: Predicting age of ovarian failure after radiation to a field that includes the ovaries. Int J Radiat Oncol Biol Phys 2005;62:738–744.

15 Lushbaugh CC, Casarett GW: The effects of gonadal irradiation in clinical radiation therapy: a review. Cancer 1976;37:1111–1125.

16 Sanders JE, Hawley J, Levy W, Gooley T, Buckner CD, Deeg HJ, Doney K, Storb R, Sullivan K, Witherspoon R, Appelbaum FR: Pregnancies following high-dose cyclophosphamide with or without high-dose busulfan or total-body irradiation and bone marrow transplantation. Blood 1996;87:3045–3052.

Acta Haematol 2014;132:400–413
DOI: 10.1159/000360199

17 Wallace WH, Shalet SM, Crowne EC, Morris-Jones PH, Gattamaneni HR: Ovarian failure following abdominal irradiation in childhood: natural history and prognosis. Clin Oncol (R Coll Radiol) 1989;1:75–79.

18 Bath LE, Critchley HO, Chambers SE, Anderson RA, Kelnar CJ, Wallace WH: Ovarian and uterine characteristics after total body irradiation in childhood and adolescence: response to sex steroid replacement. Br J Obstet Gynaecol 1999;106:1265–1272.

19 Critchley HO, Wallace WH, Shalet SM, Mamtora H, Higginson J, Anderson DC: Abdominal irradiation in childhood: the potential for pregnancy. Br J Obstet Gynaecol 1992;99:392–394.

20 Familiari G, Caggiati A, Nottola SA, Ermini M, Di Benedetto MR, Motta PM: Ultrastructure of human ovarian primordial follicles after combination chemotherapy for Hodgkin's disease. Hum Reprod 1993;8:2080–2087.

21 Oktem O, Oktay K: A novel ovarian xenografting model to characterize the impact of chemotherapy agents on human primordial follicle reserve. Cancer Res 2007;67:10159–10162.

22 Nicosia SV, Matus-Ridley M, Meadows AT: Gonadal effects of cancer therapy in girls. Cancer 1985;55:2364–2372.

23 Meirow D, Biederman H, Anderson RA, Wallace WH: Toxicity of chemotherapy and radiation on female reproduction. Clin Obstet Gynecol 2010;53:727–739.

24 Kalich-Philosoph L, Roness H, Carmely A, Fishel-Bartal M, Ligumsky H, Paglin S, Wolf I, Kanety H, Sredni B, Meirow D: Cyclophosphamide triggers follicle activation and 'burnout': AS101 prevents follicle loss and preserves fertility. Sci Transl Med 2013;5:185ra162.

25 Lee SJ, Schover LR, Partridge AH, Patrizio P, Wallace WH, Hagerty K, Beck LN, Brennan LV, Oktay K: American Society of Clinical Oncology recommendations on fertility preservation in cancer patients. J Clin Oncol 2006;24:2917–2931.

26 Harel S, Ferme C, Poirot C: Management of fertility in patients treated for Hodgkin's lymphoma. Haematologica 2011;96:1692–1699.

27 Brusamolino E, Baio A, Orlandi E, Arcaini L, Passamonti F, Griva V, Casagrande W, Pascutto C, Franchini P, Lazzarino M: Long-term events in adult patients with clinical stage Ia-IIa nonbulky Hodgkin's lymphoma treated with four cycles of doxorubicin, bleomycin, vinblastine, and dacarbazine and adjuvant radiotherapy: a single-institution 15-year follow-up. Clin Cancer Res 2006;12:6487–6493.

28 Hodgson DC, Pintilie M, Gitterman L, Dewitt B, Buckley CA, Ahmed S, Smith K, Schwartz A, Tsang RW, Crump M, Wells W, Sun A, Gospodarowicz MK: Fertility among female Hodgkin lymphoma survivors attempting pregnancy following ABVD chemotherapy. Hematol Oncol 2007;25:11–15.

29 Behringer K, Breuer K, Reineke T, May M, Nogova L, Klimm B, Schmitz T, Wildt L, Diehl V, Engert A: Secondary amenorrhea after Hodgkin's lymphoma is influenced by age at treatment, stage of disease, chemotherapy regimen, and the use of oral contraceptives during therapy: a report from the German Hodgkin's Lymphoma Study Group. J Clin Oncol 2005;23:7555–7564.

30 Elis A, Tevet A, Yerushalmi R, Blickstein D, Bairy O, Dann EJ, Blumenfeld Z, Abraham A, Manor Y, Shpilberg O, Lishner M: Fertility status among women treated for aggressive non-Hodgkin's lymphoma. Leuk Lymphoma 2006;47:623–627.

31 Seshadri T, Hourigan MJ, Wolf M, Mollee PN, Seymour JF: The effect of the hyper-CVAD chemotherapy regimen on fertility and ovarian function. Leuk Res 2006;30:483–485.

32 Grigg AP, McLachlan R, Zaja J, Szer J: Reproductive status in long-term bone marrow transplant survivors receiving busulfan-cyclophosphamide (120 mg/kg). Bone Marrow Transplant 2000;26:1089–1095.

33 Meirow D: Ovarian injury and modern options to preserve fertility in female cancer patients treated with high dose radio-chemotherapy for hemato-oncological neoplasias and other cancers. Leuk Lymphoma 1999;33:65–76.

34 Teinturier C, Hartmann O, Valteau-Couanet D, Benhamou E, Bougneres PF: Ovarian function after autologous bone marrow transplantation in childhood: high-dose busulfan is a major cause of ovarian failure. Bone Marrow Transplant 1998;22:989–994.

35 Thibaud E, Rodriguez-Macias K, Trivin C, Esperou H, Michon J, Brauner R: Ovarian function after bone marrow transplantation during childhood. Bone Marrow Transplant 1998;21:287–290.

36 Jadoul P, Donnez J: How does bone marrow transplantation affect ovarian function and fertility? Curr Opin Obstet Gynecol 2012;24:164–171.

37 Nabhan SK, Bitencourt MA, Duval M, Abecasis M, Dufour C, Boudjedir K, Rocha V, Socie G, Passweg J, Goi K, Sanders J, Snowden J, Yabe H, Pasquini R, Gluckman E: Fertility recovery and pregnancy after allogeneic hematopoietic stem cell transplantation in Fanconi anemia patients. Haematologica 2010;95:1783–1787.

38 Borgmann-Staudt A, Rendtorff R, Reinmuth S, Hohmann C, Keil T, Schuster FR, Holter W, Ehlert K, Keslova P, Lawitschka A, Jarisch A, Strauss G: Fertility after allogeneic haematopoietic stem cell transplantation in childhood and adolescence. Bone Marrow Transplant 2012;47:271–276.

39 Holm K, Nysom K, Brocks V, Hertz H, Jacobsen N, Muller J: Ultrasound B-mode changes in the uterus and ovaries and Doppler changes in the uterus after total body irradiation and allogeneic bone marrow transplantation in childhood. Bone Marrow Transplant 1999;23:259–263.

40 Spinelli S, Chiodi S, Costantini S, Van Lint MT, Raiola AM, Ravera GB, Bacigalupo A: Female genital tract graft-versus-host disease following allogeneic bone marrow transplantation. Haematologica 2003;88:1163–1168.

41 DeLord C, Treleaven J, Shepherd J, Saso R, Powles RL: Vaginal stenosis following allogeneic bone marrow transplantation for acute myeloid leukaemia. Bone Marrow Transplant 1999;23:523–525.

42 Yanai N, Shufaro Y, Or R, Meirow D: Vaginal outflow tract obstruction by graft-versus-host reaction. Bone Marrow Transplant 1999;24:811–812.

43 Corson SL, Sullivan K, Batzer F, August C, Storb R, Thomas ED: Gynecologic manifestations of chronic graft-versus-host disease. Obstet Gynecol 1982;60:488–492.

44 Hirokawa M, Sato H, Kawabata Y, Sawada K: Vaginal outflow tract obstruction associated with chronic graft-versus-host disease following allogeneic peripheral blood stem cell transplantation. Int J Hematol 2006;83:181–182.

45 Chuah C: Imatinib does not impair gonadal function. Leuk Res 2012;36:262–263.

46 Leader A, Lishner M, Michaeli J, Revel A: Fertility considerations and preservation in haemato-oncology patients undergoing treatment. Br J Haematol 2011;153:291–308.

47 Gonfloni S: Modulating c-Abl nuclear activity as a strategy to preserve female fertility. Cell Cycle 2010;9:217–218.

48 Pye SM, Cortes J, Ault P, Hatfield A, Kantarjian H, Pilot R, Rosti G, Apperley JF: The effects of imatinib on pregnancy outcome. Blood 2008;111:5505–5508.

49 Hensley ML, Ford JM: Imatinib treatment: specific issues related to safety, fertility, and pregnancy. Semin Hematol 2003;40:21–25.

50 Brougham MF, Crofton PM, Johnson EJ, Evans N, Anderson RA, Wallace WH: Anti-mullerian hormone is a marker of gonadotoxicity in pre- and postpubertal girls treated for cancer: a prospective study. J Clin Endocrinol Metab 2012;97:2059–2067.

51 Anderson RA, Cameron DA: Pretreatment serum anti-mullerian hormone predicts long-term ovarian function and bone mass after chemotherapy for early breast cancer. J Clin Endocrinol Metab 2011;96:1336–1343.

52 Meirow D, Dor J, Kaufman B, Shrim A, Rabinovici J, Schiff E, Raanani H, Levron J, Fridman E: Cortical fibrosis and blood-vessels damage in human ovaries exposed to chemotherapy. Potential mechanisms of ovarian injury. Hum Reprod 2007;22:1626–1633.

53 Blumenfeld Z: How to preserve fertility in young women exposed to chemotherapy? The role of GnRH agonist cotreatment in addition to cryopreservation of embrya, oocytes, or ovaries. Oncologist 2007;12:1044–1054.

54 Ben-Aharon I, Gafter-Gvili A, Leibovici L, Stemmer SM: Pharmacological interventions for fertility preservation during chemotherapy: a systematic review and meta-analysis. Breast Cancer Res Treat 2010;122:803–811.

55 Clowse ME, Behera MA, Anders CK, Copland S, Coffman CJ, Leppert PC, Bastian LA: Ovarian preservation by GnRH agonists during chemotherapy: a meta-analysis. J Womens Health (Larchmt) 2009;18:311–319.

56 Kim SS, Lee JR, Jee BC, Suh CS, Kim SH, Ting A, Petroff B: Use of hormonal protection for chemotherapy-induced gonadotoxicity. Clin Obstet Gynecol 2010;53:740–752.

57 Del Mastro L, Boni L, Michelotti A, Gamucci T, Olmeo N, Gori S, Giordano M, Garrone O, Pronzato P, Bighin C, Levaggi A, Giraudi S, Cresti N, Magnolfi E, Scotto T, Vecchio C, Venturini M: Effect of the gonadotropin-releasing hormone analogue triptorelin on the occurrence of chemotherapy-induced early menopause in premenopausal women with breast cancer: a randomized trial. JAMA 2011;306:269–276.

58 Behringer K, Wildt L, Mueller H, Mattle V, Ganitis P, van den Hoonaard B, Ott HW, Hofer S, Pluetschow A, Diehl V, Engert A, Borchmann P: No protection of the ovarian follicle pool with the use of GnRH-analogues or oral contraceptives in young women treated with escalated BEACOPP for advanced-stage Hodgkin lymphoma. Final results of a phase II trial from the German Hodgkin Study Group. Ann Oncol 2010;21:2052–2060.

59 Gerber B, von Minckwitz G, Stehle H, Reimer T, Felberbaum R, Maass N, Fischer D, Sommer HL, Conrad B, Ortmann O, Fehm T, Rezai M, Mehta K, Loibl S: Effect of luteinizing hormone-releasing hormone agonist on ovarian function after modern adjuvant breast cancer chemotherapy: the GBG 37 ZORO study. J Clin Oncol 2011;29:2334–2341.

60 Munster PN, Moore AP, Ismail-Khan R, Cox CE, Lacevic M, Gross-King M, Xu P, Carter WB, Minton SE: Randomized trial using gonadotropin-releasing hormone agonist triptorelin for the preservation of ovarian function during (neo)adjuvant chemotherapy for breast cancer. J Clin Oncol 2012;30:533–538.

61 Donnez J, Dolmans MM, Pellicer A, Diaz-Garcia C, Sanchez Serrano M, Schmidt KT, Ernst E, Luyckx V, Andersen CY: Restoration of ovarian activity and pregnancy after transplantation of cryopreserved ovarian tissue: a review of 60 cases of reimplantation. Fertil Steril 2013;99:1503–1513.

62 Meirow D, Levron J, Eldar-Geva T, Hardan I, Fridman E, Zalel Y, Schiff E, Dor J: Pregnancy after transplantation of cryopreserved ovarian tissue in a patient with ovarian failure after chemotherapy. N Engl J Med 2005;353:318–321.

63 Anderson RA, Hindmarsh PC, Wallace WH: Induction of puberty by autograft of cryopreserved ovarian tissue in a patient previously treated for Ewing sarcoma. Eur J Cancer 2013;49:2960–2961.

64 Ernst E, Kjaersgaard M, Birkebaek NH, Clausen N, Andersen CY: Case report: stimulation of puberty in a girl with chemo- and radiation therapy induced ovarian failure by transplantation of a small part of her frozen/thawed ovarian tissue. Eur J Cancer 2013;49:911–914.

65 Chung K, Donnez J, Ginsburg E, Meirow D: Emergency IVF versus ovarian tissue cryopreservation: decision making in fertility preservation for female cancer patients. Fertil Steril 2013;99:1534–1542.

66 Meirow D, Baum M, Yaron R, Levron J, Hardan I, Schiff E, Nagler A, Yehuda DB, Raanani H, Hourvitz A, Dor J: Ovarian tissue cryopreservation in hematologic malignancy: ten years' experience. Leuk Lymphoma 2007;48:1569–1576.

67 Rosendahl M, Schmidt KT, Ernst E, Rasmussen PE, Loft A, Byskov AG, Andersen AN, Andersen CY: Cryopreservation of ovarian tissue for a decade in Denmark: a view of the technique. Reprod Biomed Online 2011;22:162–171.

68 Dittrich R, Lotz L, Keck G, Hoffmann I, Mueller A, Beckmann MW, van der Ven H, Montag M: Live birth after ovarian tissue autotransplantation following overnight transportation before cryopreservation. Fertil Steril 2012;97:387–390.

69 Andersen CY, Rosendahl M, Byskov AG, Loft A, Ottosen C, Dueholm M, Schmidt KL, Andersen AN, Ernst E: Two successful pregnancies following autotransplantation of frozen/thawed ovarian tissue. Hum Reprod 2008;23:2266–2272.

70 Ernst E, Bergholdt S, Jorgensen JS, Andersen CY: The first woman to give birth to two children following transplantation of frozen/thawed ovarian tissue. Hum Reprod 2010;25:1280–1281.

71 Stern CJ, Gook D, Hale LG, Agresta F, Oldham J, Rozen G, Jobling T: First reported clinical pregnancy following heterotopic grafting of cryopreserved ovarian tissue in a woman after a bilateral oophorectomy. Hum Reprod 2013;28:2996–2999.

72 Abir R, Feinmesser M, Yaniv I, Fisch B, Cohen IJ, Ben-Haroush A, Meirow D, Felz C, Avigad S: Occasional involvement of the ovary in Ewing sarcoma. Hum Reprod 2010;25:1708–1712.

73 Dolmans MM, Marinescu C, Saussoy P, Van Langendonckt A, Amorim C, Donnez J: Reimplantation of cryopreserved ovarian tissue from patients with acute lymphoblastic leukemia is potentially unsafe. Blood 2010;116:2908–2914.

74 Greve T, Clasen-Linde E, Andersen MT, Andersen MK, Sorensen SD, Rosendahl M, Ralfkiaer E, Andersen CY: Cryopreserved ovarian cortex from patients with leukemia in complete remission contains no apparent viable malignant cells. Blood 2012;120:4311–4316.

75 Kim SS, Radford J, Harris M, Varley J, Rutherford AJ, Lieberman B, Shalet S, Gosden R: Ovarian tissue harvested from lymphoma patients to preserve fertility may be safe for autotransplantation. Hum Reprod 2001;16:2056–2060.

76 Meirow D, Ben Yehuda D, Prus D, Poliack A, Schenker JG, Rachmilewitz EA, Lewin A: Ovarian tissue banking in patients with Hodgkin's disease: is it safe? Fertil Steril 1998;69:996–998.

77 Meirow D, Hardan I, Dor J, Fridman E, Elizur S, Ra'anani H, Slyusarevsky E, Amariglio N, Schiff E, Rechavi G, Nagler A, Ben Yehuda D: Searching for evidence of disease and malignant cell contamination in ovarian tissue stored from hematologic cancer patients. Hum Reprod 2008;23:1007–1013.

78 Rosendahl M, Andersen MT, Ralfkiaer E, Kjeldsen L, Andersen MK, Andersen CY: Evidence of residual disease in cryopreserved ovarian cortex from female patients with leukemia. Fertil Steril 2010;94:2186–2190.

79 Rosendahl M, Timmermans Wielenga V, Nedergaard L, Kristensen SG, Ernst E, Rasmussen PE, Anderson M, Schmidt KT, Andersen CY: Cryopreservation of ovarian tissue for fertility preservation: no evidence of malignant cell contamination in ovarian tissue from patients with breast cancer. Fertil Steril 2011;95:2158–2161.

80 Dolmans MM, Jadoul P, Gilliaux S, Amorim CA, Luyckx V, Squifflet J, Donnez J, Van Langendonckt A: A review of 15 years of ovarian tissue bank activities. J Assist Reprod Genet 2013;30:305–314.

81 Bastings L, Beerendonk CC, Westphal JR, Massuger LF, Kaal SE, van Leeuwen FE, Braat DD, Peek R: Autotransplantation of cryopreserved ovarian tissue in cancer survivors and the risk of reintroducing malignancy: a systematic review. Hum Reprod Update 2013;19:483–506.

82 Grimwade D, Jovanovic JV, Hills RK, Nugent EA, Patel Y, Flora R, Diverio D, Jones K, Aslett H, Batson E, Rennie K, Angell R, Clark RE, Solomon E, Lo-Coco F, Wheatley K, Burnett AK: Prospective minimal residual disease monitoring to predict relapse of acute promyelocytic leukemia and to direct pre-emptive arsenic trioxide therapy. J Clin Oncol 2009;27:3650–3658.

83 Huang M, Li C, Liang H, Zhou J, Deng J, Liu W: Multiplex reverse transcription-polymerase chain reaction for simultaneous screening of 29 chromosomal translocations in hematologic malignancies. J Huazhong Univ Sci Technolog Med Sci 2006;26:661–663.

84 Janse F, Donnez J, Anckaert E, de Jong FH, Fauser BC, Dolmans MM: Limited value of ovarian function markers following orthotopic transplantation of ovarian tissue after gonadotoxic treatment. J Clin Endocrinol Metab 2011;96:1136–1144.

85 Donnez J, Silber S, Andersen CY, Demeestere I, Piver P, Meirow D, Pellicer A, Dolmans MM: Children born after autotransplantation of cryopreserved ovarian tissue. A review of 13 live births. Ann Med 2011;43:437–450.

86 Donnez J, Dolmans MM, Demylle D, Jadoul P, Pirard C, Squifflet J, Martinez-Madrid B, van Langendonckt A: Livebirth after orthotopic transplantation of cryopreserved ovarian tissue. Lancet 2004;364:1405–1410.

87 Pfeifer S, Goldberg J, McClure R, Lobo R, Thomas M, Widra E, Licht M, Collins J, Cedars M, Racowsky C, Vernon M, Davis O, Gracia C, Catherino W, Thornton K, Rebar R, La Barbera A: Mature oocyte cryopreservation: a guideline. Fertil Steril 2013;99:37–43.

88 Al-Inany HG, Youssef MA, Aboulghar M, Broekmans F, Sterrenburg M, Smit J, Abou-Setta AM: Gonadotrophin-releasing hormone antagonists for assisted reproductive technology. Cochrane Database Syst Rev 2011;5:CD001750.

89 Nayak SR, Wakim AN: Random-start gonadotropin-releasing hormone (GnRH) antagonist-treated cycles with GnRH agonist trigger for fertility preservation. Fertil Steril 2011;96:e51–e54.

90 Von Wolff M, Thaler CJ, Frambach T, Zeeb C, Lawrenz B, Popovici RM, Strowitzki T: Ovarian stimulation to cryopreserve fertilized oocytes in cancer patients can be started in the luteal phase. Fertil Steril 2009;92:1360–1365.

91 Meirow D, Schiff E: Appraisal of chemotherapy effects on reproductive outcome according to animal studies and clinical data. J Natl Cancer Inst Monogr 2005;21–25.

92 Bar-Joseph H, Ben-Aharon I, Rizel S, Stemmer SM, Tzabari M, Shalgi R: Doxorubicin-induced apoptosis in germinal vesicle (GV) oocytes. Reprod Toxicol 2010;30:566–572.

93 Kujjo LL, Chang EA, Pereira RJ, Dhar S, Marrero-Rosado B, Sengupta S, Wang H, Cibelli JB, Perez GI: Chemotherapy-induced late transgenerational effects in mice. PLoS One 2011;6:e17877.

94 Winther JF, Boice JD Jr, Mulvihill JJ, Stovall M, Frederiksen K, Tawn EJ, Olsen JH: Chromosomal abnormalities among offspring of childhood-cancer survivors in Denmark: a population-based study. Am J Hum Genet 2004;74:1282–1285.

95 Loren AW, Mangu PB, Beck LN, Brennan L, Magdalinski AJ, Partridge AH, Quinn G, Wallace WH, Oktay K: Fertility preservation for patients with cancer: American Society of Clinical Oncology clinical practice guideline update. J Clin Oncol 2013;31:2500–2510.

96 Lawrenz B, Jauckus J, Kupka M, Strowitzki T, von Wolff M: Efficacy and safety of ovarian stimulation before chemotherapy in 205 cases. Fertil Steril 2010;94:2871–2873.

97 Robertson AD, Missmer SA, Ginsburg ES: Embryo yield after in vitro fertilization in women undergoing embryo banking for fertility preservation before chemotherapy. Fertil Steril 2011;95:588–591.

98 Noyes N, Porcu E, Borini A: Over 900 oocyte cryopreservation babies born with no apparent increase in congenital anomalies. Reprod Biomed Online 2009;18:769–776.

99 Bedoschi GM, de Albuquerque FO, Ferriani RA, Navarro PA: Ovarian stimulation during the luteal phase for fertility preservation of cancer patients: case reports and review of the literature. J Assist Reprod Genet 2010;27:491–494.

100 Demirtas E, Elizur SE, Holzer H, Gidoni Y, Son WY, Chian RC, Tan SL: Immature oocyte retrieval in the luteal phase to preserve fertility in cancer patients. Reprod Biomed Online 2008;17:520–523.

101 Maman E, Meirow D, Brengauz M, Raanani H, Dor J, Hourvitz A: Luteal phase oocyte retrieval and in vitro maturation is an optional procedure for urgent fertility preservation. Fertil Steril 2011;95:64–67.

102 In vitro maturation: a committee opinion. Fertil Steril 2013;99:663–666.

103 Chian RC, Uzelac PS, Nargund G: In vitro maturation of human immature oocytes for fertility preservation. Fertil Steril 2013;99:1173–1181.

104 Kiserud CE, Fosså A, Holte H, Fosså SD: Post-treatment parenthood in Hodgkin's lymphoma survivors. Br J Cancer 2007;96:1442–1449.

105 Oktay K, Buyuk E, Libertella N, Akar M, Rosenwaks Z: Fertility preservation in breast cancer patients: a prospective controlled comparison of ovarian stimulation with tamoxifen and letrozole for embryo cryopreservation. J Clin Oncol 2005;23:4347–4353.

106 Knopman JM, Noyes N, Talebian S, Krey LC, Grifo JA, Licciardi F: Women with cancer undergoing ART for fertility preservation: a cohort study of their response to exogenous gonadotropins. Fertil Steril 2009;91(suppl 4):1476–1478.

107 Quintero RB, Helmer A, Huang JQ, Westphal L: Ovarian stimulation for fertility preservation in patients with cancer. Fertil Steril 2010;93:865–868.

108 Domingo J, Guillén V, Ayllón Y, Martínez M, Muñoz E, Pellicer A, Garcia-Velasco JA: Ovarian response to controlled ovarian hyperstimulation in cancer patients is diminished even before oncological treatment. Fertil Steril 2012;97:930–934.

109 Meirow D: Reproductive outcome after fertility preservation in girls and women. Hum Reprod 2013;28(suppl 1): i17–i18.

Acta Haematol 2014;132:414–422
DOI: 10.1159/000360241

Published online: September 10, 2014

Challenges for Cancer Care Delivery to Adolescents and Young Adults: Present and Future

Mathew R. Meeneghan   William A. Wood

Lineberger Comprehensive Cancer Center, University of North Carolina, Chapel Hill, N.C., USA

Key Words

Adolescents and young adults · Hematological malignancy

Abstract

Adolescents and young adults occupy a unique place within the cancer community due to the challenges they face related to disease biology, access to care, and psychosocial and socioeconomic circumstances. Efforts to define specific needs and targets for intervention in these areas are under way and evolving. This review will discuss the current and future challenges in delivering quality care to this population.

© 2014 S. Karger AG, Basel

Introduction

Cancer in the adolescent and young adult (AYA) population is the most common cause of nonaccidental death following injuries, suicide and homicide [1, 2] with up to a third of cases coming from hematological malignancies (table 1) [2, 3]. AYAs have been recognized as a distinct population within the oncology community due to the unique challenges they face. When compared to pediatric and older adult oncology patients, these 15- to 39-year-olds encounter differences in disease biology, access to care, psychosocial and socioeconomic circumstances, and issues related to long-term follow-up [4–6]. Furthermore, there have been fewer improvements in treatment of AYA cancers than have been observed in non-AYA populations, a trend that is evident across all ethnic groups and tumor types [2]. Current reports place the 5-year overall survival for AYAs with hematological malignancies between 47 and 95% [7]. There have been efforts to define specific needs and targets for intervention in order to achieve high-quality care for AYAs. The National Comprehensive Cancer Network has recently published guidelines to address this [8].

The spectrum of malignant diseases varies among different age groups. Pediatric oncological diseases are predominated by embryonal-type tumors such as Wilms' tumor, neuroblastoma, hepatoblastoma and acute lymphoblastic leukemia (ALL). In contrast, adult cancer diagnoses tend to come from epithelial origin such as breast, lung and prostate tissue. AYAs straddle these two groups, sharing overlaps in terms of age and tumor type; however, the prognosis of a given tumor type may be significantly different when compared to non-AYAs. For instance, the outcomes of AYAs with ALL are worse than those of pediatric patients [9].

Mathew R. Meeneghan
Division of Hematology/Oncology, Physicians Office Building
170 Manning Drive Campus, Box 7305
Chapel Hill, NC 27599-7305 (USA)
E-Mail meeneghan@gmail.com

Table 1. Percentage of all cancer diagnoses [adapted from Bleyer et al. 2]

Disease	Aged 15–19, %	Aged 20–29, %	Aged 30–39, %
Hodgkin's lymphoma	15	10	3
Non-Hodgkin's lymphoma	7	6	6
Acute lymphoblastic leukemia	7	2	1
Acute myeloid leukemia	5	3	1

Other papers have discussed how diverse and incompletely understood disease biology can explain how the same pathological diagnosis can have different courses in different age groups [5]. The purpose of this article is to discuss the nonpathological issues that create challenges in achieving satisfactory care delivery for AYAs with a focus on hematological malignancies.

Access to Clinical Trials and Initiation of Treatment

The main method by which the field of medicine advances is careful scientific study of disease. Detailed analysis of various interventions through clinical trials informs the medical community of the proper way to best improve outcomes. Unfortunately, cancer patients between the ages of 15 and 35 have the lowest rates of accrual to clinical trials [10]. Roughly 90% of patients under the age of 15 are managed at institutions with trials sponsored by the National Cancer Institute, and most of those patients are entered into trials. These numbers drop off rapidly for older patients. Only 20–35% of 15- to 19-year-olds are seen at such institutions, and only 10% go on trial. For 20- to 29-year-olds, less than 10% are seen at institutions with trials sponsored by the National Cancer Institute, and only 1% are actually enrolled. Including community settings, rates of enrollment for pediatric populations are around 60%. In older adults with cancer, enrollment falls in the 3–5% range [10]. The overall rate for enrollment of AYAs in clinical trials is estimated to be less than 2% [2]. Within the AYA group, clinical trial enrollment for hematological malignancies seems to worsen with age. Liu et al. [11] found that when compared to patients younger than 15 years, patients aged 15–19 were 48% less likely to enroll in leukemia trials and 62% less likely to enroll in lymphoma trials. Meanwhile patients aged 20–44 accrued to clinical trials at a rate of 91–96% lower than patients aged <15 years for all leukemias [12].

Similar evidence of poor trial enrollment has been noted for older AYAs with lymphoma [13].

Reasons for lower clinical trial enrollment are likely multifaceted. Lack of awareness of ongoing trials by treating physicians and patients and lack of willingness of patients to participate in the trials are obvious barriers. In addition, there are simply fewer trials open for the cancers that are common in this age group. Historically, there may also be lack of collaboration between pediatric and adult cooperative groups, resulting in trials designed for older or younger patients, but few specifically designed with AYAs in mind [9]. To combat this, the Children's Oncology Group Adolescent and Young Adult Initiative has been working to increase the age limits on trials that include diseases that also affect AYAs [2]. The Cancer and Leukemia Group B 10403 trial for patients aged 16–39 with newly diagnosed ALL is the first intergroup study designed specifically for AYAs [14].

There may also be economic reasons underlying the low rate of AYA trial enrollment. AYAs are the most uninsured age group, and not every clinical trial covers the complete cost of care [2]. In general, community-based physicians are less likely to enroll AYAs in clinical trials, the reasons for which are variable but may include economic disincentives. Furthermore, providers may lack adequate training in issues specific to the AYA population and thus may not recognize the particular importance of trials in this age group. AYAs may also be perceived by local physicians as a group with a higher likelihood of noncompliance and may thus be considered less suited to clinical trial enrollment [2].

Education and outreach at multiple steps may help to address gaps in enrollment of AYAs into trials [10]. AYAs should be encouraged to ask about clinical trials and to consider traveling to other facilities that have open trials, if possible, since in some instances the standard of care for the AYA population has not been defined and is thus not clear locally. Once enrolled, AYAs should be given adequate support to help them with adherence to the protocol. One example of this strategy is the Children's Oncology Group's Adolescent and Young Adult Initiative which was integral to increasing the upper limit for age in Children's Oncology Group trials as discussed above and continues to collaborate with adult cooperative groups on codevelopment of trials for Hodgkin's lymphoma (HL) and non-HL [2].

From a policy standpoint, it is important to note that the available funding for clinical trials is limited and thus may preclude developing specific trials for the AYA population. In one survey of providers and patients, both

Acta Haematol 2014;132:414–422
DOI: 10.1159/000360241

groups agreed that higher priority is needed for trials that address specific predefined topics as opposed to traditional investigator-initiated studies [15]. This type of strategic prioritization could benefit areas of need such as defining standards of care for AYA hematological malignancies. Additionally, though randomized trials remain the gold standard for developing the evidence base for AYA hematological malignancies, comparative effectiveness research studies may be a helpful and less expensive adjunct to facilitate this goal. Comparative effectiveness research compares the effectiveness of tests, treatments, procedures or other health care services in multiple formats, such as prospective data collection or systematic reviews [16]. The goal of comparative effectiveness research is to improve health care by studying 'real-world' data, which is particularly applicable to AYAs with leukemias and lymphomas as this population may be treated in both pediatric and adult settings [17].

Access to Multidisciplinary Professionals Well Versed in Specific Issues in the AYA Population

The majority of 15- to 19-year-old patients are referred to adult oncologists [10]; however, this practice pattern does vary with disease pathology. Cases of acute leukemia tend to get referred to pediatric oncologists, while lymphomas tend to get referred to adult oncologists [9]. The primary goal of treating AYAs should be achieving the best outcome. Some have argued that this may mean treating AYAs with ALL using a pediatric regimen and possibly at a pediatric center, though this is the subject of ongoing debate. In general, issues around which approach and which treatment setting are optimal for AYA hematological malignancies remain largely unresolved and deserve further specific attention [10]. In addition to making sure AYAs receive the best disease-based care possible, this group of patients also has a large and unique set of psychosocial issues that require diligent attention.

Treatment-Related Issues

Long-term effects from treatment of AYA hematological malignancies vary by specific treatment-related exposure. Cardiac toxicity is a well-described potential complication of anthracyclines [18], as is the lung toxicity associated with bleomycin used in the treatment of HL [19]. Secondary malignancies including leukemia and lung cancer have been reported after treatment of non-HL [20] and HL [21], whether from primary therapy or from subsequent hematopoietic stem cell transplantation (HSCT) [22]. Long-term infertility (see below) and endocrine dysfunction [23–25] are also prevalent. In the AYA population, physicians must consider these consequences and assume long-term survival of patients when weighing the risks and benefits of competing treatment strategies that may carry different late effect risk profiles. For any given regimen, it is imperative that patients undergo the proper and necessary pretreatment organ function screening and that meticulous detail is paid to proper dosing and supportive care to help mitigate these risks. Having noted that, AYAs tend to be better equipped to tolerate intensive therapies than their older counterparts, even if they have a higher risk of treatment-related complications than pediatric patients treated in a similar way.

Interestingly, technology may prove to be a useful ally in these situations. Patients with chronic diseases are more likely to use the Internet, and cancer patients who research their diseases online are more engaged with their physicians, ask more questions and have more of a partnership in their treatments [26]. Internet use changes how patients cope with and manage their pain [27]. Because most AYAs use smartphones [28] and are generally technology avid, these observations raise the possibility that technology could be used to facilitate communication between AYAs and providers in the areas of patient-reported symptoms or management of short- or long-term disease and treatment-related complications.

Fertility

Infertility is defined as the inability to conceive after 1 year of intercourse without contraception [29]. Unfortunately, infertility can occur as a result of treatment for several of the hematological malignancies in the AYA population. Men can have disease-related infertility, primary or secondary hormonal insufficiency, and treatment-related damage or depletion of germinal stem cells that may or may not resolve after completion of therapy [29]. For women, cancer-directed treatments can decrease primordial follicles, affect hormonal balance or interfere with the function of the ovaries, fallopian tubes, uterus or cervix even if menses do return [29]. Furthermore, premature ovarian failure not only causes infertility but can also lead to vasomotor symptoms and fatigue [30]. AYAs generally regard fertility as important, prefer biological offspring and want to have children in the fu-

Acta Haematol 2014;132:414–422
DOI: 10.1159/000360241

Table 2. Risk of infertility by treatment regimen [adapted from Lee et al. 29 and Levine et al. 32]

Risk	Treatment	Disease
High risk (>80%)	Radiation therapy ≥10 Gy to ovaries; alkylators	HL
	TBI; alkylators	BMT
	Alkylators + TBI	BMT, HL
	Cyclophosphamide ≥7.5 mg/m^2 in women <20 years old	Non-HL, ALL
	Procarbazine-containing regimens	HL
Medium risk (30–70%)	Whole abdominal or pelvic radiation 5–10 Gy; spinal radiation >25 Gy	Relapsed ALL
		Relapsed non-HL
Low risk (<20%)	Multiagent therapy	ALL
	7 + 3	AML
	CHOP (4–6 cycles)	Non-HL
	COP	Non-HL
	ABVD	HL
Very low or no risk	Vincristine	Leukemia, HL, non-HL
Unknown risk	Monoclonal antibodies, TKIs	

TBI = Total body irradiation; 7 + 3 = cytarabine and anthracycline; CHOP = cyclophosphamide, hydroxydaunorubicin, vincristine, prednisone; COP = cyclophosphamide, vincristine, prednisone; ABVD = doxorubicin, bleomycin, vinblastine, dacarbazine; TKIs = tyrosine kinase inhibitors; BMT = bone marrow transplantation; AML = acute myeloid leukemia.

ture [31, 32]. The risk of ovarian failure varies with the type of therapy, dose, duration and age of the patient, but the risk of having at least some posttreatment symptoms is significant [30]. For instance, one survey showed that following stem cell transplantation, all women have at least some postmenopausal symptoms [30].

Fortunately, there are resources available for providers to estimate the risk of infertility based on the sex of the patient and the type of cancer or regimen used. One such website is http://www.fertilehope.org/tool-bar/risk-calculator.cfm, which can be useful when having this discussion during the planning phases of treatment. Table 2 shows similar estimates in tabular form [29]. Education of the oncology medical community is one intervention that offers a chance for great improvement in the fertility preservation of AYAs undergoing cancer treatment [31]. One survey of practitioners showed that while oncologists knew the importance of fertility and were aware of potential adverse effects of alkylators and irradiation, about half of responders were unaware that risks were higher in men, that birth defects and cancer rates in children of cancer survivors are at baseline population levels, and did not know that ovarian cryopreservation is an option in the prepubertal setting. Moreover, 10% thought sperm banking was not successful enough to be worthwhile. With this knowledge gap, it is not surprising that oncologists have room for improvement when discussing fertility issues with their patients [32].

Further complicating matters, 30–60% of cancer survivors did not recall getting information about possible infertility issues even when they did receive prior counseling [32].

In addition to problems with awareness and education, there are still limitations related to the availability and efficacy of the techniques used to address fertility preservation. One obvious impediment is cost. As an example, one analysis found that sperm banking cost USD 275 for initiation followed by an ongoing USD 300 annual storage fee [31]. Access to appropriate referral sites and finding an appropriate specialist were also barriers to care [31, 32]. Some oncologists report that in a busy modern practice there simply is not enough time to address these issues, especially when there are concerns about treatment delay [32].

Finally, there are several ethical issues involved in fertility preservation. Levine et al. [32] and Jadoul and Kim [33] suggest the following examples:

(1) making sure to clarify reasonable expectations for fertility preservation;

(2) distinguish which methods of preservation are standard of care and which are experimental;

Acta Haematol 2014;132:414–422
DOI: 10.1159/000360241

(3) dealing with the consent or assent of patients under 18;

(4) whether or not to delay treatment to allow for preservation, especially experimental ones;

(5) accurate articulation of immediate and long-term financial costs;

(6) consideration of the role of long-term prognosis on the decision to conceive in the first place;

(7) cancer treatment is difficult and can affect relationships; therefore, it may not be the best time to make embryos during this major life stressor.

Keeping the above ethical questions in mind, when considering fertility preservation it is important to remember that treatment of the underlying oncological disease is paramount. Any intervention should minimize harm and avoid delay in disease-directed therapy that would worsen the prognosis. There have been multiple guidelines published on fertility issues in oncology patients [e.g. American Society of Reproductive Medicine Ethics Committee 34; American Society of Clinical Oncology fertility guidelines 35]. Regarding fertility preservation options, men are largely limited to sperm banking, which they should all be offered regardless of the risk of spermatic failure [36]. For women, options include in vitro fertilization, in vitro maturation or oopheropexy to move the ovaries out of a planned field of radiation [33]. Ovarian cortex cryopreservation is another choice that is still experimental. Which of these methods is right for a given woman will depend on the urgency of treatment, age of the patient, marital status, regimen and dose of gonadotoxic drugs [36].

Risks for infertility vary by specific hematological disease and by regimen. For example, one popular standard of care treatment for HL is doxorubicin, bleomycin, vinblastine and dacarbazine (ABVD) which poses little to no risk of premature ovarian failure. A study of 36 female HL survivors who were alive without relapse at least 3 years after completion of ABVD showed that the median time to pregnancy and 12-month pregnancy rates were statistically similar when compared to healthy controls [37]. Neither age at treatment nor the number of cycles (range 2–6) were associated with altered pregnancy rates. In contrast, more aggressive regimens like bleomycin, etoposide, doxorubicin, cyclophosphamide, vincristine, procarbazine and prednisone (BEACOPP) can be more gonadotoxic. The risk of azoospermia following BEACOPP is 90% [38] and reported rates of birth after natural fertilization by male HL survivors at <1% after BEACOPP as compared to 7.5% for non-BEACOPP regimens [39]. Likewise for females, rates of birth after BEACOPP were 6.5% compared to 16.6% for non-BEACOPP regimens. It is reasonable in most cases to delay treatment for 1 ovulatory cycle in order to cryopreserve embryos or oocytes [33]. Men can have pretreatment fertility impairment, but sperm banking should still be offered [40].

ALL and acute myeloid leukemia protocols attempt to preserve fertility by minimizing gonadotoxic medications, resulting in rates of infertility of less than 20% [31]. In chronic myeloid leukemia, imatinib is not felt to impair future fertility, but pregnancies are not advised while taking this medication [33]. Data regarding future fertility with later-generation tyrosine kinase inhibitors are sparse. Regardless, there have been pregnancies reported while taking these medications [41, 42] so AYAs taking these medications should be counseled about the risk of becoming pregnant and to discuss fertility concerns with their treating physicians.

All of the hematological malignancies discussed above may require HSCT at some point along the disease trajectory, either early for high-risk diseases or later in the event of disease relapse. HSCT itself carries a high risk of infertility. Myeloablative preparation using total body irradiation has a subsequent rate of successful pregnancy of less than 3%, while the overall rate of successful conception ranges from 0.6 to 11% depending on the study and preparative regimen used [43–47]. There is also a theoretical concern that pregnancy may lead to increased rates of disease relapse after HSCT due to the state of decreased immune surveillance, but this has not yet been clearly demonstrated by empirical data [33].

Finally, in contrast to problems with infertility are problems with unwanted fertility. If cancer patients are sexually active and do not desire pregnancy, they should be counseled that they must still use contraceptives and cannot rely on cancer treatment as a contraceptive itself [31].

Psychosocial Care

There is a recognized gap between the psychosocial needs of cancer patients and the services available to them [48]. On the supply side, very few pediatric or adult cancer centers have sufficient psychosocial support staff (e.g. social workers, psychologists, psychiatrists) with expertise in AYAs. Also lacking are centers with peer mentoring, support groups or counseling services for AYAs [9]. From a more patient-centered perspective, emotional barriers, poverty and underemployment due to illness, physical and functional limitations, and lack of knowledge can lead to underutilization of psychiatric services [49].

Psychosocial issues reported by AYAs with hematological malignancies include depression, anxiety, distress, delirium, posttraumatic stress disorder, sexual dysfunction, physical limitations, family dysfunction, strain on relationships, infertility, body image, problems with work, issues with education, hospital readmission, complications of treatment, slow recovery and other chronic issues [15, 48]. Late effects of cancer treatment include problems with memory, learning, attention, cognition, social interactions and work performance [48]. Cancer patients use multiple coping mechanisms, most of which attempt to increase hope and give the patient a sense of control over his or her disease even though in reality many disease-related issues may be outside of the patient's control [48]. It may be helpful for providers to understand this, so they can appreciate how patients cope with these potentially fatal diagnoses.

To this end the National Comprehensive Cancer Network has included in its AYA guidelines a section on psychosocial issues to help clinicians address these issues [8]. Recommendations are mostly general rather than specific, but do include suggestions such as anticipatory education on the importance of medication adherence and early referral to mental health providers for psychiatric or cognitive dysfunction or signs of substance abuse. Church young adult groups and mentors can be useful allies for patients with crises of faith or conscience. In addition, there are a variety of face-to-face and virtual support groups that can act as adjunct support networks for AYAs. Finally, providers are encouraged to simplify treatment as much as possible and have some flexibility to account for non-disease-related obligations that patients may have.

Access to Care and Socioeconomic Issues

Despite the perception that AYAs are a generally healthy population, roughly one sixth suffer from some form of chronic illnesses and have trouble paying medical bills [7]. Access to care is paramount in order to cover the illnesses from which this group suffers including hematological malignancies [6]. Treatment of these diseases is complicated, requiring multidisciplinary care and significant social support. Leukemias and lymphomas are frequently treated at tertiary care hospitals, which may require patients to stay locally even if they live hours away.

In the USA, recent slow economic growth has depressed the job market, which in turn has led to difficulties obtaining adequate insurance [6]. As a subset, AYAs are the most uninsured population, which can lead to missed care opportunities and subsequent economic burdens including tradeoffs with education and career, using up savings, delinquency on loans, building up credit card debt, delaying moving out from their parents' home, increased cohabitation, delaying marriage and sometimes difficulty paying for basic necessities like rent and food [6, 50]. Even if one has adequate insurance at the time of diagnosis, there is the risk of losing insurance if there is loss of employment during treatment or – for dependent patients – the risk of aging out of eligibility for dependent insurance [6].

American AYAs suffer an increased interval from onset of symptoms to time of diagnosis. This does not seem to be affected by race, ethnicity, age, gender, marital status or surrogate measures of socioeconomic status, but is linked to underinsurance [10]. This delay can be as long as 13 weeks and lead to a more advanced stage of disease at the time of diagnosis [51]. Furthermore, at least one study showed that despite some popular belief, AYAs do tend to purchase insurance when offered by their employers [6]. For AYAs who are unemployed or whose parents are unemployed, the only other option is private health insurance. Employer-based health insurance tends to have subsidies to defray some of the cost to employees, but independently purchased insurance does not [52]. Moreover, premiums can increase seemingly arbitrarily, and preexisting conditions can be grounds for denial of coverage.

In an effort to make medical care more available to Americans, the Patient Protection and Affordable Care Act (PPACA) is being phased in and will establish among other things an insurance exchange system in which the federal government and each state will have programs available to health care consumers. Health exchanges will offer essential services that are important to hematological malignancy patients and will likely include ambulatory care, emergency room visits, hospitalization, psychiatric care, substance abuse, chronic diseases, prescriptions and rehabilitation [53]. Another benefit from which patients with hematological malignancies will benefit is the mandate that insurances will now cover any services that occur in the course of a clinical trial but would have been covered under routine care if that patient were not on trial [54].

Another important aspect of the PPACA is mitigation of health care costs, which are inflating at an unsustainable rate. One example of a cost-cutting measure being piloted by the government is bundling payments for a given diagnosis [54, 55]. How this might work in the case of hematological malignancy is difficult to foresee due to the complex and multidisciplinary nature of the care involved. For instance, a lymphoma patient may see a surgeon, radiation oncologist and medical oncologist, and have multiple hospital admissions over a relatively short time both due to scheduled chemotherapy and complications of that therapy.

Two features of the PPACA, which will greatly impact access for AYAs and which are already in place, are the expansion of dependent insurance eligibility and the elimination of preexisting conditions. Prior to enactment, patients receiving insurance through their parents became disqualified for this option at the age of 19 or at the time of graduation from high school or college. Since September 23, 2010, all dependents are allowed to have dependent insurance until the age of 26 [56, 57]. Evidence has shown that AYAs have taken advantage of this expansion of coverage [6, 58]. While dependent insurance increased, Medicaid claims stayed stable and private self-insurance decreased [57].

The elimination of preexisting conditions means that insurance companies and exchanges cannot deny patients because of their chronic medical conditions. In addition, the Department of Health and Human Services will review premium increases to make sure they are justified. The only variables on which issue of insurance and premiums can be based are age, geography, family versus individual status and tobacco use. Prior limitations on lifetime coverage for essential services and annual limitations on nonessential services which can both be a heavy burden to the oncology population are largely eliminated or phased out. Appeals against denials of coverage have also been made easier and will involve third parties that objectively review the cases.

Conclusion

AYAs with hematological malignancies are a unique population as defined not simply by their age and pathological diagnosis, but in terms of the challenges they face with regard to adequate access to medical care, representation on clinical trials, and short- and long-term treatment effects including altered fertility. There are efforts on national and international levels to better define and address these issues from both medical and social perspectives. In the meantime, it is the duty of the oncologists who treat these individuals to recognize this and to help these patients navigate treatment as best as possible. Resources available to clinicians include published guidelines specific to AYAs [8] and sites like ClinicalTrials.gov [59] to help patients and providers identify potential clinical trials that may result in better outcomes for individual patients and, eventually, the AYA community as a whole.

References

1 Bleyer A, O'Leary M, Barr R, Ries LAG (eds): Cancer Epidemiology in Older Adolescents and Young Adults 15–29 Years of Age, Including SEER Incidence and Survival: 1975–2000. NIH Publ No 06-5767. Bethesda, National Cancer Institute, 2006.

2 Bleyer A, Budd T, Montello M: Adolescents and young adults with cancer: the scope of the problem and criticality of clinical trials. Cancer 2006;107(suppl):1645–1655.

3 Surveillance, Epidemiology, and End Results (SEER) program: Seer*Stat database: incidence-SEER 13 Regs, public-use Nov 2004 sub for expanded races (1992–2002), National Cancer Institute, DCCPS, Surveillance Research Program, Cancer Statistics Branch, released April 2005, based on the November 2004 submission. www.seer.cancer.gov (accessed November 8, 2005).

4 Adolescents and young adults with cancer. Bethesda, National Cancer Institute at the National Institutes of Health, 2013. http:// www.cancer.gov/cancertopics/aya/reports (accessed July 31, 2013).

5 Wood WA, Lee SJ: Malignant hematologic diseases in adolescents and young adults. Blood 2011;117:5803–5815.

6 Collins SR, Garber T, Doty M: Young, uninsured, and in debt: why young adults lack health insurance and how the affordable care act is helping. Findings from the Commonwealth Fund Health Insurance Tracking Survey of young adults, 2011. Commonwealth Fund 2012;14:1–24.

7 Pulte D, Gondos A, Brenner H: Trends in survival after diagnosis with hematologic malignancy in adolescence or young adulthood in the United States, 1981–2005. Cancer 2009; 115:4973–4979.

8 National Comprehensive Cancer Network: Adolescent and young adult (AYA) oncology (version 1.2012). http://www.nccn org/professionals/physician_gls/pdf/aya.pdf (accessed May 25, 2013).

9 Ramphal R, Meyer R, Schacter B, Rogers P, Pinkerton R: Active therapy and models of care for adolescents and young adults with cancer. Cancer 2011;117(suppl):2316–2322.

10 Bleyer A: Young adult oncology: the patients and their survival challenges. CA Cancer J Clin 2007;57:242–255.

11 Liu L, Krailo M, Reaman GH, Bernstein L; Surveillance, Epidemiology and End Results Childhood Cancer Linkage Group: Childhood cancer patients' access to cooperative group cancer programs: a population-based study. Cancer 2003;97:1339–1345.

12 Bleyer A, Montello M, Budd T: Young adults with leukemia in the United States: lack of clinical trial participation and mortality reduction during the last decade. JCO Meeting Abstracts July 2004, vol 22, No 14, suppl 6623. http://meeting.ascopubs.org/cgi/content/abstract/22/14_suppl/6623.

13 Bleyer A, Budd T, Montello M: Older adolescents and young adults with cancer, and clinical trials: lack of participation and progress in North America; in Bleyer A, Barr R, Albritton K, Phillips M, Siegel S (eds): Cancer in Adolescents and Young Adults. New York, Springer, 2007, pp 71–81.

14 Freyer DR, Felgenhauer J, Perentesis J; COG Adolescent and Young Adult Oncology Discipline Committee: Children's Oncology Group's 2013 blueprint for research: adolescent and young adult oncology. Pediatr Blood Cancer 2013;60:1055–1058.

15 Clinton-McHarg T, Paul C, Sanson-Fisher R, D'Este C, Williamson A: Determining research priorities for young people with haematological cancer: a value-weighting approach. Eur J Cancer 2010;46:3263–3270.

16 Effective Health Care Program: Helping you make better treatment choices: what is comparative effectiveness research. Rockville, Agency for Healthcare Research and Quality, US Department of Health and Human Services, 2013. http://www.effectivehealthcare.ahrq. gov/index.cfm/what-is-comparative-effectiveness-research1/ (accessed July 24, 2013).

17 Edge SB, Zwelling LA, Hohn DC: The anticipated and unintended consequences of the Patient Protection and Affordable Care Act on cancer research. Cancer J 2010;16:606–613

18 Singal PK, Iliskovic N, Li T, Kumar D: Adriamycin cardiomyopathy: pathophysiology and prevention. FASEB J 1997;11:931–936.

19 Sleijfer S: Bleomycin-induced pneumonitis. Chest 2001;120:617.

20 Mudie NY, Swerdlow AJ, Higgins CD, Smith P, Qiao Z, Hancock BW, Hoskin PJ, Linch DC: Risk of second malignancy after non-Hodgkin's lymphoma: a British cohort study. J Clin Oncol 2006;24:1568–1574.

21 Koontz MZ, Horning SJ, Balise R, Greenberg PL, Rosenberg SA, Hoppe RT, Advani RH: Risk of therapy-related secondary leukemia in Hodgkin lymphoma: the Stanford University experience over three generations of clinical trials. J Clin Oncol 2013;31:592–598.

22 Pedersen-Bjergaard J, Andersen MK, Christiansen DH: Therapy-related acute myeloid leukemia and myelodysplasia after high-dose chemotherapy and autologous stem cell transplantation. Blood 2000;95:3273–3279.

23 Chemaitilly W, Sklar CA: Endocrine complications in long-term survivors of childhood cancers. Endocr Relat Cancer 2010;17:R141–R159.

24 Chow E: Risk of thyroid dysfunction and subsequent thyroid cancer among survivors of acute lymphoblastic leukemia: a report from the Childhood Cancer Survivor Trial. Pediatr Blood Cancer 2009;53:432–437.

25 Brennan BM, Rahim A, Mackie EM, Eden OB, Shalet SM: Growth hormone status in adults treated for acute lymphoblastic leukaemia in childhood. Clin Endocrinol (Oxf) 1998;48:777–783.

26 Fox S: E-patients with a disability or chronic disease. Washington, Pew Research Center, October 8, 2007. http://www.pewinternet.org/ Reports/2007/EpatientsWith-a-Disability-or-Chronic-Disease.aspx (accessed July 31, 2013).

27 Fox S, Jones S: The social life of health information. Washington, Pew Research Center, June 2009. http://www.pewinternet.org/Reports/2009/8-The-Social-Life-of (accessed July 31, 2013).

28 Rainie L: Two-thirds of young adults and those with higher income are smartphone owners. Washington, Pew Research Center, September 11, 2012. http://www.pewinternet. org/Reports/2012/PIP_Smartphones_ Sept12%209%2010%2012.pdf (accessed July 31, 2013).

29 Lee SJ, Schover LR, Partridge AH, Patrizio P, Wallace WH, Hagerty K, Beck LN, Brennan LV, Oktay K: American Society of Clinical Oncology recommendations on fertility preservation in cancer patients. J Clin Oncol 2006; 24:2917–2931.

30 Tierney KD, Facione N, Padilla G, Blume K, Dodd M: Altered sexual health and quality of life in women prior to hematopoietic cell transplantation. Eur J Oncol Nurs 2007;11: 298–308.

31 Goodwin T, Oosterhuis EB, Kiernan M, Hudson MM, Dahl GV: Attitudes and practices of pediatric oncology providers regarding fertility issues. Pediatr Blood Cancer 2007;4:80–85.

32 Levine J, Canada A, Stern CJ: Fertility preservation in adolescents and young adults with cancer. J Clin Oncol 2010;28:4831–4841.

33 Jadoul P, Kim SS; ISFP Practice Committee: Fertility considerations in young women with hematological malignancies. J Assist Reprod Genet 2012;29:479–487.

34 The Ethics Committee of the American Society for Reproductive Medicine: Fertility preservation and reproduction in cancer patients. Fertil Steril 2005;83:1622–1628.

35 Loren AW, Mangu PB, Beck LN, Brennan L, Magdalinski AJ, Patridge AH, Quinn G, Wallace WH, Oktay K: Fertility preservation for patients with cancer: American Society of Clinical Oncology clinical practice guideline update. J Clin Oncol 2013;31:2500–2510.

36 ISPF Practice Committee, Kim SS, Donnez J, Barri P, Pellicer A, Patrizio P, Rosenwaks Z, Nagy P, Falcone T, Andersen C, Hovatta O, Wallace H, Meirow D, Gook D, Kim SH, Tzeng C, Suzuki S, Ishizuka B, Dolmans M: Recommendations for fertility preservation in patients with lymphoma, leukemia, and breast cancer. J Assist Reprod Genet 2012;29: 465–468.

37 Hodgson DC, Pintilie M, Gitterman L, Dewitt B, Buckley CA, Ahmed S, Smith K, Schwartz A, Tsang RW, Crump M, Wells W, Sun A, Gospodarowicz MK: Fertility among female Hodgkin lymphoma survivors attempting pregnancy following ABVD chemotherapy. Hematol Oncol 2007;25:11–15.

38 Sieniawski M, Reinecke T, Novoga L, Josting A, Pfisner B, Diehl V, Engert A: Fertility in male patients with advanced Hodgkin lymphoma treated with BEACOPP: a report of the German Hodgkin Study Group (GHSG). Blood 2008;111:71–76.

39 Behringer K, Mueller H, Goergen H, Thielen I, Eibl AD, Stumpf V, Wessels C, Wiehlpütz M, Rosenbrock J, Halbsguth T, Reiners KS, Schober T, Renno JH, von Wolff M, van der Ven K, Kuehr M, Fuchs M, Diehl V, Engert A, Borchmann P: Gonadal function and fertility in survivors after Hodgkin lymphoma treatment within the German Hodgkin Study Group HD13 to HD15 trials. J Clin Oncol 2013;31:231–239.

40 De Luyk N, Pozzato G, Ricci G, Tamaro P, Manno M, Tomei F, Trombetta C: Pre-treatment and posttreatment fertility in young male patients affected by Hodgkin and non-Hodgkin lymphoma. Arch Ital Urol Androl 2012;84:141–145.

41 Conchon M, Sanabani SS, Bendit I, Santos FM, Serpa M, Dorliac-Llacer PE: Two successful pregnancies in a woman with chronic myeloid leukemia exposed to nilotinib during the first trimester of her second pregnancy: case study. J Hematol Oncol 2009;2:42.

42 Cole S, Kantarjian H, Ault P, Cortés JE: Successful completion of pregnancy in a patient with chronic myeloid leukemia without active intervention: a case report and review of the literature. Clin Lymphoma Myeloma 2009;9: 324–327.

43 Salooja N, Szydlo RM, Socie G, Rio B, Chatterjee R, Ljungman P, Van Lint MT, Powles R, Jackson G, Hinterberger-Fischer M, Kolb HJ, Apperly JF; Late Effects Working Party of the European Group for Blood and Marrow Transplantation: Pregnancy outcomes after peripheral blood or bone marrow transplantation: a retrospective survey. Lancet 2001; 358:271–276.

44 Sanders JE, Pritchard S, Mahoney P, Amos D, Buckner CD, Witherspoon RP, Deeg HJ, Doney KC, Sullivan KM, Appelbaum FR: Growth and development following marrow transplantation for leukemia. Blood 1986;68:1129–1135.

45 Jadoul P, Anckaert E, Dewandeleer A, Steffens M, Dolmans MM, Vermylen C, Smitz J, Donnez J, Maiter D: Clinical and biologic evaluation of ovarian function in women treated by bone marrow transplantation for various indications during childhood or adolescence. Fertil Steril 2011;96:126–133.

46 Sanders JE, Hawley J, Levy W, Gooley T, Buckner CD, Deeg HJ, Doney K, Storb R, Sullivan K, Witherspoon R, Appelbaum FR: Pregnancies following high-dose cyclophosphamide with or without high-dose busulfan or total-body irradiation and bone marrow transplantation. Blood 1996;87:3045–3052.

47 Carter A, Robison LL, Francisco L, Smith D, Grant M, Baker KS, Gurney JG, McGlave PB, Weisdorf DJ, Forman SJ, Bhatia S: Prevalence of conception and pregnancy outcomes after hematopoietic cell transplantation: report from the Bone Marrow Transplant Survivor Study. Bone Marrow Transplant 2006;37: 1023–1029.

48 Koehler M, Koenigsmann M, Frommer J: Coping with illness and subjective theories of illness in adult patients with haematological malignancies: systematic review. Crit Rev Oncol Hematol 2009;69:237–257.

49 Mosher CE, Duhamel KN, Rini CM, Li Y, Isola L, Labay L, Rowley S, Papadopoulos E, Moskowitz C, Scigliano E, Grosskreutz C, Redd WH: Barriers to mental health service use among hematopoietic SCT survivors. Bone Marrow Transplant 2010;45:570–579.

50 Fry R: Young adults after the recession: fewer homes, fewer cars, less debt. Washington, Pew Research Center, February 21, 2013. http://www.pewinternet.org/files/2013/02/ Financial_Milestones_of_Young_Adults_ FINAL_2-19.pdf (accessed July 31, 2013).

51 Martin S, Ulrich C, Munsell M, Taylor S, Lange G, Bleyer A: Delays in cancer diagnosis in underinsured young adults and older adolescents. Oncologist 2007;12:816–824.

52 Schwartz K, Claxton G: The Patient Protection and Affordable Care Act: how will it affect private health insurance for cancer patients? Cancer J 2010;16:572–576.

53 Hutchins VA, Samuels MB, Lively AM: Analyzing the Affordable Care Act: essential health benefits and implications for oncology. J Oncol Pract 2013;9:73–77.

54 Bailes JS, Kamin DY, Foster SE: The Patient Protection and Affordable Care Act: exploring the potential impact on oncology practice. Cancer J 2010;16:588–592.

55 Albright HW, Moreno M, Feeley TW, Walters R, Samuels M, Pereira A, Burke TW: The implications of the 2010 Patient Protection and Affordable Care Act and the Health Care and Education Reconciliation Act on cancer care delivery. Cancer 2011;117:1564–1574.

56 Bleyer WA: Potential favorable impact of the Affordable Care Act of 2010 on cancer in young adults in the United States. Cancer J 2010;16:563–571.

57 Sommers BD, Buchmueller T, Decker SL, Carey C, Kronick R: The Affordable Care Act has led to significant gains in health insurance and access to care for young adults. Health Aff (Millwood) 2013;32:165–174.

58 Cantor J, Monheit A, DeLia D, Lloyd K: Early impact of the Affordable Care Act on health insurance coverage of young adults. Health Serv Res 2012;47:1773–1789.

59 ClinicalTrials.gov. Bethesda, National Institutes of Health, 2013. http://www.clinicaltrials.gov (accessed July 31, 2013).

Subject Index